Joint Preservation
of the Knee

Adam B. Yanke • Brian J. Cole
Editors

Joint Preservation of the Knee

A Clinical Casebook

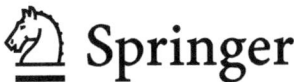 Springer

Editors
Adam B. Yanke
Department of Orthopedic
  Surgery
Rush University Medical
  Center
Chicago, IL
USA

Brian J. Cole
Department of Orthopedic
  Surgery
Rush University Medical
  Center
Chicago, IL
USA

ISBN 978-3-030-01490-2   ISBN 978-3-030-01491-9   (eBook)
https://doi.org/10.1007/978-3-030-01491-9

Library of Congress Control Number: 2018964573

This Springer imprint is published by the registered company Springer Nature Switzerland AG
The registered company address is: Gewerbestrasse 11, 6330 Cham, Switzerland

Contents

Contributors

Burak Altintas, MD Steadman Philippon Clinic, Vail, CO, USA

Luiz Felipe Ambra, MD, PhD Department of Orthopedic and Traumatology, Universidade Federal de São Paulo, São Paulo, SP, Brazil

Charles A. Baumann, BS Missouri Orthopaedic Institute, University of Missouri, Columbia, MO, USA

Adam J. Beer, BS Department of Orthopedic Surgery, Rush University Medical Center, Chicago, IL, USA

Chantelle C. Bozynski, DVM Missouri Orthopaedic Institute, University of Missouri, Columbia, MO, USA

William Bugbee, MD Joint Preservation and Cartilage Repair Service, Medical Direction of Orthopaedic Research, Division of Orthopaedic Surgery, Scripps Clinic, La Jolla, CA, USA

Jorge Chahla, MD, PhD Department of Orthopedic Surgery, Rush University Medical Center, Chicago, IL, USA

Brian J. Chilelli, MD Northwestern Medicine, Regional Medical Group Orthopaedics, Warrenville, IL, USA

David R. Christian, BS Department of Orthopedic Surgery, Rush University Medical Center, Chicago, IL, USA

Brian J. Cole, MD, MBA Department of Orthopedic Surgery, Rush University Medical Center, Chicago, IL, USA

Annabelle Davey, BS University of Vermont, College of Medicine, Burlington, VT, USA

Kyle R. Duchman, MD Department of Orthopaedic Surgery, University of Iowa Hospitals and Clinics, Iowa City, IA, USA

Michael B. Ellman, MD Panorama Orthopedics & Spine Center, Golden, CO, USA

Jack Farr, MD Cartilage Restoration Center, OrthoIndy Hospital, Indianapolis, IN, USA

Rachel M. Frank, MD Department of Orthopaedic Surgery, University of Colorado School of Medicine, Aurora, CO, USA

Katie Freeman, MD Department of Orthopedic Surgery and Rehabilitation, University of Nebraska Medical Center, Omaha, NE, USA

Andreas H. Gomoll, MD Department of Orthopedic Surgery, Hospital for Special Surgery, New York, NY, USA

Trevor R. Gulbrandsen, MD Department of Orthopaedic Surgery, University of Iowa Hospitals and Clinics, Iowa City, IA, USA

Betina B. Hinckel, MD, PhD Missouri Orthopaedic Institute, University of Missouri, Columbia, MO, USA

Drew A. Lansdown, MD Department of Orthopaedic Surgery, University of California, San Francisco School of Medicine, San Francisco, CA, USA

Christian Lattermann, MD Brigham and Women's Hospital, Harvard Medical School, Boston, MA, USA

Michael L. Redondo, MA, BS Department of Orthopedic Surgery, Rush University Medical Center, Chicago, IL, USA

Jonathan C. Riboh, MD Department of Orthopaedic Surgery, Duke University Medical Center, Durham, NC, USA

Andrew J. Riff, MD IU Health Physicians Orthopedics & Sports Medicine, Indianapolis, IN, USA

Seth L. Sherman, MD Department of Orthopaedic Surgery, University of Missouri, Columbia, MO, USA

Missouri Orthopaedic Institute, Columbia, MO, USA

Luis Eduardo Tirico, MD Knee Surgery Department, Orthopedic and Traumatology Institute, University of São Paulo Medical School, São Paulo, Brazil

Kevin C. Wang, BS Department of Orthopedics, Icahn School of Medicine at Mount Sinai, New York, NY, USA

Brian Waterman, MD Wake Forest School of Medicine, Winton-Salem, NC, USA

Adam B. Yanke, MD, PhD Department of Orthopedic Surgery, Rush University Medical Center, Chicago, IL, USA

Part I
The Knee Joint as an Organ

Chapter 1
Articular Cartilage: Structure and Restoration

Charles A. Baumann, Betina B. Hinckel,
Chantelle C. Bozynski, and Jack Farr

Function and Significance

Articular cartilage is a highly specialized (osteochondral unit) connective tissue found at the epiphyses of synovial joints. Glassy and light blue in appearance, the articular cartilage layer is 2–4 mm thick contingent on its location. Articular cartilage is composed of hyaline cartilage, which functions to protect the underlying subchondral bone and, in combination with the synovial fluid, reduce the friction between movable joints to levels less than water on ice. The articular cartilage layer also functions to redistribute the daily loads applied to the synovial joints and acts as a shock absorber. These loads are prevalent during everyday walking, jumping, running, and kneeling. During these movements, load and shear forces are being redistributed from the articular cartilage layer to the ends of long bones. Therefore, the articular cartilage layer

C. A. Baumann · B. B. Hinckel · C. C. Bozynski
Missouri Orthopaedic Institute, University of Missouri,
Columbia, MO, USA

J. Farr (✉)
Cartilage Restoration Center, OrthoIndy Hospital,
Indianapolis, IN, USA
e-mail: jfarr@orthoindy.com

© Springer Nature Switzerland AG 2019   3
A. B. Yanke, B. J. Cole (eds.), *Joint Preservation of the Knee*,
https://doi.org/10.1007/978-3-030-01491-9_1

acts as a safeguard to maintain the strength of the entire bone-cartilage interface, the osteochondral unit.

Articular cartilage lesions are one of the most consistently encountered conditions in orthopedics, leading to significant long-term sequelae. In a retrospective study of 31,516 knee arthroscopies performed, chondral lesions were reported in an astounding 19,827 (63%) patients across all age groups [1, 2]. Once osteochondral unit defects occur, many will progress to osteoarthritis (OA) dependent on a multifactorial process. OA is a very common injury and can occur because of genetic predisposition and/or can be induced by trauma, by obesity/immobility, and through normal wear and tear. OA may cause pain and serious disability, decreasing the quality of life for those it affects. As OA progresses, bone spurs form, and inflammation leads to further degeneration of the articular cartilage. This ultimately leads to painful bone-on-bone interactions and a vicious cycle of continual and worsening damage. Radiographically, more than 80% of people above the age of 65 have signs of OA in at least one joint of the hand, hip, knee, or spine [3]. The associated annual costs for the treatment of OA and inflammatory arthritis exceed $100 billion dollars in the United States, and healthcare costs account for ~2% of the US gross domestic product [3–6].

Understanding the normal function and structure of articular cartilage is required to adequately understand chondral lesions and the osteochondral unit in its diseased state. Moreover, understanding normal function and anatomy of the articular cartilage may lead to improved operative and non-operative treatments. Because of the complex structure of articular cartilage, restoration to its normal state is difficult to achieve. Artificial constructs have yet to satisfactorily replicate the effectiveness of the osteochondral unit, thus highlighting the importance of preserving its original structure and continuing research aimed at improving current conservative and surgical treatments.

Structure of the Osteochondral Unit

Cartilage Structure

The preservation of articular cartilage is critical to maintain the osteochondral unit's function. Articular cartilage is aneural, alymphatic, and avascular, which limits its regenerative healing capacity. Due to the avascular nature of articular cartilage, the cartilage must receive nutrients and oxygen by diffusion from the synovial fluid and the subchondral bone.

Articular cartilage is composed of an extracellular matrix (ECM) and chondrocytes. The ECM is mainly composed of water, collagens, and proteoglycans, although there are also other proteins, glycoproteins, and lipids found in sparse concentrations [7]. If one includes the surrounding pericellular matrix of chondrocytes, this is referred to as the chondron [8]. Articular cartilage has low chondrocyte cellularity, and the chondrocytes are encapsulated within a dense matrix, further reducing its capacity to regenerate. The structure of articular cartilage is represented in Fig. 1.1.

Extracellular Matrix

The largest component of the ECM is water, contributing ~65–80% of its wet weight. Traversing through the zones of cartilage, the water content decreases from ~80% at the superficial zone to ~65% at the deep zone [2, 9]. Water's main function is to hydrate the proteoglycans, which along with water molecules themselves expands the collagen network, lubricates the joint, and aids in the flow of nutrition to the cartilage. Water is maintained in the matrix by the proteoglycans and collagens. Electrolytes including potassium, sodium, calcium, and chloride are also dissolved in the water [7]. The water content of articular cartilage generally diminishes over the lifetime but rises to ~90% in those with OA. An increase in the water content of articular cartilage leads to decreases in strength and increases in the permeability of the cartilage layer.

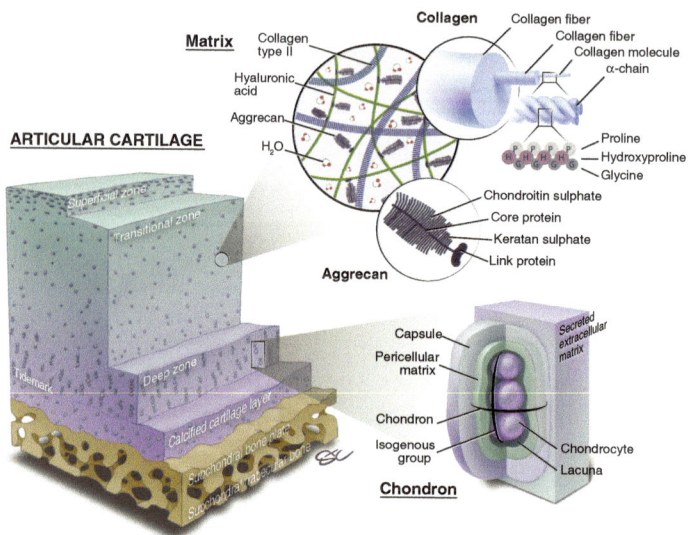

FIGURE 1.1 Structure of the osteochondral unit and the unit's individual components

The second largest component of the ECM is collagen. Collagen is a fibrous tough structural protein found throughout the body, namely, the connective tissues. Collagen develops its tensile strength from its sophisticated triple-helix structure. Composed of three polypeptides wound together by hydrogen bonds, collagen forms a tight right-handed triple helix. Each polypeptide is primarily comprised of a repeating trimer of amino acids: glycine, proline, and hydroxyproline. This repeating trimer forms a left-handed helical structure formed by hydrogen bonds [10]. The predominant collagen found in articular cartilage is Type II collagen, ~95% [9]. Little attention has been paid to other collagen fibers present in articular cartilage; Types IV, VI, IX, X, XI, XII, XIII, and XIV. The monitoring of the breakdown of these collagens could generate new biomarkers to further understand disease progression and elucidate improved therapeutic treatments [11]. Collagen is dispersed throughout the ECM, and its distribution is dependent on regional differences of the articular cartilage (articular cartilage zones). Moreover, the collagen organization at the apical surface of a chondron is denser than that on the basal side [12]. Collagen is found associated and crosslinked with proteoglycans, forming the structural unit of the ECM.

Proteoglycans are found throughout the connective tissues, and their negative charges help attract water to the articular cartilage, further strengthening the matrix. In articular cartilage, the most prevalent proteoglycan and the largest in size is aggrecan. Proteoglycans are proteins covalently attached to glycosaminoglycans (GAGs), long repetitive dimers of a hexosamine and a uronic acid. The major GAGs attached to the aggrecan link protein are chondroitin sulfate and keratin sulfate. Another GAG highly important to the function and structure of articular cartilage is hyaluronic acid (HA). HA is extremely large and does not form covalent attachments to proteins; therefore, it is not a formal constituent of proteoglycans. However, HA serves an important function by forming non-covalent complexes with proteoglycans via proteoglycan link proteins. Together, HA and proteoglycans, such as aggrecan, form extensive proteoglycan-HA aggregates. These aggregates bind to the surface of collagen II fibers via their side chains, linking all the constituents of the ECM forming the strong backbone of articular cartilage.

Chondrocytes

Chondrocytes are the viable cells of cartilage and they reside in lacunae. These spheroidal cells contribute to only ~5% of the articular cartilage volume [13]. Chondrocytes are formed in clusters among one another, known as isogenous groups, and the cell's metabolism is critical for the preservation of the ECM. Due to the hypoxic nature of the cartilage, much of the metabolism is anaerobic [2]. Originating from mesenchymal stem cells, chondroblasts form and secrete the collagens and proteoglycans of the ECM. Once chondroblasts are completely engulfed by their secreted matrix, they are referred to as chondrocytes. The surrounding ECM protects the chondro-cytes from the forces and friction applied to the joint. Growth factors and cytokines play a critical role in the control of chondrogenesis, directing the differentiation of mesenchymal stem cells into mature chondrocytes. Essential growth factors for chondrogenesis include insulin-like growth factor 1 (IGF-1), members of the fibroblast growth factor (FGF) family, and members of the transforming growth factor-beta (TGF-ß) superfamily, which includes the bone morphogenic proteins (BMP) [14]. This chondrogenesis is termed appositional growth and occurs near the apical surface of the articular cartilage in the superficial zone. Load on the articular carti-lage allows for chondrocyte maturation, differentiation, and proliferation [15].

When a defect is perceived by the osteochondral unit, chondroblasts migrate to locations of cartilage injury where chondrocytes are damaged. Chondrocytes at the site of injury can then divide and form chondroblasts that will secrete a surrounding matrix and heal the injured cartilage. Ultimately, these chondroblasts will become chondrocytes. Chondrocytes and chondroblasts, however, have an extremely limited ability to replicate or regenerate. Mitotic rates in the adult chondrocyte are at levels 1/20th of those found in the epiphyseal growth plate during development, resulting in an inadequate healing capacity for articular cartilage [16]. Immune responses against chondrocytes are limited due to the aneural and alymphatic nature of articular cartilage. Furthermore, the ECM of articular cartilage guards against major histocompatibility complex (MHC) I antigen recogni-tion of host cells [17].

Zones

Articular cartilage can be separated into four anatomically and functionally distinct zones: superficial, transitional, deep, and the calcified cartilage layer (CCL). Collectively these zones function in syncytium to provide the highly specialized functions of articular cartilage.

The superficial zone, also known as the tangential fiber zone, is the outermost zone of the cartilage and is in immediate contact with the synovial fluid of articular joints. This zone can be further divided into the lamina splendens and the cellular layer. Preservation of the lamina splendens is required to maintain the integrity of the entire joint as it provides the friction-free surface that allows for joint mobility. The cellularity in the superficial zone is more robust, and the chondrocytes are flatter relative to more basal zones [8]. The superficial zone has the highest collagen and water content. It comprises 10–20% of the thickness of the cartilage, and the collagen fibers in this zone are highly organized [18]. These fibers are arranged parallel to the surface of the joint in order to resist shear forces from friction produced by motion between the articular surfaces [9].

Immediately beneath the superficial zone is the transitional or middle zone. In this layer, collagen fibers are much thicker and are organized obliquely [9]. As its name implies, the transitional zone is a transition point between the highly specialized superficial and deep zones. The chondrons in the transitional zone are less prominent than the apical superficial zone, and the cells are more spheroidal [8]. The transitional zone accounts for ~50% of the depth of the cartilage and by nature is responsible for resistance to compressive forces. The transitional zone has higher levels of proteoglycans and less collagen content than the superficial layer. As mentioned above, the water content of the transitional layer is less than that of the superficial layer and is more than that of the deep layer.

Basal to the transitional zone is the deep zone, also called the radial fiber zone. In the deep zone, the collagen fibers are organized perpendicular to the surface to provide the greatest resistance to compressive forces applied to the joints. Chondrocytes are arranged in columnar orientation, parallel to the collagen fibers and perpendicular to the tidemark. The chondrons in this layer are scarcer and are more elongated in shape. The deep zone accounts for ~35% of the depth of the cartilage. The water content in the deep zone is the lowest of the zones, ~65%. The deep zone has the largest proteoglycan content and the largest diameter of collagen fibrils.

The calcified cartilage layer is a thin layer, ~20 to ~250 microns, located directly above the subchondral bone and below the deep zone [19]. The CCL anchors the cartilaginous zones to the subchondral bone and serves as a transitional buffer to compensate for the discontinuity of stiffness between the cartilage and subchondral bone [20, 21]. The thickness and intermediate stiffness of the CCL aid in the transfer of load by reducing the stress concentrations between the articular cartilage and the subchondral bone. The CCL has undulating vascularity, and the cellularity in this level is extremely low; thus, there are trace amounts of metabolism present [7]. A tidemark is present that delimits the CCL from the deep zone. The tidemark acts to inhibit vascular penetration of the above zones [22]. This tidemark can be clearly seen histologically by most stains, including hematoxylin and eosin.

Subchondral Bone

Although the subchondral bone is not a constituent of articular cartilage, together, they form the osteochondral unit. Therefore, subchondral bone is incredibly important for the functioning of articular cartilage and the pathogenesis of OA [23]. In severe abnormalities of the cartilage, such as in an International Cartilage Repair Society (ICRS) grade 4 lesion, the subchondral bone is affected yet is still habitually neglected in basic science reviews of articular cartilage. Further, some conditions that affect the entire osteochondral unit, such as osteochondritis dissecans (OCD) and spontaneous osteonecrosis, originate in the subchondral bone and progress to the articular cartilage [24]. Thus, to fully understand the structure of articular cartilage and the entire osteochondral unit, the subchondral bone must be appreciated.

The subchondral bone is separated from the CCL by the cement line and can be further separated into the subchondral bone plate and subchondral trabecular bone.

The subchondral bone plate is a thin bone layer that separates the CCL from the marrow spaces of the subchondral trabecular bone. Composed of cortical bone, the subchondral bone plate is nonporous and strong [25].

The trabecular bone of the subchondral bone operates as a shock absorber for the rest of the long bone and functions to retain the shape of the joint. The trabecular bone has higher metabolism than the subchondral bone plate. Additionally, the trabecular bone has bone marrow present. The bone marrow of trabecular bone houses mesenchymal stem cells (MSCs) with chondrogenic potential [26].

Vascular channels run from the marrow of the trabecular layer to the CCL. As mentioned earlier, the tidemark inhibits vascular penetration of the apical zones [22]. Apical diffusion then allows for nourishment of the avascular cartilage layers not receiving nourishment from the synovial fluid. Additionally, trabecular bone is responsible for the nourishment of the subchondral bone plate [27]. While the articular cartilage is limited in its immune response, the subchondral bone is not. The subchondral bone expresses MHC antigens [17].

Aging

With normal aging, the articular cartilage structure develops a host of changes. Although the incidence of OA increases exponentially with age, the symptoms of normal aging are not synonymous with the symptoms seen in OA. What exactly facilitates articular cartilage changes is not yet fully understood. Chondrocyte levels remain mostly unchanged with aging; however, there is a reported loss of chondrocytes from more superficial layers and a rise in chondrocyte levels closer to the subchondral bone. In addition, there is a reported thinning of the CCL with age, and the ECM typically experiences a loss of water and, as such, an intrinsic gain in stiffness [19]. Considering these changes, the entire osteochondral unit is more susceptible to damage, has a reduced ability to bear loads of the joint, and has an increased likelihood for the development of OA.

Chondral Lesions

As time has passed, it has become increasingly evident that chondral lesions must be evaluated from a perspective considering the entire osteochondral unit, rather than solely the articular cartilage [24]. Lesions of the articular cartilage provide a challenge to clinicians as it is difficult to resurface the joint. However, in young active patients, resurfacing of the defect is desirable to reduce pain levels, improve function, and increase activities and sports levels. Additionally, it may prevent the early onset of OA and avert serious disability.

The treatment plan for chondral lesions is principally determined by the size of the defect and the grading of the lesion but is also predicated on the experiences of the physician.

The International Cartilage Repair Society (ICRS) Hyaline Cartilage Lesion Classification System is the international standard for classifying the severity of chondral lesions [28, 29]. An ICRS grade 0 lesion is when the articular cartilage surface is normal. Grade 1 lesions are nearly normal; however, there may be slight indentations of the articular cartilage surface, and the cartilage may have superficial fissures. ICRS Grade 2 lesions are abnormal and extend to <50% of the depth of the cartilage, into the middle zone. Lesions of Grade 3 extend to >50% of the depth of the cartilage, which can go down to the calcified layer or subchondral bone (but not through the subchondral bone). Blisters are included in Grade 3. Grade 4 are lesions that go through the subchondral bone. The distinction between Grade 3 and 4 lesions is that Grade 4 lesions traverse through the subchondral bone [28, 29]. Figure 1.2 displays a schematic diagram, and Fig. 1.3 displays corresponding arthroscopic imagery of cartilage lesions to help further clarify the ICRS classification of cartilage lesions.

Imaging

Magnetic resonance imaging (MRI) is a useful and noninvasive tool to assess and diagnose chondral lesions. In MRI, one is also able to visualize the health of the soft tissue and the

ICRS Grade 0 - Normal

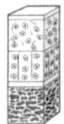

ICRS Grade 1 - Nearly normal
Superficial lesions. Soft indentation (A) and/or superficial fissures and cracks (B)

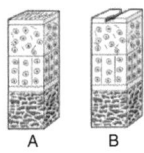

ICRS Grade 2 - abnormal
Lesions extending down to <50% of cartillage depth

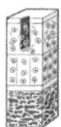

ICRS Grade 3 - Severely abnormal
Cartilage defects extending down >50% of cartilage depth (A) as well as down to calcified layer
(B) and down to but not through the subchondral bone (C). Blisters are included in this Grade (D)

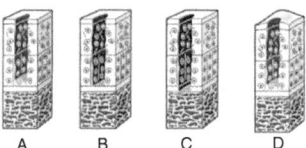

ICRS Grade 4 - Severely abnormal

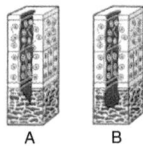

FIGURE 1.2 ICRS articular cartilage injury classification system. (Image kindly provided and reprinted with permission by the International Cartilage Repair Society)

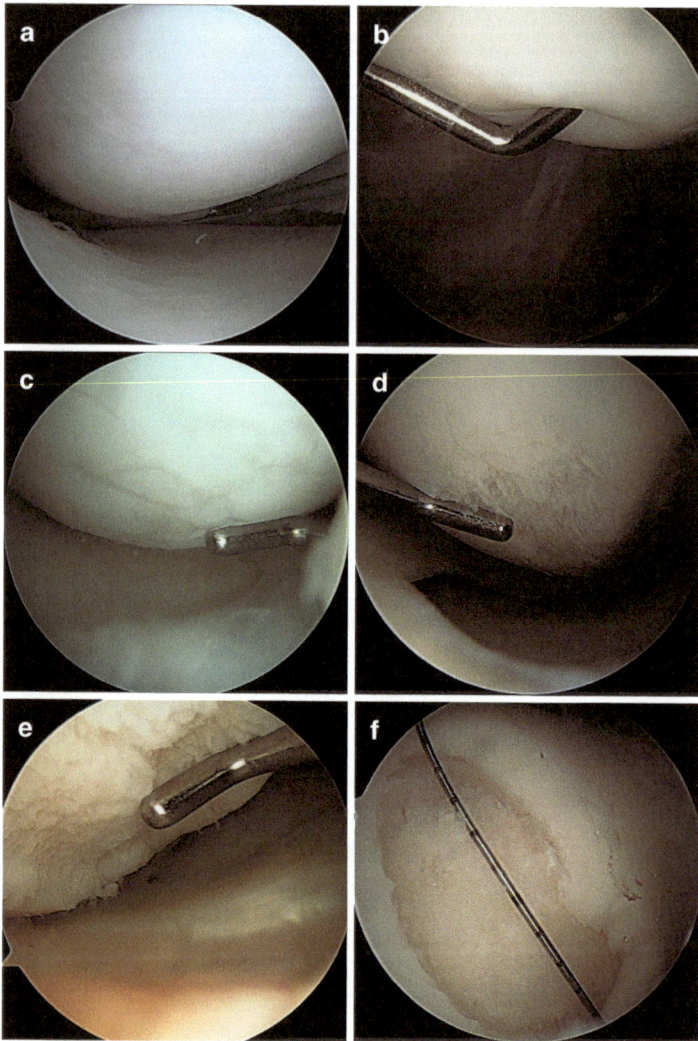

FIGURE 1.3 Representative arthroscopic images of the ICRS articular cartilage injury classification system. (**a**) Grade 0, (**b**) Grade 1A, (**c**) Grade 1B, (**d**) Grade 2, (**e**) Grade 3A, (**f**) Grade 3B, (**g**) Grade 3C, (**h**) Grade 3D, (**i**) Grade 4AB

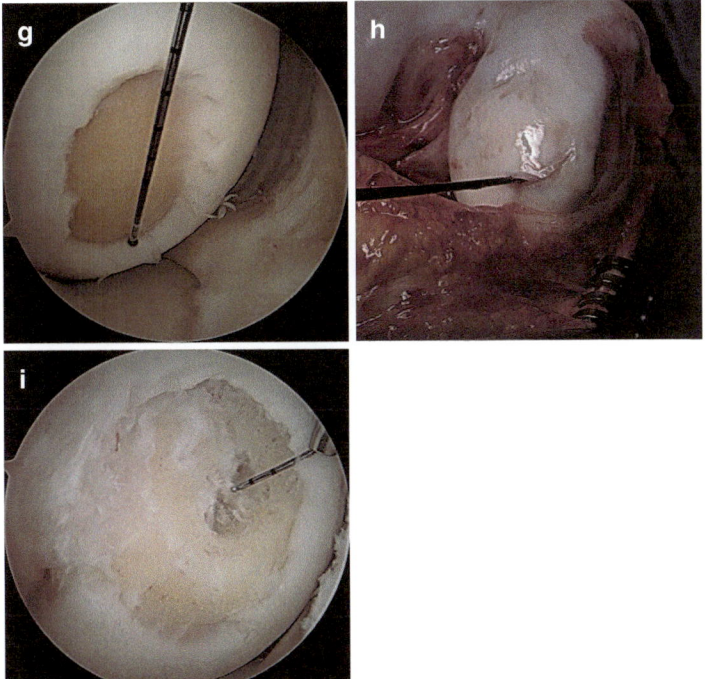

FIGURE 1.3 (continued)

subchondral bone [7]. Two-dimensional (2D) standard spin-echo (SE) and 2D gradient-recalled echo (GRE) sequences, 2D fast SE sequences, and three-dimensional (3D) SE and GRE sequences of MRI are used to assess the location, depth, and length of cartilage lesions in patients [31]. The ICRS suggests utilizing fast SE imaging for the evaluation of cartilage repair [30]. Newer 3D fast SE sequencing has not replaced the gold-standard 2D fast SE or 2D fast SE in combination with 3D GRE methods [31]. With these techniques, clinicians can clearly envision the morphology of the joint of interest and assess the progression of OA. However, the identification and evaluation of deeper lesions, grades 3 and 4, may be more precise than grades 1 and 2 that can be missed. Further, MRI can often underestimate the median defect area. On average, defects are ~65% larger than measured by MRI [32]. Most treatment algorithms are dependent on the size of cartilage defects and as such have adverse effects on the choice of treatment for clinicians [32].

The organization of collagen and GAG content can be determined by using certain MRI protocols. Since the normal collagen and proteoglycan organization is known throughout the zones, clinicians can make educated assessments about the health of their patients. When the cartilage degenerates, changes in GAG are among the first detectable manifestations [33]. To assess proteoglycan content and collagen organization and arrangement, clinicians can use a variety of methods such as T2 mapping, delayed gadolinium-enhanced MRI of the cartilage, T1ρ imaging, and sodium imaging [7, 31]. T1ρ has been shown to be the best method at assessing changes in GAG and proteoglycan content, although sodium imaging and delayed gadolinium-enhanced MRI of the cartilage may also be effective [33–35]. T2 imaging of articular cartilage detects changes in collagen content, because these images represent interactions that occur between water molecules and surrounding macromolecules. Increased interactions will result in decreased T2 levels. Another study reported that T1ρ and T2 values are significantly higher for ICRS grade 1 cartilage lesions than for those with grade 0 (normal) [33].

Perhaps with further discovery and enhancement of techniques, earlier and perhaps reversible signs of degeneration will become more apparent. The reduction of artifacts, decrease in scan time, improvement in lesion sizing, and enhancement in sensitivity of MRI will allow for improved efficacy and utility of this imaging technique [36]. Moreover, the continued and increased usage of MRI techniques such as T1ρ could detect early degeneration of the articular cartilage ECM, even before defects appear on the surface of the articular cartilage.

Macroscopic and Microscopic Evaluations

For macroscopic evaluation of articular joint tissues, staining with India ink allows pathologists to measure the depth of cartilage lesions. India ink adheres to fissured cartilage and can

be easily seen in comparison to the surrounding normal cartilage (i.e., cartilage that does not retain the India ink stain) [37].

For microscopic evaluation of articular cartilage/bone, tissues are sectioned approximately 3 mm in thickness and fixed
in 10% neutral buffered formalin (ratio of 10:1 for fixative
and specimen, respectively). Once the sections are properly
fixed (24–72 h depending on tissue size and bone density), the
bone samples are decalcified. A commonly used solution that
is gentle to the tissue and maintains cellular detail is a solution of 10% ethylenediaminetetraacetic acid (EDTA) in
phosphate-buffered saline (pH 7.2–7.4). The bone samples are
kept in 10% EDTA solution till softened (approximately
2–6 weeks based on tissue size, thickness, and bone density,
solution changed three times a week) and then embedded in
paraffin. To speed up the decalcification process, decalcifying
solution can be replaced every day. Once the tissues are pro-
cessed, there are many histochemical stains available to visualize healthy and degenerative articular cartilage. Each
method serves a specific purpose and has its own advantages.
Perhaps the most widely used stain in histology is hematoxylin
and eosin (H&E). Hematoxylin is a basic dye that stains
purple/blue. Hematoxylin attaches to negatively charged elements of the tissue (basophilic), such as the DNA of the
chondrocyte. Eosin is an acidic dye that stains pink. Eosin
attaches to positively charged elements of the tissue (acidophilic), which includes collagen. H&E stains the nuclei of
articular cartilage basophilic and the ECM acidophilic. Areas
with high proteoglycan content in the ECM stain bluer due to
being highly sulfated and having more negative charges [37].
The orientation of the collagen fibers in the ECM changes
the visual orientation of stained chondrocytes, thereby making the individual cartilage zones visible. By using H&E staining, the health of the tissue can be determined by comparing
the surface, zones, and staining intensity to baseline (Fig. 1.4).

Another method to visualize the cartilage is to use either
Safranin O or Toluidine Blue staining. Safranin O and
Toluidine Blue stain proteoglycans and GAG. When using this
method, histologists can compare normal articular cartilage to
the staining of the patient of interest. By comparing against a

control, a diseased cartilage will have reduced staining of proteoglycans and GAG (Fig. 1.4).

Collagen content and organization can be easily seen with
the use of picrosirius red. Picrosirius red staining utilizes
polarized light microscopy. Using polarized light microscopy,
the color and light visualized are reflective of the collagen
organization, alignment, size, and concentration (Fig. 1.4).
Therefore, disruptions of the normal collagen arrangement
can be seen by comparing the cartilage section to that of a
normal articular cartilage section.

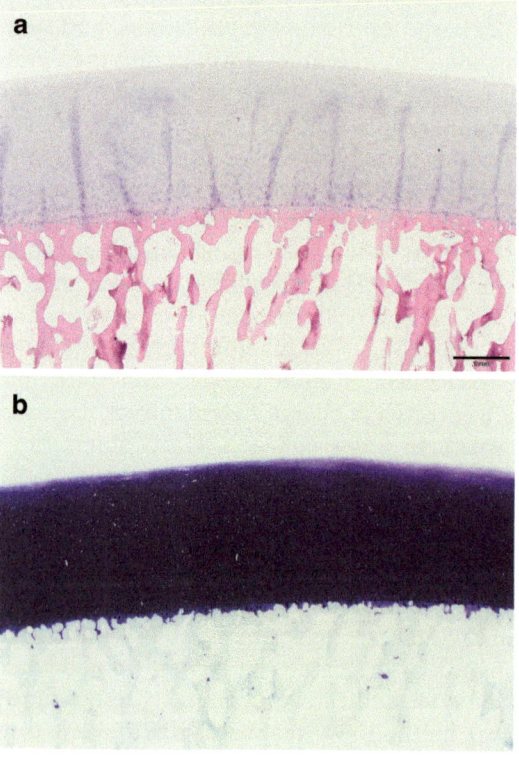

FIGURE 1.4 Histological photomicrographs (2×) of human femoral
condyle. (**a**) Hematoxylin and eosin, (**b**) Toluidine Blue, (**c**)
Picrosirius Red (polarized), and (**d**) Safranin O; scale bar, 1 mm

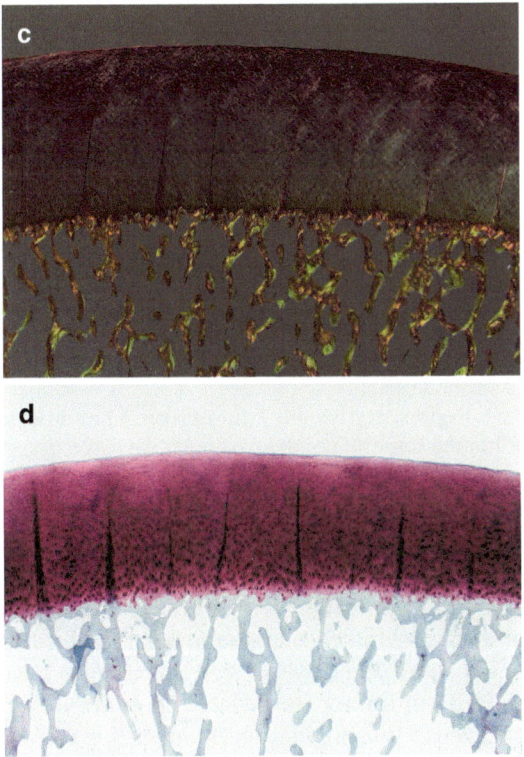

FIGURE 1.4 (continued)

The health of the osteochondral unit can be further illuminated by assessing the viable chondrocyte density (VCD) of the articular cartilage via fluorescent microscopy. Of clinical interest, the long-term success of operative treatments such as osteochondral allograft (OCA) transplantation is largely dependent on the viability of the chondrocytes of OCAs at the time of implantation [38, 39]. To assess chondrocyte viability, the tissue of interest can be stained for fluorescence using two stains that stain for live and dead cells, respectively, and subsequently imaged using fluorescent microscopy. To determine the VCD using fluorescent microscopy, a homogeneous mixture of the live stain calcein acetoxymethyl (Calcein AM), phosphate-buffered saline (PBS), and either the dead stain SYTOX Blue

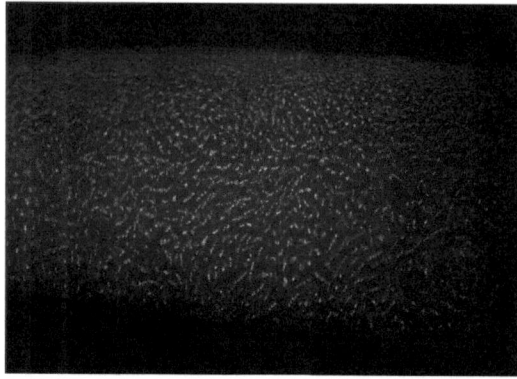

FIGURE 1.5 Representative (4×) fluorescent chondrocyte viability image of human femoral condyle articular cartilage tissue

(Life Technologies) or the dead stain ethidium homodimer (ETH) can be applied to the tissue of interest. Nonviable cells do not retain Calcein AM as their cell membranes have become weakened and permeable. Neither SYTOX Blue nor Calcein AM is able to cross intact cell membranes; therefore, these dead stains stain chondrocytes whose cell membranes have become compromised but do not stain viable chondrocytes with intact cell membranes. Utilizing these techniques, live cells stain green and dead cells stain red. Photographs can then be taken of the osteochondral unit using fluorescent microscopy, and relative chondrocyte viability can be subsequently visualized, as seen in Fig. 1.5. VCD is found by dividing the number of viable green cells by the area of the cartilage of interest. OA cartilage and cartilage with lesions have dramatically reduced VCD levels compared to those of healthy articular cartilage. This application has been of significant value in assessing articular cartilage in the laboratory, particularly in improving the storage protocols of OCAs for transplantation [40].

Summary

Articular cartilage functions as a specialized connective tissue (osteochondral unit) at the epiphyses of synovial joints. Composed of hyaline cartilage, articular cartilage functions to reduce the friction between movable joints and acts as a shock absorber. Disorders of articular cartilage are some of the most commonly encountered conditions in orthopedics. Appreciating the normal function and structure of articular cartilage is essential to understanding articular cartilage in its diseased state.

References

1. Curl WW, Krome J, Gordon ES, Rushing J, Smith BP, Poehling GG. Cartilage injuries: a review of 31,516 knee arthroscopies. Arthroscopy. 1997;13:456–60.
2. Alford JW, Cole BJ. Cartilage restoration, part 1: basic science, historical perspective, patient evaluation, and treatment options. Am J Sports Med. 2005;33(2):295–306.
3. Loeser RF. Age-related changes in the musculoskeletal system and the development of osteoarthritis. Clin Geriatr Med. 2010;26(3):371–86.
4. Jeffries MA, Donica M, Baker LW, Stevenson ME, Annan AC, Humphrey MB. Genome-wide DNA methylation study identifies significant epigenomic changes in osteoarthritic cartilage. Arthritis Rheumatol. 2014;66(10):2804–15.
5. Pop T, Szczygielska D, Drubicki M. Epidemiology and cost of conservative treatment of patients with degenerative joint disease of the knee and hip. Ortopedia Traumatologia Rehabilitacja. 2007;9(4):405–12.
6. Felson DT, Lawrence RC, Dieppe PA, Hirsch R, Helmick CG, Jordan JM, Kington RS, Lane NE, Nevitt MC, Zhang Y, Sowers M, McAlindon T, Spector TD, Poole AR, Yanovski SZ, Ateshian G, Sharma L, Buckwalter JA, Brandt KD, Fries JF. Osteoarthritis: new insights. Part 1: the disease and its risk factors. Ann Internal Med. 2000;133(8):635–46.
7. Sophia Fox AJ, Bedi A, Rodeo SA. The basic science of articular cartilage: structure, composition, and function. Sports Health. 2009;1(6):461–8.
8. Youn I, Choi JB, Cao L, Setton LA, Guilak F. Zonal variations in the three-dimensional morphology of the chondron measured in situ using confocal microscopy. Osteoarthr Cartil. 2006;14:889–97.
9. Cohen NP, Foster RJ, Mow VC. Composition and dynamics of articular cartilage: structure, function, and maintaining healthy state. J Orthop Sports Phys Ther. 1998;28(4):203–15.

10. Shoulders MD, Raines RT. Collagen structure and stability. Annu Rev Biochem. 2009;78:929–58.
11. Luo Y, Sinkeviciute D, He Y, Karsdal M, Henrotin Y, Mobasheri A, Önnerfjord P, Bay-Jensen A. The minor collagens in articular cartilage. Protein Cell. 2017;8:560. https://doi.org/10.1007/s13238-017-0377-7.
12. Wilson W, Driessen NJB, van Donkelaar CC, Ito K. Mechanical regulation of the chondron collagen fiber network structure. Trans Orthop Res Soc. 2006;31:1520.
13. Bhosale AM, Richardson JB. Articular cartilage: structure, injuries and review of management. Br Med Bull. 2008;87(1):77–95.
14. Danišovič L, Varga I, Polák S. Growth factors and chondrogenic differentiation of mesenchymal stem cells. Tissue Cell. 2012;44(2):69–73.
15. Brady MA, Waldman SD, Ethier CR. The application of multiple biophysical cues to engineer functional neocartilage for treatment of osteoarthritis. Part II: signal transduction. Tissue Eng Part B Rev. 2015;21(1):20–33.
16. Mankin HJ. Mitosis in articular cartilage of immature rabbits. Clin Orthop Relat Res. 1964;34:170–83.
17. Lattermann C, Romine SE. Osteochondral allografts: state of the art. Clin Sports Med. 2009;28(2):285–301.
18. Pearle AD, Warren RF, Rodeo SA. Basic science of articular cartilage and osteoarthritis. Clin Sports Med. 2005;24(1):1–12.
19. Hoemann CD, Lafantaiseie-Favreau CH, Lascau-Coman V, Chen G, Guzmán-Morales J. The cartilage-bone interface. J Knee Surg. 2012;25(2):85–97.
20. Norrdin RW, Kawcak CE, Capwell BA, McIlwraith CW. Calcified cartilage morphometry and its relation to subchondral bone remodeling in equine arthrosis. Bone. 1999;24(2):109–14.
21. Hwang J, Kyubwa EM, Bae WC, Bugbee WD, Masuda K, Sah RL. In vitro calcification of immature bovine articular cartilage: formation of a functional zone of calcified cartilage. Cartilage. 2010;1(4):287–97.
22. Langworthy MJ, Nelson FRT, Coutts RD. Basic science. In: Cole BJ, Malek MM, editors. Articular cartilage lesions: a practical guide to assessment and treatment. New York: Springer; 2004. p. 3–12.
23. Finnilä MA, Thevenot J, Aho OM, Tiitu V, Rautiainen J, Sl K, Nieminen MT, Pritzker K, Valkealahti M, Lehenkari P, Saarakkala S. Association between subchondral bone structure

and osteoarthritis histopathological grade. J Orthop Res. 2016; https://doi.org/10.1002/jor.23312.

24. Gomoll AH, Farr J. The osteochondral unit. In: Farr J, Gomoll AH, editors. Cartilage restoration: practical clinical applications. New York: Springer; 2014. p. 9–16.

25. Li G, Yin J, Gao J, Cheng TS, Pavlos NJ, Zhang C, Zheng MH. Subchondral bone in osteoarthritis: insight into risk factors and microstructural changes. Arthritis Res Ther. 2013;15(6):223.

26. Wang Y, Yuan M, Guo Q, Lu S, Peng J. Mesenchymal stem cells for treating articular cartilage defects and osteoarthritis. Cell Transplant. 2015;24:1661–78.

27. Kawcak CE, McIlwraith CW, Norrdin RW, Park RD, James SP. The role of subchondral bone in joint disease: a review. Equine Vet J. 2001;33(2):120–6.

28. van der Meijden OA, Gaskill TR, Millett PJ. Glenohumeral joint preservation: a review of management options for young, active patients with osteoarthritis. Arthroscopy. 2010;26(5):685–96.

29. Brittberg M, Winalski CS. Evaluation of cartilage injuries and repair. J Bone Joint Surg Am. 2003;85-A Suppl 2:58–69.

30. Bobic V. ICRS articular cartilage imaging committee. ICRS MR imaging protocol for knee articular cartilage. Zollikon: International Cartilage Repair Society; 2000.

31. Crema MD, Roemer FW, Marra MD, Burstein D, Gold GE, Eckstein F, Baum T, Mosher TJ, Carrino JA, Guermazi A. Articular cartilage in the knee: current MR imaging techniques and applications in clinical practice and research. Radiographics. 2011;31(1):37–61.

32. Gomoll AH, Yoshioka H, Watanabe A, Dunn JC, Minas T. Preoperative measurement of cartilage defects by MRI underestimates lesion size. Cartilage. 2011;2(4):389–93.

33. Nishioka H, Hirose J, Nakamura E, Okamoto N, Karasugi T, Taniwaki T, Okada T, Yamashita Y, Mizuta H. Detecting ICRS grade 1 cartilage lesions in anterior cruciate ligament injury using T1ρ and T2 mapping. Eur J Radiol. 2013;82(9):1499–505.

34. Duvvuri U, Reddy R, Patel SD, Kaufman JH, Kneeland JB, Leigh JS. T1rho-relaxation in articular cartilage: effects of enzymatic degradation. Magn Reson Med. 1997;38(6):863–7.

35. Akella SV, Regatte RR, Gougoutas AJ, Borthakur A, Shapiro EM, Kneeland JB, Leigh JS, Reddy R. Proteoglycan-induced changes in T1rho-relaxation of articular cartilage at 4T. Magn Reson Med. 2001;46(3):419–23.

36. Braun HJ, Gold GE. Advanced MRI of articular cartilage. Imaging Med. 2011;3(5):541–55.

37. Schmitz N, Laverty S, Kraus VB, Aigner T. Basic methods in histopathology of joint tissues. Osteoarthr Cartil. 2010;18:113–6.

38. Allen RT, Robertson CM, Pennock AT, Bugbee WD, Harwood FL, Wong VW, Chen AC, Sah RL, Amiel D. Analysis of stored osteochondral allografts at the time of surgical implantation. Am J Sports Med. 2005;33(10):1479–84.

39. Gross AE, Kim W, Las Heras F, Backstein D, Safir O, Pritzker KP. Fresh osteochondral allografts for posttraumatic knee defects: long-term follow-up. Clin Orthop Relat Res. 2008;466(8):1863–70.

40. Cook JL, Stoker AM, Stannard JP, Kuroki K, Cook CR, Pfeiffer FM, Bozynski C, Hung CT. A novel system improves preservation of osteochondral allografts. Clin Orthop Relat Res. 2014;472(11):3404–14.

Chapter 2
Meniscus: Biomechanics and Biology

Michael B. Ellman and Jorge Chahla

Introduction

In the United States, a meniscal tear is the most common diagnosis among patients undergoing knee arthroscopy [1, 2]. Clinically, patients with meniscal deficiency or tears have been shown to progress to early joint degeneration and osteoarthritis [1, 2], revealing the essential chondroprotective role of this structure in the knee joint. The meniscus optimizes load transmission across the knee by increasing joint congruency, thereby increasing contact area and decreasing point loading. Further, the menisci serve as important shock absorbers in the knee, as meniscal tissue is more elastic than articular cartilage and absorbs stress caused by impact loading [3]. The menisci also help to stabilize the knee joint [1], as the medial and lateral menisci function as secondary stabilizers for anterior-posterior translation and rotatory motion, respectively.

While early treatment of meniscal tears focused primarily on the removal of the injured tissue, recent attention on detrimental long-term consequences following partial or total meniscectomy has led to increased attempts at meniscus

M. B. Ellman (✉)
Panorama Orthopedics & Spine Center, Golden, CO, USA

J. Chahla
Department of Orthopedic Surgery, Rush University Medical Center, Chicago, IL, USA

© Springer Nature Switzerland AG 2019   25
A. B. Yanke, B. J. Cole (eds.), *Joint Preservation of the Knee*,
https://doi.org/10.1007/978-3-030-01491-9_2

repair whenever possible. Although meniscal repairs have a higher reoperation rate than meniscectomy, repairs have been reported to result in better long-term patient-reported outcomes, improved activity levels, and slower progression to osteoarthritis [4–6]. Therefore, understanding and preserving meniscal integrity are crucial to maintain the long-term health of the knee joint.

The purpose of this chapter is to describe the (i) anatomy of the menisci with an emphasis on anatomic root attachments, (ii) microstructure and biology of meniscal tissue, and (iii) biomechanical properties of meniscal tissue and their clinical relevance following meniscal injury.

Anatomy

The medial meniscus is a semilunar sheet of fibrocartilage localized between the medial femoral and medial tibial condyle (Fig. 2.1). It covers up to 60% of the articular surface of the medial tibial condyle, with an average width of 9–10 mm and average thickness of 3–5 mm [7]. The medial meniscus has a strong attachment to the surrounding structures (medial collateral ligament (MCL), posteromedial capsule) and therefore is less mobile than the lateral meniscus.

The lateral meniscus is more circular and covers a larger portion of the articular surface than the medial meniscus (up to 70%) (Fig. 2.1). The average width of the lateral meniscus is 10–12 mm, with an average thickness of 4–5 mm. The meniscus itself is grooved laterally for the popliteus tendon, which separates the meniscus from the fibular collateral ligament (FCL).

There are several supplemental attachments to the menisci that may play a role in stabilization of meniscal tissue. The transverse intermeniscal ligament connects the medial and lateral menisci anteriorly. The coronary ligaments connect the menisci to the capsule posteriorly and are stronger on the medial side than the lateral side, helping to explain the increased rigidity of the medial meniscus compared with the

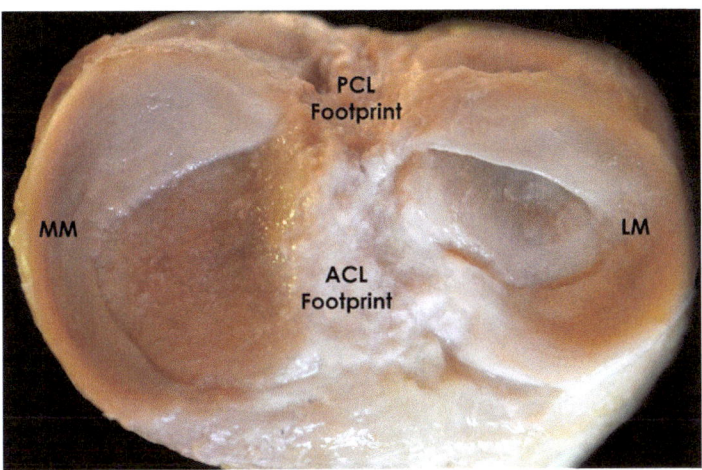

FIGURE 2.1 Axial view of cadaveric right knee demonstrating the anatomy of the medial meniscus (MM) and lateral meniscus (LM) in relation to the ACL and PCL footprint. The medial meniscus is semilunar in shape, while the lateral meniscus is more circular and covers a larger portion of the articular surface

lateral meniscus. Finally, the meniscofemoral ligaments originate from the posterior horn of the lateral meniscus (Fig. 2.2a, b). They are composed of two distinct ligamentous structures, the ligament of Humphrey, which lies anterior to the PCL (Fig. 2.2a), and the ligament of Wrisberg, posterior to the PCL (Fig. 2.2a, b). These structures help to stabilize the posterior horn of the lateral meniscus.

The menisci are anchored to the bone anteriorly and posteriorly by their strong root attachments. The clinical importance of maintaining meniscal root integrity has been well-documented in the literature. In a biomechanical study, Allaire et al. reported a significant 25% increase in medial compartment contact pressure following a PMMR tear [8]. Several other studies have corroborated these findings [9, 10], as a complete root tear biomechanically simulates a meniscectomized knee, thereby increasing the risk for (often rapid) progression of osteoarthritis. A thorough knowledge of the

a
Hemi-Sectioned
Femur
ALB
PMB
pMFL
aMFL
LM
b
Wrisberg
ALB
LM
PMB

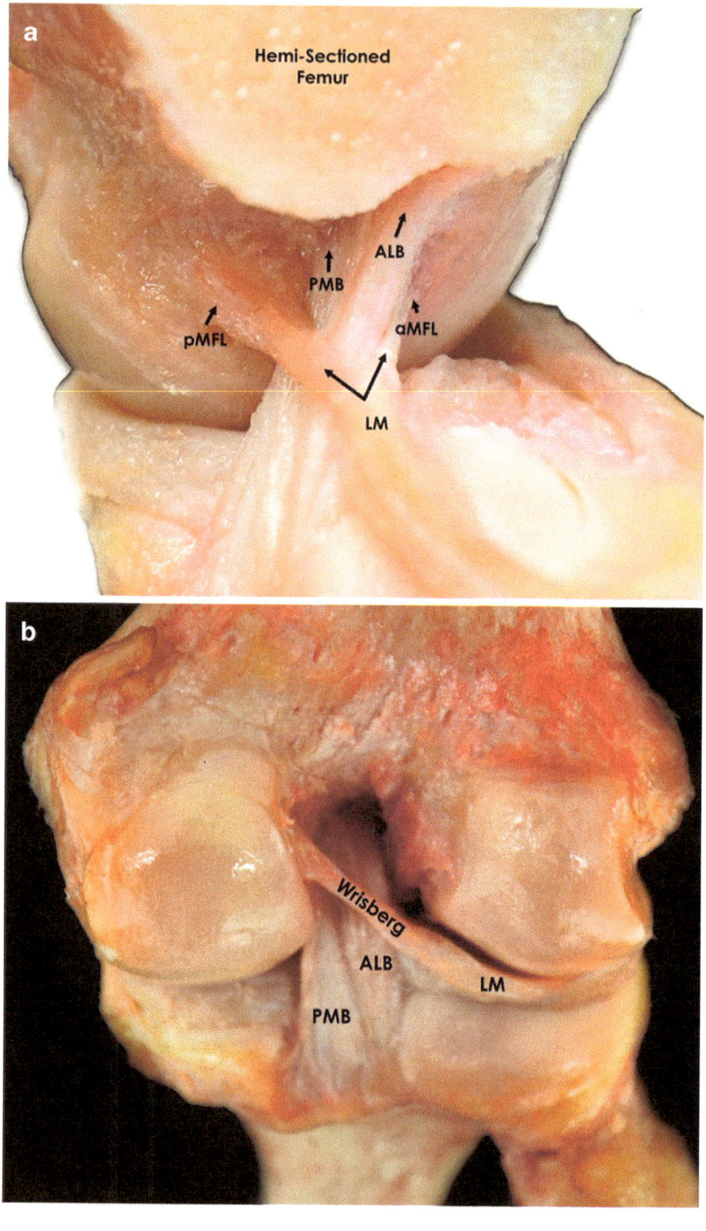

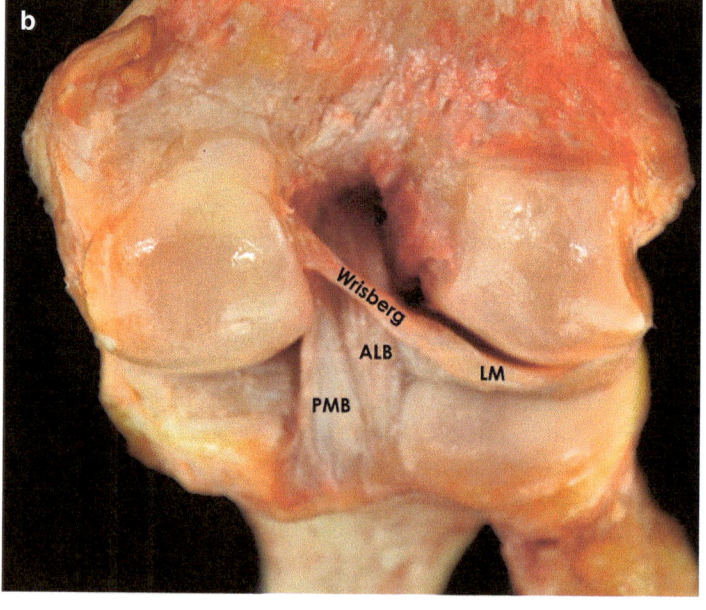

FIGURE 2.2 (a) Cadaveric sagittal hemisection of the right knee demonstrating anatomy of anterior meniscofemoral ligament (aMFL, aka ligament of Humphrey) and posterior meniscofemoral ligament (pMFL, aka ligament of Wrisberg) arising from posterior horn of lateral meniscus (LM). The PCL is present with a clear distinction between the anterolateral bundle (ALB) fibers and posteromedial bundle (PMB) fibers. (b) Posterior view of cadaveric right knee demonstrating ligament of Wrisberg originating from posterior horn of lateral meniscus (LM), traversing posterior to the two bundles of the PCL (anterolateral bundle (ALB) and posteromedial bundle (PMB), and attaching the posterolateral aspect of the medial femoral condyle

precise anatomical location and area of each root is vital for the surgeon to successfully perform anatomic meniscal root repairs.

The structural properties of the four meniscal roots have also been described in the literature [11], with each root containing strong, central fibers as well as peripheral, supplemental fibers that increase the surface area, strength, and stiffness of each root (Table 2.1). Anatomically, the medial tibial eminence (MTE) apex is the most reproducible osseous landmark for identification of the posterior medial meniscal root (PMMR) attachment (Fig. 2.3a). The center of the PMMR is approximately 10 mm posterior and 1 mm lateral to the MTE [12]. The most proximal PCL tibial attachment fibers (located 8 mm lateral from the center of the PMMR) and the medial tibial plateau articular cartilage inflection point (4 mm lateral to the root) are two other consistent landmarks to identify the root attachment (Fig. 2.3a).

The posterior lateral meniscal root (PLMR) attachment can also be identified using the apex of the lateral tibial eminence (LTE), which is the most consistent landmark (Fig. 2.3b). The center of the PLMR is consistently found to be 4 mm medial and 1.5 mm posterior to the LTE. According to Johannsen et al. [12], the center of the PLMR is located 4 mm medial to the lateral tibial plateau articular cartilage edge and 13 mm anterior to the most proximal edge of the posterior cruciate ligament (PCL) tibial attachment (Fig. 2.3b).

TABLE 2.1 Structural properties of the meniscal roots with and without sectioning of the supplemental root attachment fibers

Root	Native	Sectioned
Attachment area, mm^2		
AM	101.7 (82.4–120.9)	57.0 (49.4–64.5)
PM	68.0 (59.1–76.9)	41.6 (35.3–47.8)
AL	99.5 (83.1–116.0)	N/A
PL	83.1 (63.6–102.7)	57.7 (47.3–68.0)
Ultimate failure strength, N		
AM	655.5 (487.2–823.8)	469.1 (240.7–697.4)
PM	513.8 (388.4–639.1)	267.9 (206.6–329.2)
AL	652.8 (528.2–777.3)	608.4 (434.2–782.6)
PL	509.0 (392.0–625.9)	419.4 (288.9–549.8)
Stiffness, N/mm		
AM	124.9 (101.4–148.3)	103.7 (75.4–132.0)
PM	122.7 (95.1–150.3)	80.7 (71.1–90.2)
AL	151.1 (123.9–178.4)	136.8 (108.4–165.2)
PL	128.7 (104.1–153.3)	117.2 (89.8–144.7)

The anterior medial meniscal root has the largest native area and ultimate failure strength

AL anterior lateral, *AM* anterior medial, *PL* posterior lateral, *PM* posterior medial meniscal root; data reported as mean (95% confidence interval)

These findings help the surgeon when identifying the proper anatomic location during a meniscal root repair.

Microstructure/Biology

Understanding the microstructure of the meniscus helps to explain its complex biomechanical properties and function. The meniscus is mainly comprised of water (up to 75%) and

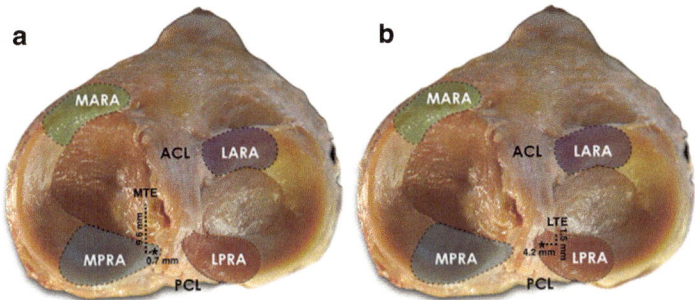

FIGURE 2.3 Cadaveric images (superior axial view) demonstrating the anatomical landmarks to identify (**a**) medial meniscus posterior root attachment and (**b**) lateral meniscus posterior root attachment in a right knee. MTE medial tibial eminence, LTE lateral tibial eminence, MARA medial meniscus anterior root attachment, LARA lateral meniscus anterior root attachment, MPRA medial meniscus posterior root attachment, LPRA lateral meniscus posterior root attachment

collagen (20–25%, 90% type I) and a minority of other elements including proteoglycans, matrix glycoproteins, and elastin [13–17].

Each meniscus is composed of three layers (Fig. 2.4). A more superficial layer is in direct contact with the articular surface and is composed of randomly oriented collagen fibers mixed with a lubricating layer of proteoglycans, allowing for a low frictional surface [18, 19]. Deep to this layer is the middle stratum, which is composed of a lamellar layer containing collagen fibers extending radially (externally), with internal fibers intersecting at various angles, creating a mesh to provide rigidity to the tissue [19]. Finally, the inner layer is composed of large circumferential fibers, with the majority located in the internal and external circumference of the menisci because the middle portion experiences more uniform compressive stress and minimal radial stress (Fig. 2.4) [20, 21]. These circumferential fibers undergo significant tensile or "hoop" stresses when axially loaded [20, 22–25].

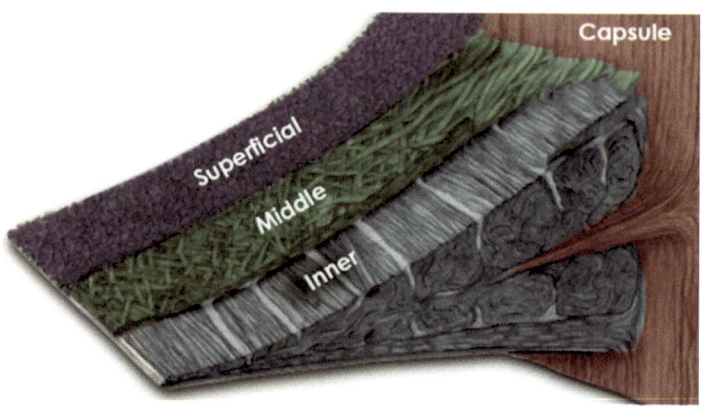

FIGURE 2.4 Schematic illustration showing the different layers of the menisci. The superficial layer contains disorganized fibers, the lamellar layer contains peripherally oriented radial fibers with an internal interconnecting meshwork, and the deep/inner layer contains large circumferential oriented bundles intermingling with radial tie fibers

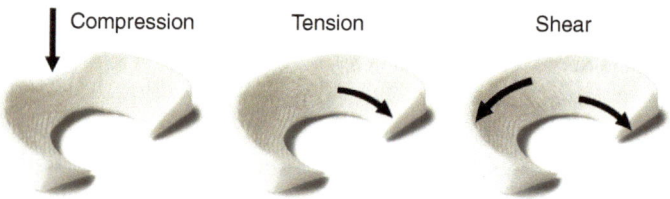

FIGURE 2.5 Illustration demonstrating application of load, including compression, tension, and shear stress to meniscal tissue

Biomechanical Properties

Several unique biomechanical principles contribute to the complex function of the menisci. These include viscoelasticity, permeability, creep, stress relaxation, ultimate tensile load, and shear stiffness, with each principle playing a vital role in the biomechanical response of meniscal tissue to compression, tension, and shear stresses (Fig. 2.5).

- *Viscoelasticity*: Due to the unique three-layered anatomy described above, the tissue properties of the menisci change throughout an applied load; i.e., they exhibit both viscous and elastic properties. This transition occurs in a time-dependent fashion, beginning in the elastic phase and shifting to the viscous phase during loading. The elastic phase is due to the meniscus collagenous-proteoglycan structure. Conversely, the viscous phase is due to its permeability and water content [20, 26, 27]. When a compressive load is applied to the menisci, the elastic phase initiates, with the meniscal tissue exhibiting an elastic response and compressing the menisci. Simultaneously, fluid extrudes slowly, which accommodates the compressive load without excess deformation, hence beginning the viscous phase [28, 29]. Under compression, meniscal permeability determines the rate at which fluid is extruded. Meniscal permeability is much lower than articular cartilage, allowing for slow extrusion and helping to maintain meniscal shape and integrity during axial loads [27, 28, 30]. Thus, menisci maintain their load-bearing capacity during gait by resisting fluid loss [17, 31, 32], which inhibits compression and helps to maintain their shape.
- *Response to Compression*: Creep and stress relaxation are two related characteristics of viscoelastic behavior [28]. After the initial load is applied and fluid is extruded from the menisci, the compressive load is resisted, known as "creep." [20, 28] This results in a diminished rate of compression over time. When the menisci are compressed and held, the tissue relaxes, and the load required to maintain the given compression decreases. This is referred to as "stress relaxation." Further, when a compressive load is applied to the menisci, an axial load redistributes "hoop stresses" to the circumferential fibers of the menisci, extending to their attachments on the tibia and femur [20, 23–25]. As the femur compresses down, the menisci extrude peripherally due to their wedge shape, causing a radially oriented tangential force [33]. This peripheral extrusion is prevented by the anterior and posterior meniscal root attachments, as

described above. When a root tear occurs clinically, these forces are unopposed, resulting in a functionally meniscectomized state with a significant increase in contract stress occurring in the respective compartment [8] and thereby increasing the risk of progression to osteoarthritis.

- *Response to Tension*: When menisci undergo tensile forces (stretching forces), elongation occurs relatively fast because collagen fibers are relaxed [34]. After the initial phase, there is a linear relationship between elongation and the load applied, followed by a drastic decrease in elongation as fibers begin to fail and tear [35]. The maximum load the menisci can maintain in tension before failure is referred to as the ultimate tensile load. The tensile properties can change depending on the location of the menisci.

- *Response to Shear*: Shear stiffness is defined as the capacity of the meniscus to resist a change of its shape. In this regard, menisci have a lower shear stiffness compared to the articular cartilage and bone, thereby allowing the menisci to maintain optimal congruency between the tibia and the femur through a full range of motion, ensuring equal load distribution [20].

In Vivo Biomechanics

Synchronized motion of the menisci during knee range of motion allows for a maximum congruency over the articulating surfaces, thereby decreasing contact stress within the joint and optimizing congruency and stability [36]. For example, the translation of the lateral meniscus is twice that of the medial meniscus [37], with greater translation of the anterior horns compared to the posterior horns. This is critical because the femoral condyles' articulating shape with the menisci changes during flexion and extension, causing the anterior and posterior horns to drift apart during full extension and closer together during flexion [27]. The anterior horns allow movement to accommodate this, while the posterior horns are more secure and stable, restricting excess movement [36]. Approximately 85% of the weight-bearing load is transmitted in knee flexion with the horns closer together, while 50% is transmitted in extension with the horns further apart [3]. Further, during internal rotation of the tibia, the lateral meniscus translates posteriorly, while the medial meniscus translates anteriorly [38]. These reciprocal functions allow the menisci to maximize contact area with the articular surfaces, reduce point stresses, and avoid chondral damage or injury over time [27].

Clinically, patients with lateral meniscal deficiency demonstrate worse outcomes compared to patients with medial meniscal deficiency [1, 2]. This may be a consequence of the less congruent, more convex articular surfaces of the lateral femoral condyle and lateral tibial plateau, as well as the greater degree of translation of the lateral meniscus, suggesting a crucial role of the lateral meniscus in maintaining lateral joint integrity [24, 37]. Further, the lateral meniscus absorbs 70% of load while the medial meniscus only 50% [3], again helping to elucidate the clinical significance of the lateral meniscus.

The aforementioned differences in translation of each meniscus may also help to explain the role of the menisci as secondary stabilizers within the knee joint. The medial meniscus is an important secondary restraint to anterior tibial translation [28, 39, 40]. This can be explained by the decreased mobility of the medial meniscus, as the medial meniscus is less mobile with approximately 50% translation compared to the lateral meniscus and therefore is more stable in an anterior-posterior direction. The medial meniscus is also postulated to have a "wedge" effect created by compression on the posterior horn during loading, further preventing anterior displacement [41]. The joint stabilizing capability of the medial meniscus is most apparent in ACL-deficient knees. Following medial meniscectomy in the ACL-deficient knee, there is a significant increase in anterior tibial translation after an anterior tibial load is applied, compared to ACL-deficient knees with an intact medial meniscus [41, 42]. These findings corroborate the vital role of the medial meniscus as a secondary stabilizer of anterior-posterior translation of the knee.

In contrast, due to its increased mobility and translation, the lateral meniscus is thought to play a lesser role in anterior-posterior stabilization [41, 43, 44], but it has been found to play a greater role in anterolateral rotatory stability [45]. The lateral meniscus has also been suggested to play an important secondary role in restraining combined axial and rotatory loads [45].

Conclusion

The meniscus plays an integral role in the knee with several chondroprotective and stabilizing functions. A thorough understanding of meniscal anatomy, biology, and biomechanics is vital to understand the complex structure and function of the medial and lateral menisci.

References

1. Raber DA, Friederich NF, Hefti F. Discoid lateral meniscus in children. Long-term follow-up after total meniscectomy. J Bone Joint Surg Am. 1998;80:1579–86.
2. McNicholas MJ, Rowley DI, McGurty D, Adalberth T, Abdon P, Lindstrand A, Lohmander LS. Total meniscectomy in adolescence. A thirty-year follow-up. J Bone Joint Surg Br. 2000;82:217–21.
3. Messner K, Gao J. The menisci of the knee joint. Anatomical and functional characteristics, and a rationale for clinical treatment. J Anat. 1998;193(Pt 2):161–78.
4. Starke C, Kopf S, Petersen W, Becker R. Meniscal repair. Arthroscopy. 2009;25:1033–44.
5. Vaquero J, Forriol F. Meniscus tear surgery and meniscus replacement. Muscles Ligaments Tendons J. 2016;6:71–89.
6. Yoon KH, Park KH. Meniscal repair. Knee Surg Relat Res. 2014;26:68–76.
7. LaPrade RF, Arendt EA, Getgood A, Faucett SC. The menisci: a comprehensive review of their anatomy, biomechanical function and surgical treatment. Berlin/Heidelberg: Springer; 2017.

8. Allaire R, Muriuki M, Gilbertson L, Harner CD. Biomechanical consequences of a tear of the posterior root of the medial meniscus. Similar to total meniscectomy. J Bone Joint Surg Am. 2008;90:1922–31.

9. Bhatia S, Civitarese DM, Turnbull TL, LaPrade CM, Nitri M, Wijdicks CA, LaPrade RF. A novel repair method for radial tears of the medial meniscus: biomechanical comparison of Transtibial 2-tunnel and double horizontal mattress suture techniques under cyclic loading. Am J Sports Med. 2016;44:639–45.

10. LaPrade CM, Jansson KS, Dornan G, Smith SD, Wijdicks CA, LaPrade RF. Altered tibiofemoral contact mechanics due to lateral meniscus posterior horn root avulsions and radial tears can be restored with in situ pull-out suture repairs. J Bone Joint Surg Am. 2014;96:471–9.

11. Ellman MB, LaPrade CM, Smith SD, Rasmussen MT, Engebretsen L, Wijdicks CA, LaPrade RF. Structural properties of the meniscal roots. Am J Sports Med. 2014;42:1881–7.

12. Johannsen AM, Civitarese DM, Padalecki JR, Goldsmith MT, Wijdicks CA, LaPrade RF. Qualitative and quantitative anatomic analysis of the posterior root attachments of the medial and lateral menisci. Am J Sports Med. 2012;40:2342–7.

13. Wirth CJ. The meniscus—structure, morphology and function. Knee. 1994;1:171–2.

14. Tissakht M, Ahmed AM. Tensile stress-strain characteristics of the human meniscal material. J Biomech. 1995;28:411–22.

15. Djurasovic M, Aldridge JW, Grumbles R, Rosenwasser MP, Howell D, Ratcliffe A. Knee joint immobilization decreases aggrecan gene expression in the meniscus. Am J Sports Med. 1998; 26:460–6.

16. Fox AJ, Wanivenhaus F, Burge AJ, Warren RF, Rodeo SA. The human meniscus: a review of anatomy, function, injury, and advances in treatment. Clin Anat. 2015;28:269–87.

17. Sweigart MA, Zhu CF, Burt DM, DeHoll PD, Agrawal CM, Clanton TO, Athanasiou KA. Intraspecies and interspecies comparison of the compressive properties of the medial meniscus. Ann Biomed Eng. 2004;32:1569–79.

18. Schumacher BL, Schmidt TA, Voegtline MS, Chen AC, Sah RL. Proteoglycan 4 (PRG4) synthesis and immunolocalization in bovine meniscus. J Orthop Res. 2005;23:562–8.

19. Petersen W, Tillmann B. Collagenous fibril texture of the human knee joint menisci. Anat Embryol (Berl). 1998;197:317–24.

20. Andrews SJ, Adesida AB, Abusara Z, Shrive NG. Current concepts on structure-function relationships in the menisci. Connect Tissue Res. 2017;58:271–81.
21. Petersen W, Tillmann B. Funktionelle anatomie der menisken des kniegelenks kollagenfasertextur und biomechanik. Arthroskopie. 1998;11:133–5.
22. Zhu W, Chern KY, Mow VC. Anisotropic viscoelastic shear properties of bovine meniscus. Clin Orthop Relat Res. 1994;306:34–45.
23. Shrive NG, O'Connor JJ, Goodfellow JW. Load-bearing in the knee joint. Clin Orthop Relat Res. 1978;131:279–87.
24. Fairbank TJ. Knee joint changes after meniscectomy. J Bone Joint Surg Br. 1948;30B:664–70.
25. Bullough PG, Munuera L, Murphy J, Weinstein AM. The strength of the menisci of the knee as it relates to their fine structure. J Bone Joint Surg Br. 1970;52:564–7.
26. Fithian DC, Kelly MA, Mow VC. Material properties and structure-function relationships in the menisci. Clin Orthop Relat Res. 1990;252:19–31.
27. Proctor CS, Schmidt MB, Whipple RR, Kelly MA, Mow VC. Material properties of the normal medial bovine meniscus. J Orthop Res. 1989;7:771–82.
28. McDermott ID, Masouros SD, Amis AA. Biomechanics of the menisci of the knee. Curr Orthop. 2008;22:193–201.
29. Spilker RL, Donzelli PS, Mow VC. A transversely isotropic biphasic finite element model of the meniscus. J Biomech. 1992;25:1027–45.
30. Favenesi J, Shaffer J, Mow V. Biphasic mechanical properties of knee meniscus. Trans Orthop Res Soc. 1983;8:57.
31. Joshi MD, Suh JK, Marui T, Woo SL. Interspecies variation of compressive biomechanical properties of the meniscus. J Biomed Mater Res. 1995;29:823–8.
32. Hacker S, Woo S, Wayne J, Kwan M. Compressive properties of the human meniscus. Tran Annu Meet Orthop Res Soc. 1992:627.
33. Kummer B. 38. Anatomie und Biomechanik des Kniegelenksmeniscus. Langenbecks Arch Chir. 1987;372:241–6.
34. Viidik A. Functional properties of collagenous tissues. Int Rev Connect Tissue Res. 1973;6:127–215.
35. Butler DL, Grood ES, Noyes FR, Zernicke RF. Biomechanics of ligaments and tendons. Exerc Sport Sci Rev. 1978;6:125–81.
36. Vedi V, Williams A, Tennant SJ, Spouse E, Hunt DM, Gedroyc WM. Meniscal movement. An in-vivo study using dynamic MRI. J Bone Joint Surg Br. 1999;81:37–41.

37. Aagaard H, Verdonk R. Function of the normal meniscus and consequences of meniscal resection. Scand J Med Sci Sports. 1999;9:134–40.
38. Bylski-Austrow DI, Ciarelli MJ, Kayner DC, Matthews LS, Goldstein SA. Displacements of the menisci under joint load: an in vitro study in human knees. J Biomech. 1994;27:421425–3431.
39. Bargar WL, Moreland JR, Markolf KL, Shoemaker SC, Amstutz HC, Grant TT. In vivo stability testing of post-meniscectomy knees. Clin Orthop Relat Res. 1980;150:247–52.
40. Arno S, Hadley S, Campbell KA, Bell CP, Hall M, Beltran LS, Recht MP, Sherman OH, Walker PS. The effect of arthroscopic partial medial meniscectomy on tibiofemoral stability. Am J Sports Med. 2013;41:73–9.
41. Levy IM, Torzilli PA, Warren RF. The effect of medial meniscectomy on anterior-posterior motion of the knee. J Bone Joint Surg Am. 1982;64:883–8.
42. Allen CR, Wong EK, Livesay GA, Sakane M, Fu FH, Woo SL. Importance of the medial meniscus in the anterior cruciate ligament-deficient knee. J Orthop Res. 2000;18:109–15.
43. Lerer D, Umans H, Hu M, Jones M. The role of meniscal root pathology and radial meniscal tear in medial meniscal extrusion. Skelet Radiol. 2004;33:569–74.
44. Thompson WO, Thaete FL, Fu FH, Dye SF. Tibial meniscal dynamics using three-dimensional reconstruction of magnetic resonance images. Am J Sports Med. 1991;19:210–5; discussion 215–6.
45. Musahl V, Citak M, O'Loughlin PF, Choi D, Bedi A, Pearle AD. The effect of medial versus lateral meniscectomy on the stability of the anterior cruciate ligament-deficient knee. Am J Sports Med. 2010;38:1591–7.

Chapter 3
Coronal and Axial Alignment: The Effects of Malalignment

Luiz Felipe Ambra, Andreas H. Gomoll, and Jack Farr

Introduction

The normal knee joint can support a lifetime of repetitive load, generally, without the development of degenerative changes. Excessive stress, which exceeds the tolerance of articular cartilage, disrupts articular homeostasis leading to deterioration of the articular cartilage. In physiological condition, the load applied to the knee joint is distributed across the compartments. Any deviation of the knee alignment, referred to as malalignment, negatively affects load distribution. Improper load distribution reduces the knee joint's ability to accommodate physiological forces which may cause damage to the articular cartilage.

L. F. Ambra
Department of Orthopedic and Traumatology, Universidade
Federal de São Paulo, São Paulo, SP, Brazil

A. H. Gomoll
Department of Orthopedic Surgery, Hospital for Special Surgery,
New York, NY, USA

J. Farr (✉)
Cartilage Restoration Center, OrthoIndy Hospital,
Indianapolis, IN, USA
e-mail: jfarr@orthoindy.com

© Springer Nature Switzerland AG 2019   41
A. B. Yanke, B. J. Cole (eds.), *Joint Preservation of the Knee*,
https://doi.org/10.1007/978-3-030-01491-9_3

Cartilage lesions are one of the most challenging pathologies to manage successfully. When conservative treatment fails to relieve symptoms and recover functional limitations, surgery is usually recommended to treat both the cartilage defect and any underlying anatomic abnormalities. Despite these lesions being technically easily accessible, the analysis of concomitant pathologies is difficult; therefore, a rational approach to systematically evaluate and identify pathologic deviation of the knee alignment is required to plan specific treatment that addresses each pathologic component.

Imaging

Radiographic exams are the first step to evaluate knee alignment. A standard knee series includes a weight-bearing anteroposterior (AP) view in full extension, a posterior-anterior view in flexion (PA Rosenberg), full-length hip-to-ankle alignment radiograph, true lateral view, and axial view with 45° or 30° of flexion.

Standard weight-bearing AP and Rosenberg views allow evaluation of femorotibial pathology. A standing hip-to-ankle alignment radiograph is the most accurate method to evaluate mechanical axis of the lower extremity. In a neutrally aligned knee, it is defined as a line from the center of the femoral head to the center of the ankle joint, passing across the center of the knee joint. By definition, if the line is off-center at the knee toward the lateral compartment, it is valgus alignment, and if toward the medial compartment, it is varus alignment (Fig. 3.1).

True lateral view with superposition of both femoral condyles is usually taken with an angle of flexion of 20°. This incidence allows evaluation of tibial slope, patellar height (Insall-Salvati; Caton-Deschamps; Blackburne-Peel), patellar tilt, and trochlear morphology (Dejour classification).

Low flexion axial radiograph allows assessment of trochlea and patella morphology and the position of the patella relative to the trochlea. The difficulty with this technique is that images are not taken near full extension where the troch-

FIGURE 3.1 A long-length radiograph showing valgus alignment on the right and neutral alignment on the left

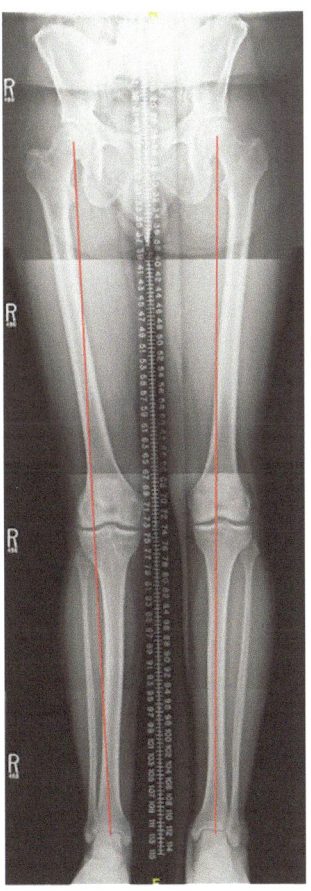

lea is most shallow. As the knee flexes, the trochlear groove deepens, and the patella slides medially, becoming more congruent with the femoral sulcus. Hence, trochlear dysplasia, patellar tilt, or subluxation are underestimated on the axial view due to the flexion required to obtain this incidence.

Computed tomography (CT) exam provides valuable information regarding the anatomy and kinematics of the knee joint, mainly the patellofemoral joint (PFJ). Allowing a true axial view of the PFJ, this exam can image in different degrees of flexion, letting one accurately define the anatomy and relationship between the patella and the femoral trochlea. Another important contribution of CT is the ability to create overlapping images, allowing assessment of torsional deformities, such as femoral anteversion (FA) and external tibial torsion, as well as measurements of tibial tubercle-trochlear groove (TT-TG) and/or tibial tubercle-posterior cruciate ligament (TT-PCL) distance.

Magnetic resonance imaging (MRI) is the most complete imaging technique. This exam allows for the simultaneous evaluation of all the structures that constitute the knee joint, distinguishing the different tissues. MRI exams can better evaluate articular morphology as well as meniscal and ligament tearing, chondral and osteochondral lesions, rotational deformities, and patellar alignment.

Table 3.1 summarizes clinical exams and imaging studies used to evaluate patellofemoral joint disorders and underlying comorbidities.

Tibiofemoral Alignment and Cartilage Lesions

During a normal gait, knee reaction forces reach three times the body weight, increasing to six times the body weight during higher activity levels. In a normally aligned knee, approximately 60% of the weight-bearing force is transmitted through the medial compartment, the adduction moment being the primary contributing factor to an increased medial joint reaction force [1]. Biomechanical studies have demonstrated that varus and valgus alignment increase medial and lateral load, respectively [2, 3]. Accordingly, malalignment has been recognized as an independent risk factor for development and progression of knee osteoarthritis (OA) [4, 5]. After 18 months of follow-up, a valgus-aligned knee was five times more likely to present progression of lateral compartment OA compared with knees of neutral alignment; similarly, a varus-aligned knee increases risk of medial OA progression by a factor of 4.

TABLE 3.1 Preoperative considerations for cartilage restoration

Consideration	Clinical exam/imaging study	Objective evaluation
Coronal alignment	Valgus and varus alignment	Inspection on physical examination, mechanical axis view radiograph
Axial alignment	External tibial torsion increased femoral neck anteversion	Thigh-foot angle; CT or MRI version study hip/ knee/ankle
	Lateralized patellar force vector	Q angle; CT or MRI measurement of TT-TG and TT-PCL
		Patellar tilt
Sagittal alignment	Increased patellar height	True lateral with loading flexion radiographic, CT or MRI measurement of patella alta (Insall-Salvati, Caton-Deschamps, or Blackburne-Peel ratio)
	Tibial slope	True lateral view radiographic, CT or MRI
Patellofemoral morphology	Trochlear dysplasia	Radiographic crossing sign, trochlear boss, CT/ MRI findings (Dejour classification)

Patellofemoral Alignment and Cartilage Lesions

Clinically, extensor mechanism alignment can be assessed measuring Q angle. Described as the direction of the quadriceps force and the patellar tendon reaction force, this angle determines the lateral vector of the extensor mechanism force. Despite the widely discussed potential for inaccuracy of the clinical measurement of the Q angle, a theoretical understanding of the influence of extensor mechanism alignment is crucial to comprehend the influence of anatomical abnormalities on patellofemoral contact forces.

Patellofemoral malalignment is a complex pathology with a wide spectrum of clinical presentation. Several features can influence the Q angle and, consequently, the PF reaction forces. No single factor may be the sole defining etiology, as patellofemoral malalignment is most frequently the result of an association of anatomic abnormalities. Therefore, a global understanding of the pathology is crucial to tailor the most suitable approach in each case.

Coronal Alignment

Both valgus and varus alignment may contribute to modification of the contact stresses in the PFJ [6, 7]. Valgus alignment increases the Q angle, which leads to an increment increase in the lateral vector of the quadriceps force, thereby overloading the lateral side of the PFJ. Conversely, varus alignment tends to reduce the Q angle, shifting the quadriceps force medially, therefore, increasing the contact stress on the medial side of the PFJ [8]. Cahue et al. prospectively showed that valgus alignment was associated with lateral PF OA progression; likewise, varus alignment increased the risk for medial PF OA progression [9].

Axial Alignment

Evaluation of the patellofemoral alignment in the axial plane can be challenging and should be evaluated carefully to understand the true source of abnormality. The tibial tubercle-trochlear groove (TT-TG) distance is one of the most used parameters for the measurement of patellofemoral alignment, being largely correlated with Q angle [10, 11]. This measurement assesses the mediolateral distance between the center of the patellar tendon insertion at the tibial tubercle and the deepest point of the trochlear groove (Fig. 3.2). The TT-TG

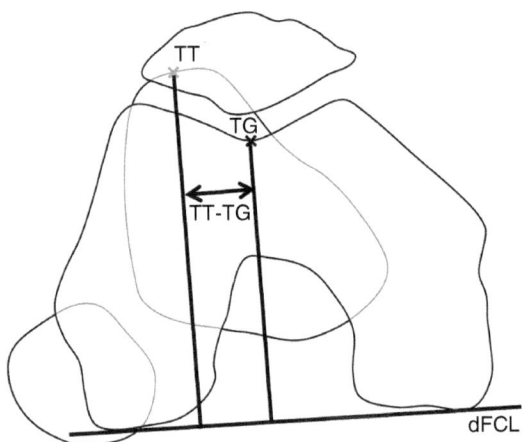

FIGURE 3.2 TT-TG measurement. Images from the trochlear groove and tibial tubercle are superimposed. Trochlear groove location is determined at the level where the posterior cortex of the femoral condyles is well defined. The trochlear line is drawn perpendicular to the posterior condylar axis, tangential to the posterior femoral condyles (dFCL), and passing through the deepest point of the trochlear groove (TG). Tibial tubercle image is selected at the level of the most anterior point of the tibial tuberosity. A line crossing through the center of the tibial tubercle (TT) is drawn perpendicular to the posterior femoral axis. The distance between these two parallel lines is the TT-TG distance. (Copyright © 2012 American Orthopaedic Society for Sports Medicine. Reprinted from Seitlinger et al. [15] with permission from SAGE publications)

distance can be measured with ease using both MRI and CT; however, the values resultant from these two techniques may not be interchangeable. Due to discrepancies in knee flexion during image acquisition, MRI exams tend to underestimate the TT-TG distance when compared with CT and should be taken into consideration during surgical planning [12].

Traditionally, a TT-TG distance of greater than 20 mm is considered pathologic, representing an excessive lateral position of the TT in relation to the trochlea, and has been accepted as the threshold for recommendation of distal realignment [13]. However, a large TT-TG must be interpreted carefully. Other conditions such as trochlear dysplasia, distal femoral internal rotation, or tibial external rotation may lead to increased TT-TG distance; each should be evaluated to determine the site of potential treatment [14, 15]. Tensho et al., compared the influence of trochlea medialization, tibial tubercle lateralization, and knee rotation, and found that knee rotation is the most important factor influencing TT-TG distance [16].

Tibial tubercle-posterior cruciate ligament (TT-PCL) distance was introduced as an adjunct measurement to evaluate the TT position [15]. This parameter is assessed by measuring the distance between the medial margin of the PCL and the midpoint of the TT at the level of the patellar tendon attachment (Fig. 3.3), normal values being less than 24 mm. As it is referenced to the tibia, this parameter is independent of trochlear morphology and femoral rotation. Therefore, femoral rotation abnormalities should be investigated in patients with a TT-TG distance more than 20 mm and normal TT-PCL distance.

The Q angle is also influenced by the rotational interaction between the femur and tibia. Lateral rotation of the tibia in relation to the femur moves the tibial tubercle (TT) laterally, resulting in an increase in the Q angle [17, 18]. Similarly, increased femoral anteversion leads to internal rotation of the distal femur, moving the patella medially, thereby, increasing the Q angle [19, 20].

During normal gait, the knee joint axis rotates externally, in relation to the pelvis, during the swing phase, and moves internally during the stance phase. The increment of the femoral anteversion leads to an abnormal internally rotated gait. While the body is moving forward, the knee joint axis is pointing medially. This leads to an increased internal rotation of the knee joint axis during stance phase, causing excessive lateral forces on the patella. This excessive lateralization increases tension on the MPFL and pressure on the lateral side of the patellofemoral joint while unloading the medial side. Hence, increased FA

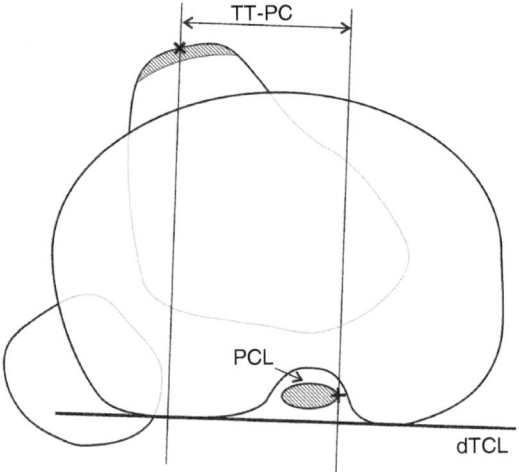

FIGURE 3.3 TT-PCL measurement. Proximal tibia (below the joint and above the head of the fibula) and patellar tendon insertion (most inferior slice in which the ligament could still be clearly identified) images are superimposed. The TT-PCL distance is the mediolateral distance between the medial border of the posterior cruciate ligament (PCL) and the center of the insertion of the patellar tendon. Both lines are drawn perpendicular to a posterior tibial condyles reference line (dTCL), tangential to the proximal tibia below the joint and above the head of the fibula. (Copyright © 2012 American Orthopaedic Society for Sports Medicine. Reprinted from Seitlinger et al. [15] with permission from SAGE publications)

results in abnormal lateral patellofemoral pressure and the tendency for lateral subluxation.

Several techniques have been described to assess rotational alignment of the inferior limb. Femoral, tibial, and knee torsion can be assessed by overlapping axial cuts from the femoral head, base of the femoral neck or lesser trochanter, the knee joint (either tangent to the posterior condyles or between the medial and lateral epicondyles), the proximal tibia at the joint, and the ankle joint. Either CT or MRI studies can provide similar measurements. Femoral anteversion can be measured by drawing a line from the center of the femoral neck to the femoral head and distally either along the transepicondylar axis (mean value 7.4°) or the tangent of the posterior femoral condyles (mean value 13.1°). These values differ by about 6°, with a range of 11° of retroversion to 22° of anteversion (Fig. 3.4) [21].

Numerous studies have highlighted the importance of tibial torsion on patellar tracking [17, 22]. There is no consensus concerning the measurement techniques to determine the tibial torsion. Thus, the lack of a standardized method to measure tibial torsion is a major stumbling block to determining a pathologic threshold for this abnormality. Both MRI and CT studies have been demonstrated as reliable reproducible methods to assess tibial torsion [23, 24]. The measurement is taken from two superimposed axial images: one of the proximal tibial epiphysis right above the proximal end of the fibula and the other tangent to the talar dome. This is the angle between the line tangent to the posterior tibial plateau rim and the bimalleolar axis as drawn through the centers of the anteroposterior aspect of the lateral and medial malleoli [24, 25].

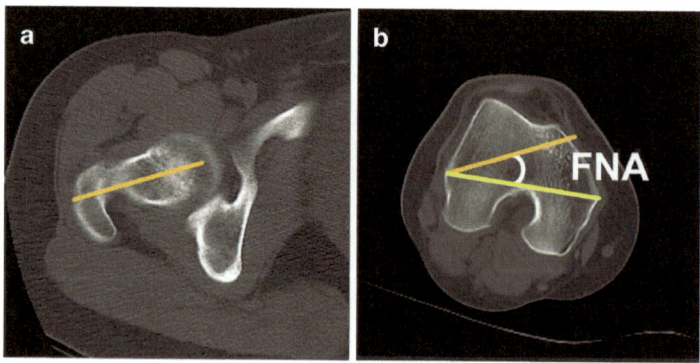

FIGURE. 3.4 Femoral neck anteversion (FNA) measurement using transepicondylar axis. (a) Orange line demonstrates femoral neck axis, connecting the center of the femoral head and the center of the femoral neck. (b) Yellow line shows transepicondylar axis, connecting the medial and lateral epicondyles

Biomechanical studies have shown the influence of both tibial and femoral rotation on patellofemoral contact pressure. Lee et al. demonstrated that increased external tibial rotation resulted in a lateral shift of the patella, thus increasing the pressure on the lateral facet [17]. A comparison of patients with chronic patellofemoral symptoms and asymptomatic controls showed that symptomatic patients presented significant increased external tibial torsion compared to controls [22]. Moreover, a biomechanical study analyzing PF contact pressures demonstrated that if a torsional and an angular deformity coexist, the rotatory component causes greater PF changes [26]. Takai et al. have evaluated femoral and tibial torsion in patients with unicompartmental PF arthrosis and demonstrated the high correlation between PF arthrosis and increased femoral anteversion (23° of femoral anteversion in the PF OA group versus 9° of anteversion in the control group) [27]. Similarly, Lerat has found an increased risk for patellar chondropathy in patients with increased internal femoral torsion [28].

Patellar tilt and subluxation are additional factors that indicate PF malalignment and have been associated with deterioration of PF cartilage laterally. Patellar position can be easily assessed using axial radiographs or axial images from MRI or CT; however, the source of this incongruence is multifactorial and requires a deeper evaluation. In addition to the rotational deviation described earlier, a laxity or weakness of medial soft tissue restraints, such as the MPFL and vastus medialis, and/or a lateral tethering lead to an overload of the lateral facet. In this case, physical evaluation demonstrates a decrease in medial-lateral patellar translation.

Sagittal Alignment

The position of the patella in the sagittal axis is an additional factor influencing patellofemoral tracking. Essentially, patella alta or infera must be evaluated using an identified index. The main indexes currently used in the literature are Insall-Salvati,

Caton-Deschamps, and Blackburne-Peel. All imaging techniques (lateral view radiographs, MRI, and CT) have demonstrated reliable and reproducible methods for measurement and can be interchangeable when assessing patellar height [29]. Mehl et al., in a case control study comparing patients with cartilage defects and normal controls, found that 67% of patients with a chondral lesion showed a pathologic Insall-Salvati index of >1.2, while this ratio was only 25.6% of the control group [30]. Additionally, an observational study of patients with osteoarthritis showed a significant association between patellar alignment and cartilage loss in both lateral and medial sides [31].

Patellofemoral Geometry

In addition to patellofemoral alignment, but no less significant, the contour of the trochlea and the patella is an important contributor to the patellofemoral contact force and consequently a risk factor for patellofemoral cartilage lesions. The geometry of the trochlea has been recognized as a risk factor for the development of cartilage lesions of the PF joint. Several studies have correlated patellofemoral cartilage loss with flat or shallow trochlea [31–33]. Historically, trochlea morphology was mainly assessed using axial radiography or CT using bone landmarks. However, bone reference may not reproduce the articular cartilage surface, and investigation with MRI is advisable [34].

Summary

In conclusion, identification and correction of underlying abnormal patellofemoral alignment is crucial for successful cartilage repair in the patellofemoral joint. Patients with full-thickness cartilage defects of the patella frequently demonstrate a high number of co-pathologies in association. Therefore, these pathologies must be identified accurately and considered carefully when planning surgical treatment of patellofemoral cartilage defects.

References

1. Hsu RW, Himeno S, Coventry MB, Chao EY. Normal axial alignment of the lower extremity and load-bearing distribution at the knee. Clin Orthop Relat Res. 1990;255:215–27.
2. Tetsworth K, Paley D. Malalignment and degenerative arthropathy. Orthop Clin North Am. 1994;25(3):367–77.
3. McKellop HA, Llinás A, Sarmiento A. Effects of tibial malalignment on the knee and ankle. Orthop Clin North Am. 1994;25(3):415–23.
4. Sharma L, Chmiel JS, Almagor O, Felson D, Guermazi A, Roemer F, Lewis CE, Segal N, Torner J, Cooke TD, Hietpas J, Lynch J, Nevitt M. The role of varus and valgus alignment in the initial development of knee cartilage damage by MRI: the MOST study. Ann Rheum Dis. 2013;72(2):235–40. https://doi.org/10.1136/annrheumdis-2011-201070.
5. Tanamas S, Hanna FS, Cicuttini FM, Wluka AE, Berry P, Urquhart DM. Does knee malalignment increase the risk of development and progression of knee osteoarthritis? A systematic review. Arthritis Rheum. 2009;61(4):459–67. https://doi.org/10.1002/art.24336.
6. Weinberg DS, Tucker BJ, Drain JP, Wang DM, Gilmore A, Liu RW. A cadaveric investigation into the demographic and bony alignment properties associated with osteoarthritis of the patellofemoral joint. Knee. 2016;23(3):350–6. https://doi.org/10.1016/j.knee.2016.02.016.
7. McWalter EJ, Cibere J, MacIntyre NJ, Nicolaou S, Schulzer M, Wilson DR. Relationship between varus-valgus alignment and patellar kinematics in individuals with knee osteoarthritis. J Bone Joint Surg Am. 2007;89(12):2723–31. https://doi.org/10.2106/JBJS.F.01016.
8. Schön SN, Afifi FK, Rasch H, Amsler F, Friederich NG, Arnold MP, Hirschmann MT. Assessment of in vivo loading history of the patellofemoral joint: a study combining patellar position, tilt, alignment and bone SPECT/CT. Knee Surg Sports Traumatol Arthrosc. 2013;22(12):3039–46. https://doi.org/10.1007/s00167-013-2698-2.
9. Cahue S, Dunlop D, Hayes K, Song J, Torres L, Sharma L. Varus-valgus alignment in the progression of patellofemoral osteoarthritis. Arthritis Rheum. 2004;50(7):2184–90. https://doi.org/10.1002/art.20348.

10. Ho CP, James EW, Surowiec RK, Gatlin CC, Ellman MB, Cram TR, Dornan GJ, LaPrade RF. Systematic technique-dependent differences in CT versus MRI measurement of the tibial tubercle-trochlear groove distance. Am J Sports Med. 2015;43(3):675–82. https://doi.org/10.1177/0363546514563690.
11. Dickschas J, Harrer J, Bayer T, Schwitulla J, Strecker W. Correlation of the tibial tuberosity–trochlear groove distance with the Q-angle. Knee Surg Sports Traumatol Arthrosc. 2016;24(3):915–20. https://doi.org/10.1007/s00167-014-3426-2.
12. Camp CL, Stuart MJ, Krych AJ, Levy BA, Bond JR, Collins MS, Dahm DL. CT and MRI measurements of tibial tubercle-trochlear groove distances are not equivalent in patients with patellar instability. Am J Sports Med. 2013;41(8):1835–40. https://doi.org/10.1177/0363546513484895.
13. Dejour H, Walch G, Nove-Josserand L, Guier C. Factors of patellar instability: an anatomic radiographic study. Knee Surg Sports Traumatol Arthrosc. 1994;2(1):19–26.
14. Daynes J, Hinckel B, Farr J. Tibial tuberosity—posterior cruciate ligament distance. J Knee Surg. 2016;29(06):471–7. https://doi.org/10.1055/s-0035-1564732.
15. Seitlinger G, Scheurecker G, Hogler R, Labey L, Innocenti B, Hofmann S. Tibial tubercle-posterior cruciate ligament distance: a new measurement to define the position of the tibial tubercle in patients with patellar dislocation. Am J Sports Med. 2012;40(5):1119–25. https://doi.org/10.1177/0363546512438762.
16. Tensho K, Akaoka Y, Shimodaira H, Takanashi S, Ikegami s KH, Saito N. What components comprise the measurement of the tibial tuberosity-trochlear groove distance in a patellar dislocation population? J Bone Joint Surg Am. 2015;97(17):1441–8. https://doi.org/10.2106/JBJS.N.01313.
17. Lee TQ, Yang BY, Sandusky MD, McMahon PJ. The effects of tibial rotation on the patellofemoral joint: assessment of the changes in in situ strain in the peripatellar retinaculum and the patellofemoral contact pressures and areas. J Rehabil Res Dev. 2001;38(5):463–9.
18. Hefzy MS, Jackson WT, Saddemi SR. Effects of tibial rotations on patellar tracking and patello-femoral contact areas. J Biomed Eng. 1992;14(4):329–43.
19. Lee TQ, Anzel SH, Bennett KA, Pang D, Kim WC. The influence of fixed rotational deformities of the femur on the patellofemoral contact pressures in human cadaver knees. Clin Orthop Relat Res. 1994;302:69–74.

20. van Kampen A, Huiskes R. The three-dimensional tracking pattern of the human patella. J Orthop Res. 1990;8(3):372–82. https://doi.org/10.1002/jor.1100080309.
21. Yoshioka Y, Cooke TDV. Femoral anteversion: assessment based on function axes. J Orthop Res. 1987;5(1):86–91. https://doi.org/10.1002/jor.1100050111.
22. Cooke TDV, Price N, Fisher B, Hedden D. The inwardly pointing knee. An unrecognized problem of external rotational malalignment. Clin Orthop Relat Res. 1990;260:56–60. https://doi.org/10.1097/00003086-199011000-00011.
23. Basaran SH, Ercin E, Bayrak A, Cumen H, Bilgili MG, Inci E, Avkan MC. The measurement of tibial torsion by magnetic resonance imaging in children: the comparison of three different methods. Eur J Orthop Surg Traumatol. 2015;25(8):1327–32. https://doi.org/10.1007/s00590-015-1694-2.
24. Folinais D, Thelen P, Delin C, Radier C, Catonne Y, Lazennec JY. Measuring femoral and rotational alignment: EOS system versus computed tomography. Orthop Traumatol Surg Res. 2013;99(5):509–16. https://doi.org/10.1016/j.otsr.2012.12.023.
25. Reikerås O, Høiseth A. Torsion of the leg determined by computed tomography. Acta Orthop Scand. 1989;60(3):330–3.
26. Fujikawa K, Seedhom BB, Wright V. Biomechanics of the patello-femoral joint. Part I: a study of the contact and the congruity of the patello-femoral compartment and movement of the patella. Eng Med. 1983;12(1):3–11.
27. Takai S, Sakakida K, Yamashita F, Suzu F, Izuta F. Rotational alignment of the lower limb in osteoarthritis of the knee. Int Orthop. 1985;9(3):209–15.
28. Lerat JL, Moyen B, Bochu M, Galland O. Femoropatellar pathology and rotational and torsional abnormalities of the inferior limbs: the use of CT scan. In: Müller W, Hackenbruch W, editors. Surgery and arthroscopy of the knee. Berlin: Springer; 1988. p. 61–5. https://doi.org/10.1007/978-3-642-72782-5_11.
29. Lee PP, Chalian M, Carrino JA, Eng J, Chhabra A. Multimodality correlations of patellar height measurement on X-ray, CT, and MRI. Skelet Radiol. 2012;41(10):1309–14. https://doi.org/10.1007/s00256-012-1396-3.
30. Mehl J, Feucht MJ, Bode G, Dovi-Akue D, Südkamp NP, Niemeyer P. Association between patellar cartilage defects and patellofemoral geometry: a matched-pair MRI comparison of patients with and without isolated patellar cartilage defects. Knee Surg Sports Traumatol Arthrosc. 2016;24(3):838–46. https://doi.org/10.1007/s00167-014-3385-7.

31. Kalichman L, Zhang Y, Niu J, Goggins J, Gale D, Felson DT, Hunter D. The association between patellar alignment and patellofemoral joint osteoarthritis features an MRI study. Rheumatology. 2007;46(8):1303–8. https://doi.org/10.1093/rheumatology/kem095.

32. Ali SA, Helmer R, Terk MR. Analysis of the patellofemoral region on MRI: association of abnormal trochlear morphology with severe cartilage defects. AJR Am J Roentgenol. 2010;194(3):721–7. https://doi.org/10.2214/AJR.09.3008.

33. Tsavalas N, Katonis P, Karantanas AH. Knee joint anterior malalignment and patellofemoral osteoarthritis: an MRI study. Eur Radiol. 2012;22(2):418–28. https://doi.org/10.1007/s00330-011-2275-3.

34. Salzmann GM, Weber TS, Spang JT, Imhoff AB, Schöttle PB. Comparison of native axial radiographs with axial MR imaging for determination of the trochlear morphology in patients with trochlear dysplasia. Arch Orthop Trauma Surg. 2009;130(3):335–40. https://doi.org/10.1007/s00402-009-0912-y.

Chapter 4
The Role of Synovium and Synovial Fluid in Joint Hemostasis

Michael L. Redondo, David R. Christian, and Adam B. Yanke

Synovium and Synovial Fluid

Synovium

All diarthrodial joints are lined by synovium which is a specialized connective tissue that plays a significant role in maintaining the intra-articular environment. The synovium is made up of two distinct layers: the outer layer called the subintima and the inner layer called the intima. The subintima is thicker (up to 5 mm), denser, and less cellular consisting of fibrous connective tissue, adipose tissue, and areolar connective tissue. The intima lines the joint cavity and consists of synoviocytes with a thickness between one and four cells [1]. Synoviocytes have been categorized into types A and B which are derived from macrophages and fibroblasts, respectively. Typically, the intima has a superficial layer of type A synoviocytes with type B synoviocytes directly below. In normal, healthy synovium type A cells are the minority, while type B synoviocytes predominate [2].

M. L. Redondo · D. R. Christian · A. B. Yanke (✉)
Department of Orthopedic Surgery, Rush University
Medical Center, Chicago, IL, USA
e-mail: Adam.yanke@rushortho.com

© Springer Nature Switzerland AG 2019   57
A. B. Yanke, B. J. Cole (eds.), *Joint Preservation of the Knee*,
https://doi.org/10.1007/978-3-030-01491-9_4

The function of normal synovium is to maintain homeostasis within the intra-articular environment, and it achieves this through maintenance of the synovial surface, lubrication of the articular surface, and maintenance of synovial fluid [2]. Maintenance of the synovial surface is important to ensure that it remains non-adherent to the joint components and is believed to be achieved through production of hyaluronate and lubricin by the type B synoviocytes [2]. Lubrication of the articular surface achieved through the synthesis of glycoproteins, specifically lubricin, by the synoviocytes which localizes to both the superficial articular surface and synovial intima creating a low-friction environment within the joint. The synovium also functions as a selective membrane to maintain the components and volume of synovial fluid, which provides nutrients to chondrocytes in the avascular extracellular matrix. The production of hyaluronate increases the viscosity of the synovial fluid creating additional cushioning between articular surfaces [2]. When healthy, the synovium selectively allows smaller molecules such as electrolytes and cytokines to diffuse between the synovial fluid and underlying vasculature, but inhibits transport of larger glycoproteins such as hyaluronate [2, 3].

Synovial Fluid

As previously mentioned, synovial fluid functions as a pool of nutrients and regulatory cytokines as well as a biological lubricant. Synovial fluid function is integral to the progression of OA, and diminished synovial fluid quality has been correlated to the progression of OA in humans [4]. A primary lubricant molecule in synovial fluid is hyaluronic acid (HA), a large polymer of repeating disaccharides of N-acetylglucosamine and glucuronic acid connected by β-linkages [5]. The friction-lowering properties of HA are dependent on its concentration and molecular mass. Lower molecular weight HA diminishes synovial fluid's viscoelastic properties [4]. As OA progresses, the concentration of HA shifts toward its lower molecular weight equivalent, reducing the mechanical protection imparted by synovial fluid [4]. Though the average native molecular weight of HA is 3–4 million Da, HA injection preparations currently exist for both low and high molecular weight HA (0.5–7 million Da) [6].

Intra-articular HA injections have been used for many years as a treatment for OA and are believed to reduce symptoms of OA through anti-inflammatory and chondroprotective mechanisms [4]. Currently, experts suggest that higher molecular weight HA is more effective at inducing these mechanisms than lower molecular weight HA. Higher molecular weight HA more effectively binds to cluster of differentiation 44 (CD44) and inhibits the expression of interleukin (IL)-1β, consequently reducing the synthesis of catabolic enzymatic known to aid in the destruction of articular cartilage [4, 5]. The HA-CD44 binding pathway additionally augments chondroprotection through decreased apoptosis of chondrocytes, slowing degeneration and preserving the matrix. Furthermore, several studies have observed an anti-inflammatory effect from HA injections through decreased synthesis of IL-8, IL-6, prostaglandin-E$_2$ (PGE$_2$), and tumor necrosis factor-alpha (TNFα), in addition to the decrease in IL-1β [4, 5].

The synovium and synovial fluid are altered in the setting of osteoarthritis. Cartilage debris activates an inflammatory cascade inducing hyperplasia, increased vascularization, and increased migration of immune cells, specifically macrophages and T cells, within the synovium [1–3, 7–9]. As this occurs, the permeability of the synovium changes, resulting in decreased synovial fluid concentrations of both hyaluronate and lubricin, which correlates with increased concentrations of hyaluronate in the serum of patients with osteoarthritis [3, 10]. Additionally, the synovium becomes pro-inflammatory as the new influx of immune cells release inflammatory mediators into the joint space. Chondrocytes then become activated to produce matrix metalloproteinases that degrade the cartilage. This in turn increases the concentration of cartilage debris, which propagates the inflammatory cycle [1].

The intra-articular environment is similarly impacted in the setting of hemarthrosis [11]. When blood enters the joint, the iron present catalyzes the formation of reactive oxygen species that damage the cartilage and stimulate chondrocyte apoptosis [12]. Simultaneously, red blood cells are broken down releasing hemosiderin which accumulates in the synovium inducing synovial hyperplasia and increased vascularization. Macrophages and other immune cells migrate into the synovium and produce of pro-inflammatory cytokines which further inhibit the function of chondrocytes leading to damage of the articular cartilage [12]. While this process may not always manifest clinically in a patient with single, acute hemarthrosis, this mechanism is well documented in the basic science literature. Additionally, this is observed in patients with hemophilia who experience repeated hemarthrosis and develop severe joint pathology called hemophilic arthropathy [12]. The clinical effects of acute trauma and likely hemarthrosis, however, may be observed in the literature describing anterior cruciate ligament (ACL) rupture and the development of post-traumatic osteoarthritis (PTOA). It has been observed that there is an increase in the prevalence of osteoarthritis in patients who have experienced an ACL rupture, and increased time from rupture to surgical intervention has been identified as a risk factor for development of post-traumatic osteoarthritis [13]. This data suggests that episodes of trauma may have lasting effects on the intra-articular environment and acute intervention such as aspiration and possible injection may be important in preventing the development of future osteoarthritis. As previously mentioned, a single or repetitive hemarthrosis can lead to devastating cartilage, synovium, and bone damage and may contribute to PTOA [12, 14–16]. Several methods to prevent blood-induced cartilage damage have been proposed. Post-traumatic knee hemarthrosis aspiration has been recently proposed as a method disrupting the inflammatory cascade and blood-driven chondrocyte death [17, 18]. Recently, joint lavage and viscosupplementation have been reported to improve knee function and stability in patients with blood-derived hemophilic arthropathy [17]. Arthrocentesis or lavage is a promising technique and warrants further investigation.

Synovial Biomarkers

Many of the items present in the synovial fluid can function as biomarkers of overall joint health. These biomarkers can include inflammatory cytokines, metalloproteinases, proteases, and degradation products of cartilage [19–21]. Biomarkers isolated from the blood, urine, or synovial fluid of patients can be helpful in elucidating normal processes, pathology, or responses to therapeutic intervention. In the field of orthopedics, the integration of biomarkers into the diagnostic workup and treatment decision-making process is being explored for a variety of pathologies, especially osteoarthritis and focal cartilage lesions [19, 21]. Despite the advancements in preoperative imaging and diagnosis techniques, preoperative MRI only has a sensitivity of 45% for the identification of chondral lesions in the knee [22]. Studies have reported associations between protein biomarkers and preoperative radiographic findings, MRI, and preoperative pain [23–25]. Additionally, serum biomarkers such IL-1Ra have recently been suggested to predict radiographic progression of knee OA [26]. Thus, further investigation of several protein biomarkers may be helpful tools for identification and qualification cartilage damage preoperatively.

Cytokine biomarkers have been largely investigated due to their known involvement in the inflammatory cascade [1]. Of the pro-inflammatory cytokines involved in the cartilage degeneration cascade, IL-6 and IL-1 have been extensively described. Increased concentrations of IL-1 and IL-6 have been established in the synovial fluid, synovial membrane, cartilage, and subchondral bone of osteoarthritis patient [1]. Also, these cytokines have synergistic effects on inflammatory cascades that increase inflammation and cartilage degradation [1, 23]. IL-6 has a well-profiled role in the production of acute-phase reactants and is integral to the induction and maintenance of chronic inflammation [27]. Also, authors have hypothesized IL-6 may have a major role in persistently painful joints due to its ability to sensitize C pain fibers innervating the knee joint [28, 29]. Strauss et al. [23] examined synovial fluid samples from 81 patients undergoing knee arthroscopy in order to correlate the contents with cartilage pathology and outcomes. In this study, the authors reported that IL-6 concentration was among the strongest predictors of more severe cartilage lesions and was correlated with worse outcomes on preoperative Visual Analog Scale, Lysholm, and Knee injury and Osteoarthritis Outcome Score – physical function – as well as continued pain at final follow-up [23].

The role of IL-1 in the progression of OA has been extensively studied, especially pertaining to its role in post-traumatic OA [1]. Several authors have identified IL-1 an integral mediator of acute inflammation after joint trauma [25, 26, 30, 31]. Intra-articular IL-1 concentrations increase after cartilage trauma and correlate to the severity of cartilage degradation via the promotion of extracellular matrix metalloproteases [1]. In a study by Attur et al. [25], synovial fluid analysis revealed that smaller concentrations of IL-1B in the synovial fluid of patients with preexisting OA were associated with decreased risk of radiologic severity, greater joint space width, and lower IL-6 and IL-10 concentrations.

Acute Intervention Following Traumatic Knee Injury

As the loss of normal articular hyaline cartilage is irreversible, timely intervention to disrupt cartilage degradation pathways is imperative. Kraus et al. characterized the initial cartilage degradation pathway as an initial wave of proteoglycan loss followed by subsequent collagen loss within the first month after injury acute ACL injury [32]. Several experts advocate the need for early intervention after acute knee trauma to disrupt the synovial fluid or synovium inflammatory cascade [1, 32, 33]. IL-1 is a frequent target to modify the environment of the post-traumatic knee and attempt to prevent PTOA. IL-1 receptor antagonist (IL-1Ra) inhibits IL-1 function by binding competitively to the IL-1 receptor [26, 30, 34]. In the mouse model, intra-articular injection of IL-1Ra resulted inhibition of IL-1 levels, significantly reduced cartilage degeneration, and synovial inflammation following articular fracture [34]. In a recent randomized pilot, 11 patients with acute ACL injury were administered intra-articular IL-1Ra or saline injection 2 weeks after injury [32]. The IL-1Ra injection groups displayed less knee pain and improved function as well as reduced IL-1a concentrations, a pro-inflammatory cytokine known to lead to cartilage degeneration. Other intra-articular early interventions have also been described. In a recent randomized controlled trial, Lattermann et al. [33] compared no intervention after acute ACL rupture to the use of corticosteroid injections (CSI) in an attempt to disrupt the progressive inflammatory cascade. In the control group, these authors identified that cartilage degeneration biomarkers consistently increase during the 5 weeks after ACL injury, highlighting the early degenerative process and its rapid progression. The administration of intra-articular CSI within the first several days after the ACL rupture resulted in smaller levels of chondrodegenerative biomarkers, such as CTX-II, in the synovial fluid. The aforementioned literature suggests that CSI and other intra-articular therapies may be valuable tools for prevention of PTOA.

Conclusion

Synovium and synovial fluid have a large impact of homeostasis of joints. As the primary source of nutrients for chondrocytes, the biologic milieu contained within the synovial fluid can have long-lasting effects on overall joint health. Further understanding the complex interaction of cartilage, bone, synovial fluid, and the synovium will help clinicians approach the knee as an organ and not tissues functioning in isolation. As more knowledge is elucidated on the importance of joint microenvironment, future work on early interventions or screening may be pivotal in prevention of PTOA and improving clinical outcomes.

References

1. Mathiessen A, Conaghan PG. Synovitis in osteoarthritis: current understanding with therapeutic implications. Arthritis Res Ther. 2017;19(1):18. PubMed PMID: 28148295. Pubmed Central PMCID: PMC5289060. Epub 2017/02/02. eng.
2. Smith MD. The normal synovium. Open Rheumatol J. 2011;5:100–6. PubMed PMID: 22279508. Pubmed Central PMCID: PMC3263506. Epub 2011/12/30. eng.
3. Scanzello CR, Goldring SR. The role of synovitis in osteoarthritis pathogenesis. Bone. 2012;51(2):249–57. PubMed PMID: 22387238. Pubmed Central PMCID: PMC3372675. Epub 2012/02/22. eng.
4. Altman RD, Manjoo A, Fierlinger A, Niazi F, Nicholls M. The mechanism of action for hyaluronic acid treatment in the osteoarthritic knee: a systematic review. BMC Musculoskelet Disord. 2015;16:321. PubMed PMID: 26503103. Pubmed Central PMCID: PMC4621876. Epub 2015/10/26. eng.
5. Temple-Wong MM, Ren S, Quach P, Hansen BC, Chen AC, Hasegawa A, et al. Hyaluronan concentration and size distribution in human knee synovial fluid: variations with age and cartilage degeneration. Arthritis Res Ther. 2016;18:18. PubMed PMID: 26792492. Pubmed Central PMCID: PMC4721052. Epub 2016/01/21. eng.
6. Gigis I, Fotiadis E, Nenopoulos A, Tsitas K, Hatzokos I. Comparison of two different molecular weight intra-articular injections of hyaluronic acid for the treatment of knee osteoarthritis. Hippokratia. 2016;20(1):26–31. PubMed PMID: 27895439. Pubmed Central PMCID: PMC5074393. eng.
7. Manferdini C, Paolella F, Gabusi E, Silvestri Y, Gambari L, Cattini L, et al. From osteoarthritic synovium to synovial-derived cells characterization: synovial macrophages are key effector cells. Arthritis Res Ther. 2016;18:83. PubMed PMID: 27044395. Pubmed Central PMCID: PMC4820904. Epub 2016/04/04. eng.

8. Klein-Wieringa IR, de Lange-Brokaar BJ, Yusuf E, Andersen SN, Kwekkeboom JC, Kroon HM, et al. Inflammatory cells in patients with Endstage knee osteoarthritis: a comparison between the synovium and the infrapatellar fat pad. J Rheumatol. 2016;43(4):771–8. PubMed PMID: 26980579. Epub 2016/03/15. eng.

9. Moradi B, Rosshirt N, Tripel E, Kirsch J, Barié A, Zeifang F, et al. Unicompartmental and bicompartmental knee osteoarthritis show different patterns of mononuclear cell infiltration and cytokine release in the affected joints. Clin Exp Immunol. 2015;180(1):143–54. PubMed PMID: 25393692. Pubmed Central PMCID: PMC4367102. eng.

10. Goldberg RL, Huff JP, Lenz ME, Glickman P, Katz R, Thonar EJ. Elevated plasma levels of hyaluronate in patients with osteoarthritis and rheumatoid arthritis. Arthritis Rheum. 1991;34(7):799–807. PubMed PMID: 2059228. eng.

11. Swärd P, Frobell R, Englund M, Roos H, Struglics A. Cartilage and bone markers and inflammatory cytokines are increased in synovial fluid in the acute phase of knee injury (hemarthrosis) – a cross-sectional analysis. Osteoarthr Cartil. 2012;20(11):1302–8. PubMed PMID: 22874525. Epub 2012/08/05. eng.

12. Roosendaal G, Lafeber FP. Pathogenesis of haemophilic arthropathy. Haemophilia. 2006;12(Suppl 3):117–21. PubMed PMID: 16684006. eng.

13. Cinque ME, Dornan GJ, Chahla J, Moatshe G, LaPrade RF. High rates of osteoarthritis develop after anterior cruciate ligament surgery: an analysis of 4108 patients. Am J Sports Med. 2017;46:2011–9. https://doi.org/10.1177/0363546517730072. PubMed PMID: 28982255. Epub 2017/09/01. eng.

14. Hooiveld M, Roosendaal G, Vianen M, van den Berg M, Bijlsma J, Lafeber F. Blood-induced joint damage: longterm effects in vitro and in vivo. J Rheumatol. 2003;30(2):339–44. PubMed PMID: 12563692. eng.

15. Hakobyan N, Enockson C, Cole AA, Sumner DR, Valentino LA. Experimental haemophilic arthropathy in a mouse model of a massive haemarthrosis: gross, radiological and histological changes. Haemophilia. 2008;14(4):804–9. PubMed PMID: 18422608. Epub 2008/04/12. eng.

16. Jansen NW, Roosendaal G, Wenting MJ, Bijlsma JW, Theobald M, Hazewinkel HA, et al. Very rapid clearance after a joint bleed in the canine knee cannot prevent adverse effects on cartilage and synovial tissue. Osteoarthr Cartil. 2009;17(4):433–40. PubMed PMID: 18922705. Epub 2008/10/14. eng.

17. Rezende MU, Andrusaitis FR, Silva RT, Okazaki E, Carneiro JD, Campos GC, et al. Joint lavage followed by viscosupplementation and triamcinolone in patients with severe haemophilic arthropathy: objective functional results. Haemophilia. 2017;23(2):e105–15. PubMed PMID: 27860135. Epub 2016/11/16. eng.

18. Wang JH, Lee JH, Cho Y, Shin JM, Lee BH. Efficacy of knee joint aspiration in patients with acute ACL injury in the emergency department. Injury. 2016;47(8):1744–9. PubMed PMID: 27262773. Epub 2016/05/18. eng.

19. Patra D, Sandell LJ. Recent advances in biomarkers in osteoarthritis. Curr Opin Rheumatol. 2011;23(5):465–70. PubMed PMID: 21720244. eng.

20. Henrotin Y. Osteoarthritis year 2011 in review: biochemical markers of osteoarthritis: an overview of research and initiatives. Osteoarthr Cartil. 2012;20(3):215–7. PubMed PMID: 22261406. Epub 2012/01/13. eng.

21. Kraus VB. Biomarkers in osteoarthritis. Curr Opin Rheumatol. 2005;17(5):641–6. PubMed PMID: 16093846. eng.

22. Figueroa D, Calvo R, Vaisman A, Carrasco MA, Moraga C, Delgado I. Knee chondral lesions: incidence and correlation between arthroscopic and magnetic resonance findings. Arthroscopy. 2007;23(3):312–5. PubMed PMID: 17349476. eng.

23. Cuéllar VG, Cuéllar JM, Kirsch T, Strauss EJ. Correlation of synovial fluid biomarkers with cartilage pathology and associated outcomes in knee arthroscopy. Arthroscopy. 2016;32(3):475–85. PubMed PMID: 26524935. Epub 2015/10/30. eng.

24. Orita S, Koshi T, Mitsuka T, Miyagi M, Inoue G, Arai G, et al. Associations between proinflammatory cytokines in the synovial fluid and radiographic grading and pain-related scores in 47 consecutive patients with osteoarthritis of the knee. BMC Musculoskelet Disord. 2011;12:144. PubMed PMID: 21714933. Pubmed Central PMCID: PMC3144455. Epub 2011/06/30. eng.

25. Attur M, Wang HY, Kraus VB, Bukowski JF, Aziz N, Krasnokutsky S, et al. Radiographic severity of knee osteoarthritis is conditional on interleukin 1 receptor antagonist gene variations. Ann Rheum Dis. 2010;69(5):856–61. PubMed PMID: 19934104. Pubmed Central PMCID: PMC2925146. Epub 2009/11/23. eng.

26. Attur M, Statnikov A, Samuels J, Li Z, Alekseyenko AV, Greenberg JD, et al. Plasma levels of interleukin-1 receptor antagonist (IL1Ra) predict radiographic progression of symptomatic knee osteoarthritis. Osteoarthr Cartil. 2015;23(11):1915–24. PubMed PMID: 26521737. Pubmed Central PMCID: PMC4630783. eng.

27. Hunter CA, Jones SA. IL-6 as a keystone cytokine in health and disease. Nat Immunol. 2015;16(5):448–57. PubMed PMID: 25898198. eng.

28. Samad TA, Moore KA, Sapirstein A, Billet S, Allchorne A, Poole S, et al. Interleukin-1beta-mediated induction of Cox-2 in the CNS contributes to inflammatory pain hypersensitivity. Nature. 2001;410(6827):471–5. PubMed PMID: 11260714. eng.

29. Anderson GD, Hauser SD, McGarity KL, Bremer ME, Isakson PC, Gregory SA. Selective inhibition of cyclooxygenase (COX)-2 reverses inflammation and expression of COX-2 and interleukin 6 in rat adjuvant arthritis. J Clin Invest. 1996;97(11):2672–9. PubMed PMID: 8647962. Pubmed Central PMCID: PMC507355. eng.

30. Attur M, Belitskaya-Lévy I, Oh C, Krasnokutsky S, Greenberg J, Samuels J, et al. Increased interleukin-1β gene expression in peripheral blood leukocytes is associated with increased pain and predicts risk for progression of symptomatic knee osteo-arthritis. Arthritis Rheum. 2011;63(7):1908–17. PubMed PMID: 21717421. Pubmed Central PMCID: PMC3128429. eng.

31. Catterall JB, Stabler TV, Flannery CR, Kraus VB. Changes in serum and synovial fluid biomarkers after acute injury (NCT00332254). Arthritis Res Ther. 2010;12(6):R229. PubMed PMID: 21194441. Pubmed Central PMCID: PMC3046542. Epub 2010/12/31. eng.

32. Kraus VB, Birmingham J, Stabler TV, Feng S, Taylor DC, Moorman CT, et al. Effects of intraarticular IL1-Ra for acute anterior cruciate ligament knee injury: a randomized controlled pilot trial (NCT00332254). Osteoarthr Cartil. 2012;20(4):271–8. PubMed PMID: 22273632. Epub 2012/01/10. eng.

33. Lattermann C, Jacobs CA, Proffitt Bunnell M, Huston LJ, Gammon LG, Johnson DL, et al. A multicenter study of early anti-inflammatory treatment in patients with acute anterior cruciate ligament tear. Am J Sports Med. 2017;45(2):325–33. PubMed PMID: 28146402. Epub 2016/10/07. eng.

34. Furman BD, Mangiapani DS, Zeitler E, Bailey KN, Horne PH, Huebner JL, et al. Targeting pro-inflammatory cytokines follow-ing joint injury: acute intra-articular inhibition of interleukin-1 following knee injury prevents post-traumatic arthritis. Arthritis Res Ther. 2014;16(3):R134. PubMed PMID: 24964765. Pubmed Central PMCID: PMC4229982. Epub 2014/06/25. eng.

Chapter 5
Defining Failure in Articular Cartilage Surgery

Drew A. Lansdown, Kevin C. Wang, and Brian J. Cole

Introduction

Injury to the articular cartilage remains a difficult problem for patients and a challenging condition for orthopedic surgeons. Chondral lesions are commonly encountered in knee arthroscopy, with full-thickness lesions noted in more than 60% of knee arthroscopies [1, 2]. Additionally, osteoarthritis is one of the leading causes of worldwide disability, and the utilization of total knee arthroplasty continues to rise to attempt to address this condition.

Multiple treatment options are available to address articular cartilage lesions, and there has been great progress in developing novel cartilage restoration techniques.

D. A. Lansdown
Department of Orthopaedic Surgery, University of California, San Francisco School of Medicine, San Francisco, CA, USA

K. C. Wang
Department of Orthopedics, Icahn School of Medicine at Mount Sinai, New York, NY, USA

B. J. Cole (✉)
Department of Orthopedic Surgery, Rush University Medical Center, Chicago, IL, USA
e-mail: brian.cole@rushortho.com

© Springer Nature Switzerland AG 2019   69
A. B. Yanke, B. J. Cole (eds.), *Joint Preservation of the Knee*,
https://doi.org/10.1007/978-3-030-01491-9_5

Microfracture remains an option for initial treatment for many lesions and is frequently used as a comparative therapy in clinical trials [3, 4]. This procedure involves penetrating the subchondral bone to stimulate a healing response with fibrocartilage. In 1994, Brittberg et al. published and popularized autologous chondrocyte implantation [5]. This technology utilizes a patient's native chondrocytes expanded in culture and then reimplanted to restore hyaline cartilage to an injured area. Novel matrix-associated autologous chondrocyte implantation (MACI) techniques have been introduced recently in an attempt to improve upon the results of ACI [6]. Osteochondral autograft transfer (OATS) and osteochondral allograft implantation are further treatment options that allow for the restoration of both the bone and cartilage at the site of a defect [7, 8]. Numerous other novel therapeutics including surface allograft transplantation are early in the clinical adoption cycle or in development to address symptomatic chondral injuries.

Successful and sustained treatment of symptomatic chondral lesions, however, remains elusive in many cases. As new therapeutic options are introduced, it becomes even more important to have consistent and clear goals for treating cartilage injuries and to understand what outcome tools are available to determine which treatments will lead to excellent long-term outcomes. Additionally, the current level of evidence of the majority of the cartilage repair literature is limited at best [9]. The purpose of this chapter is to review current standards for defining treatment failure and explore methods that will be used in future studies to determine success and failure of cartilage restoration procedures.

Objective Endpoints

Clinical Definitions of Failure

Survival analysis is frequently used to evaluate cartilage restoration procedures with conversion to total knee arthroplasty or reoperation utilized as the endpoint in disease treatment. Sterett et al. reported 91% survival of microfracture and high tibial osteotomy at a mean follow-up of 7 years [10]. While conversion to TKA is easy to measure and objective, this may not capture all patients who are unsatisfied, symptomatic, or persistently limited in function after cartilage restoration procedures. Bae et al. followed a cohort of 134 knees following microfracture of symptomatic chondral lesions and defined failure as conversion to TKA or pain scores worse than the preoperative value or less than 60. With this more stringent definition of failure, success of microfracture was 88.8% at 5 years, 67.9% at 10 years, and 45.6% at 12 years after surgery [11].

Pestka et al. evaluated patients treated with ACI and compared patients with and without a prior history of microfracture. Failure in this study was defined as reoperation of any kind, with patients who had a prior microfracture having a significantly higher failure rate (25% vs 3.6%; $p = 0.024$). Patient satisfaction levels, however, showed no difference between these groups, with 25.9% of patients with prior microfracture reporting unsatisfactory results compared to 28.6% of patients without a history of prior microfracture [12]. Reoperation is an important outcome after cartilage restoration, but it is imperative to incorporate other variables to capture patient satisfaction, symptoms, and function. Additionally, understanding patient goals and expectations is necessary in interpreting conversion to TKA as a measure of failure as some patients may be satisfied with a procedure that bridges them to replacement, while others have goals of longer-term joint preservation with a desire for more complete symptom relief.

Histologic Evaluation of Cartilage Repair

Histologic assessment of cartilage repair can determine if repair tissue has similar biochemical and structural composition to native cartilage. An ideal repair technique would reproduce the complex architecture of articular cartilage, including the appropriate levels of collagen, water, and glycosaminoglycans, as well as the interaction between the cartilage and subchondral bone. Animal studies are often used to test possible cartilage restoration procedures with a major advantage being the ability to perform histologic analysis on cartilage repair tissue. A biopsy during second-look arthroscopy may also be used in clinical studies; however this is an invasive procedure and may even damage the area of cartilage repair. The International Cartilage Repair Society (ICRS) has also provided recommendations on specific variables to control when performing histologic analysis of cartilage repair tissue [13]. These variables include the location of the biopsy sample, timing of recovery, processing methodology, staining method, and blind comparison to a control group.

After obtaining a cartilage sample in either a preclinical model or from arthroscopic biopsy, different stains are available to differentiate the types of tissue present at the repair site. Hematoxylin and eosin (H&E) staining is commonly used, with dark pink staining representing mineralized collagen and light pink staining signifying fibrous tissue [14]. Safranin O staining is used to determine the presence of proteoglycans [15]. Tissue stained with toluidine blue shows collagen matrix as blue and glycosaminoglycans as purple [16].

The stained samples are then evaluated with various scoring systems, including the Pineda system, O'Driscoll system, and ICRS-1 and ICRS-2 systems. The Pineda system rates four features, including defect fill, osteochondral junction integrity, matrix stain, and morphology of the cells [17]. The O'Driscoll system includes a rating of the tissue surface on regularity and integrity, thickness, integration with surrounding tissue, cellularity and cell clustering, and degenerative changes in surrounding tissue [18]. The ICRS rating systems include evaluation of the tissue surface, matrix, cellularity, cell viability, subchondral bone, and mineralization. For ICRS-1, the components are rated from 0 to 3, while ICRS-2 uses a continuous VAS rating from 0 to 100 [19, 20]. The use of these scoring systems in both animal and human cartilage trials allows for a consistent reporting of outcomes and evaluation of parameters linked to successful and sustained clinical results.

Macroscopic scoring systems have been developed to evaluate the gross appearance of cartilage restoration procedures at the time of second-look arthroscopy. One scale is the

ICRS score. This score ranges from 0 to 12 and includes three categories rated as 0–4: amount of defect fill, integration with adjacent cartilage, and macroscopic appearance of the repair tissue [21]. A second score is the Oswestry Arthroscopy Score, which is scored from 0 to 10. Components of this score include graft fill, integration with adjacent cartilage, surface appearance, graft color, and stiffness of repair tissue [22]. Van den Borne et al. reviewed the reproducibility and validity of both measurements and found both scoring systems to be reproducible methods for evaluating cartilage restoration procedures [23].

While histologic and macroscopic appearance of cartilage repair tissue would intuitively predict clinical outcomes, defining failure based on these measures alone is insufficient. For instance, Knutsen et al. compared microfracture and ACI in a randomized trial and found no correlation between histologic appearance of repair tissue from a biopsy at 2 years after surgery and clinical outcomes or failure (23% in both groups), defined in this study as reoperation for a symptomatic defect before the final follow-up of 5 years [24]. In comparing microfracture and ACI, Saris et al. reported better histologic appearance of ACI at 1 year postoperative [25], though in a follow-up report on the same cohort, Vanlauwe et al. showed no difference between clinical outcomes between the groups at 5 years after surgery [26]. Finally, Gudas et al. reported on the ICRS macroscopic score at second-look arthroscopy in a randomized controlled trial comparing OATS and microfracture [27]. There was no difference in the clinical outcomes for groups with low-grade or high-grade ICRS scores. Future research will define which histologic and macroscopic properties are able to predict success and failure after cartilage repair procedures.

Subjective Outcomes

Patient-reported outcomes are an attractive metric to use when defining procedure-specific success and failure. These scores are collected in the form of survey questions and can be obtained at both scheduled follow-up visit and remotely through electronic- or telephone-based surveys. General health-related quality of life scores, such as the Short Form (SF)-36, are often collected to follow patients after cartilage restoration procedures, in addition to joint-specific scores and activity ratings. Patient-reported outcome measures help focus the definition of success and failure on the patient's perceived benefit from any intervention.

Joint-specific scores evaluate the symptoms, function, and level of disability and may better isolate the effects of a chondral injury and its treatment. The International Knee Documentation Committee (IKDC) Subjective Knee Form is a joint-specific outcome tool used to evaluate symptoms and function in the setting of knee ligament, meniscus, and chondral injury [28]. The IKDC score ranges from 0 to 100, with higher scores reflecting better knee function. The Knee Injury and Osteoarthritis Outcome Score (KOOS) is a second knee-specific score that is validated in measuring knee symptoms and function for osteoarthritis, meniscal injuries, and ligamentous injuries. The KOOS encompasses five subscores, including scores for activities of daily living, sports and recreation function, pain, symptoms, and knee-related quality of life. This score is also reported from 0 to 100, with higher scores reflecting better outcomes and function.

The Lysholm score was originally described to measure functional outcomes after knee ligament injury and has been validated to monitor cartilage repair procedures, as well [29, 30]. In a meta-analysis of cartilage repair studies that included the results of 61 studies and 3987 operations, the Lysholm score was the most frequently reported clinical outcome score [9]. This score may be monitored prior to and after treatment, and a Lysholm score <64 has been described as a marker of clinical failure [31]. The WOMAC (Western Ontario and McMaster Universities Osteoarthritis Index) also measures function and symptoms as a result of knee conditions [32]. This survey has been tested most in the setting of osteoarthritis though it was shown to have similar responsiveness as the IKDC Subjective Knee Form in a group of chondral injury patients [33]. Other scores, such as the HSS and Cincinnati scores, are also utilized to monitor the response to treatment of articular cartilage injuries.

These various survey instruments show different responses in patients after cartilage restoration procedures. Ebert et al. compared responses to the KOOS, SF-36, Tegner, and Lysholm outcome measures 5 years after matrix-induced autologous chondrocyte transplantation [34]. The KOOS sports and quality of life sub-scores were the most responsive scores that showed the best correlation with a patient satisfaction. The Tegner score and SF-36 had the lowest responsiveness in this patient cohort. Hambly and Griva compared the KOOS and IKDC in patients with a history of knee articular cartilage repair surgery [35]. The IKDC Subjective Knee Form was found to perform better than the KOOS in this heterogeneous patient population. In general, the IKDC Subjective Knee Form should be recorded and reported in clinical trials on the treatment of articular cartilage injuries.

In addition to measuring patient symptoms and function, defining patient activity levels is also important when interpreting results from cartilage-resurfacing studies. Multiple activity scales are used, including the Tegner activity score and Marx activity rating scale. The Tegner activity score is a 0–10 scale that asks patients to rate their level of function, ranging from disability due to a knee condition to competing in elite-level sports. The Marx activity rating scale has four domains and asks patients to rate their ability to participate in running, cutting, pivoting, and decelerating. The use of activity ratings, both before and after cartilage restoration procedures, can reflect how successful a procedure is at restoring patients to a desired level of function.

For athletes, return to play and return to prior performance rates may provide even more guidance regarding the optimal treatment. Krych et al. performed a meta-analysis to evaluate return to play rates for various cartilage procedures. In this evaluation of 44 studies, osteochondral autograft transfer (OATS) showed the highest rate of return at 92%, while microfracture had the lowest rate at 58%. The rate for

ACI was 82% and for osteochondral allograft was 88%. Additionally, OATS patients returned the quickest following the procedure, at a mean of 5.2 months, as compared to 9.1 months for microfracture, 9.6 months for osteochondral allografts, and 11.8 months for ACI. The overall return to sport rate in this study including 2549 patients was 76%. When treating an athletic patient, the definition of failure may become even more stringent with return to play as the primary criterion. Related to that endpoint is the fact that many athletes withdraw from sports for a variety of reasons unrelated to their clinical outcome and true return to play frequency may be underestimated.

Imaging-Based Endpoints

Imaging modalities can allow for a noninvasive and objective assessment after cartilage repair procedures. Magnetic resonance imaging (MRI) is commonly used in clinical trials to provide an in vivo assessment after cartilage procedures. This imaging modality is attractive as there is no ionizing radiation used and there is excellent soft tissue contrast. Additionally, multiple quantitative imaging techniques have been developed and applied specifically to cartilage to evaluate the biochemistry and microscopic structure of repair tissue.

First, MR images may be evaluated in a semiquantitative method. One such scoring system commonly utilized is the magnetic resonance observation of cartilage repair tissue (MOCART) system. This scoring system has excellent interobserver agreement and includes evaluation of defect fill, integration with surrounding tissue, surface integrity, signal intensity, subchondral bone status, the presence of adhesions, and degree of synovitis [36]. Studies have demonstrated correlations of the MOCART score with a VAS pain score [37, 38], with the KOOS [38, 39], and with IKDC scores. However a recent systematic review found inconsistent relationships of MOCART with clinical outcomes, perhaps because of the multiple components of the scoring system [40]. For instance, defect fill alone has been shown to be correlated with clinical outcomes after microfracture [41, 42].

Multiple quantitative imaging sequences offer the ability to probe the biochemical and structural makeup of tissue. First, delayed gadolinium-enhanced magnetic resonance imaging of cartilage (dGEMRIC) utilizes intravenous gadolinium contrast material to measure the proteoglycan content in the cartilage. A preinjection scan is completed, followed by the administration of contrast material, a period of exercise, and a re-scan of the affected joint. Due to the negative charge of gadolinium, the results of this scan give a direct measurement of proteoglycan content. The dGEMRIC relaxation rate has been correlated with IKDC, Lysholm, and KOOS scores after treatment of chondral lesions with osteochondral allograft and ACI [43, 44].

Multiparametric MR sequences, such as T1rho and T2 mapping, can also provide detailed information on the biochemical composition of the cartilage without exogenous contrast. The T1rho relaxation time is proportional to the proteoglycan content in the tissue and has been used to monitor changes in the composition of cartilage repair tissue [45, 46]. T2 mapping provides information on the collagen structure of cartilage and repair tissue [45]. There have been variable reports on whether T2 mapping values are correlated with subjective outcome scores after different cartilage repair surgeries [43, 44, 47, 48].

While the relationships between imaging parameters and clinical outcomes are not fully defined, there is great potential for these studies to serve as objective, noninvasive biomarkers for success and failure after cartilage repair procedures. Characterizing the macroscopic and microscopic properties of repair tissue through MRI can provide an alternative to second-look arthroscopy and biopsy. These imaging techniques offer the possibility for an earlier definition of the likelihood success or failure of new repair procedures before the deterioration of clinical function.

Conclusions

Defining success and failure is a complex question with regard to outcomes after cartilage restoration surgery. Failure may be variably defined as subsequent surgery, progression to arthroplasty, lack of improvement in outcome measures, lack of hyaline-like repair tissue, or poor appearance on imaging studies. When designing and reporting on clinical trials for cartilage injuries, multiple definitions of failure should be included. Early endpoints should encompass factors such as imaging parameters that may be predictive of long-term function, while longer-term studies may focus more on reoperation rates, ability to meet predefined outcome score thresholds, and conversion to arthroplasty surgery. All trials should incorporate patient-reported outcome measures, activity measures, and satisfaction scores to gauge whether patient-defined goals are met with specific procedures. Once this information is widely available, surgeons can better counsel and provide guidance on success and failure rates based on specific patient goals.

References

1. Curl WW, Krome J, Gordon ES, Rushing J, Smith BP, Poehling GG. Cartilage injuries: a review of 31,516 knee arthroscopies. Arthroscopy J Arthroscopic Relat Surg. 1997;13:456–60.
2. Hjelle K, Solheim E, Strand T, Muri R, Brittberg M. Articular cartilage defects in 1,000 knee arthroscopies. Arthroscopy J Arthroscopic Relat Surg. 2002;18:730–4.
3. Steadman JR, Briggs KK, Rodrigo JJ, Kocher MS, Gill TJ, Rodkey WG. Outcomes of microfracture for traumatic chondral defects of the knee: average 11-year follow-up. Arthroscopy J Arthroscopic Relat Surg. 2003;19:477–84.
4. Mithoefer K, McAdams T, Williams RJ, Kreuz PC, Mandelbaum BR. Clinical efficacy of the microfracture technique for articular cartilage repair in the knee: an evidence-based systematic analysis. Am J Sports Med. 2009;37:2053–63.
5. Brittberg M, Lindahl A, Nilsson A, Ohlsson C, Isaksson O, Peterson L. Treatment of deep cartilage defects in the knee

with autologous chondrocyte transplantation. N Engl J Med. 1994;331:889–95.

6. Kon E, Verdonk P, Condello V, et al. Matrix-assisted autologous chondrocyte transplantation for the repair of cartilage defects of the knee. Am J Sports Med. 2009;37:156S–66S.

7. Gudas R, Kalesinskas RJ, Kimtys V, et al. A prospective randomized clinical study of mosaic osteochondral autologous transplantation versus microfracture for the treatment of osteochondral defects in the knee joint in young athletes. Arthroscopy J Arthroscopic Relat Surg. 2005;21:1066–75.

8. Bugbee WD, Convery FR. Osteochondral allograft transplantation. Clin Sports Med. 1999;18:67–75.

9. Jakobsen RB, Engebretsen L, Slauterbeck JR. An analysis of the quality of cartilage repair studies. J Bone Joint Surg Am. 2005;87:2232–9.

10. Sterett WI, Steadman JR, Huang MJ, Matheny LM, Briggs KK. Chondral resurfacing and high tibial osteotomy in the varus knee: survivorship analysis. Am J Sports Med. 2010;38:1420–4.

11. Bae DK, Song SJ, Yoon KH, Heo DB, Kim TJ. Survival analysis of microfracture in the osteoarthritic knee—minimum 10-year follow-up. Arthroscopy J Arthroscopic Relat Surg. 2013;29:244–50.

12. Pestka JM, Bode G, Salzmann G, Südkamp NP, Niemeyer P. Clinical outcome of autologous chondrocyte implantation for failed microfracture treatment of full-thickness cartilage defects of the knee joint. Am J Sports Med. 2012;40:325–31.

13. Hoemann C, Kandel R, Roberts S, et al. International Cartilage Repair Society (ICRS) recommended guidelines for histological endpoints for cartilage repair studies in animal models and clinical trials. Cartilage. 2011;2:153–72.

14. Gilmore R, Palfrey A. A histological study of human femoral condylar articular cartilage. J Anat. 1987;155:77.

15. Rosenberg L. Chemical basis for the histological use of safranin O in the study of articular cartilage. J Bone Joint Surg Am. 1971;53:69–82.

16. Henderson I, Tuy B, Connell D, Oakes B, Hettwer W. Prospective clinical study of autologous chondrocyte implantation and correlation with MRI at three and 12 months. Bone Joint J. 2003;85:1060–6.

17. Pineda S, Pollack A, Stevenson S, Goldberg V, Caplan A. A semiquantitative scale or histologic grading of articular cartilage repair. Cells Tissues Organs. 1992;143:335–40.

80   D. A. Lansdown et al.

18. O'Driscoll SW, Keeley FW, Salter RB. Durability of regenerated articular cartilage produced by free autogenous periosteal grafts in major full-thickness defects in joint surfaces under the influence of continuous passive motion. A follow-up report at one year. J Bone Joint Surg Am. 1988;70:595–606.
19. Mainil-Varlet P, Aigner T, Brittberg M, et al. Histological assessment of cartilage repair. J Bone Joint Surg Am. 2003;85:45–57.
20. Mainil-Varlet P, Van Damme B, Nesic D, Knutsen G, Kandel R, Roberts S. A new histology scoring system for the assessment of the quality of human cartilage repair: ICRS II. Am J Sports Med. 2010;38:880–90.
21. Brittberg M, Peterson L. Introduction of an articular cartilage classification. ICRS Newsl. 1998;1:5–8.
22. Smith GD, Taylor J, Almqvist KF, et al. Arthroscopic assessment of cartilage repair: a validation study of 2 scoring systems. Arthroscopy J Arthroscopic Relat Surg. 2005;21:1462–7.
23. Van Den Borne M, Raijmakers N, Vanlauwe J, et al. International Cartilage Repair Society (ICRS) and Oswestry macroscopic cartilage evaluation scores validated for use in Autologous Chondrocyte Implantation (ACI) and microfracture. Osteoarthr Cartil. 2007;15:1397–402.
24. Knutsen G, Drogset JO, Engebretsen L, et al. A randomized trial comparing autologous chondrocyte implantation with microfracture. J Bone Joint Surg. 2007;89:2105–12.
25. Saris DB, Vanlauwe J, Victor J, et al. Characterized chondrocyte implantation results in better structural repair when treating symptomatic cartilage defects of the knee in a randomized controlled trial versus microfracture. Am J Sports Med. 2008;36:235–46.
26. Vanlauwe J, Saris DB, Victor J, Almqvist KF, Bellemans J, Luyten FP. Five-year outcome of characterized chondrocyte implantation versus microfracture for symptomatic cartilage defects of the knee: early treatment matters. Am J Sports Med. 2011;39:2566–74.
27. Gudas R, Gudaitė A, Pocius A, et al. Ten-year follow-up of a prospective, randomized clinical study of mosaic osteochondral autologous transplantation versus microfracture for the treatment of osteochondral defects in the knee joint of athletes. Am J Sports Med. 2012;40:2499–508.
28. Irrgang JJ, Anderson AF, Boland AL, et al. Development and validation of the international knee documentation committee subjective knee form. Am J Sports Med. 2001;29:600–13.

29. Lysholm J, Gillquist J. Evaluation of knee ligament surgery results with special emphasis on use of a scoring scale. Am J Sports Med. 1982;10:150–4.
30. Kocher MS, Steadman JR, Briggs KK, Sterett WI, Hawkins RJ. Reliability, validity, and responsiveness of the Lysholm knee scale for various chondral disorders of the knee. JBJS. 2004;86:1139–45.
31. Knutsen G, Drogset JO, Engebretsen L, et al. A randomized multicenter trial comparing autologous chondrocyte implantation with microfracture: long-term follow-up at 14 to 15 years. J Bone Joint Surg Am. 2016;98:1332–9.
32. McConnell S, Kolopack P, Davis AM. The Western Ontario and McMaster Universities Osteoarthritis Index (WOMAC): a review of its utility and measurement properties. Arthritis Care Res. 2001;45:453–61.
33. Greco NJ, Anderson AF, Mann BJ, et al. Responsiveness of the International Knee Documentation Committee subjective knee form in comparison to the Western Ontario and McMaster Universities Osteoarthritis Index, modified Cincinnati Knee Rating System, and Short Form 36 in patients with focal articular cartilage defects. Am J Sports Med. 2010;38:891–902.
34. Ebert JR, Smith A, Wood DJ, Ackland TR. A comparison of the responsiveness of 4 commonly used patient-reported outcome instruments at 5 years after matrix-induced autologous chondrocyte implantation. Am J Sports Med. 2013;41:2791–9.
35. Hambly K, Griva K. IKDC or KOOS? which measures symptoms and disabilities most important to postoperative articular cartilage repair patients? Am J Sports Med. 2008;36:1695–704.
36. Marlovits S, Striessnig G, Resinger CT, et al. Definition of pertinent parameters for the evaluation of articular cartilage repair tissue with high-resolution magnetic resonance imaging. Eur J Radiol. 2004;52:310–9.
37. Dhollander A, Huysse W, Verdonk P, et al. MRI evaluation of a new scaffold-based allogenic chondrocyte implantation for cartilage repair. Eur J Radiol. 2010;75:72–81.
38. Marlovits S, Singer P, Zeller P, Mandl I, Haller J, Trattnig S. Magnetic resonance observation of cartilage repair tissue (MOCART) for the evaluation of autologous chondrocyte transplantation: determination of interobserver variability and correlation to clinical outcome after 2 years. Eur J Radiol. 2006;57:16–23.

39. Robertson W, Fick D, Wood D, Linklater J, Zheng M, Ackland T. MRI and clinical evaluation of collagen-covered autologous chondrocyte implantation (CACI) at two years. Knee. 2007;14:117–27.

40. de Windt TS, Welsch GH, Brittberg M, et al. Is magnetic resonance imaging reliable in predicting clinical outcome after articular cartilage repair of the knee? A systematic review and meta-analysis. Am J Sports Med. 2013;41:1695–702.

41. Mithoefer K, Williams RJ, Warren RF, et al. The microfracture technique for the treatment of articular cartilage lesions in the knee. J Bone Joint Surg Am. 2005;87:1911–20.

42. Kreuz PC, Steinwachs MR, Erggelet C, et al. Results after microfracture of full-thickness chondral defects in different compartments in the knee. Osteoarthr Cartil. 2006;14:1119–25.

43. Tadenuma T, Uchio Y, Kumahashi N, et al. Delayed gadolinium-enhanced MRI of cartilage and T2 mapping for evaluation of reparative cartilage-like tissue after autologous chondrocyte implantation associated with Atelocollagen-based scaffold in the knee. Skelet Radiol. 2016;45:1357–63.

44. Brown DS, Durkan MG, Foss EW, Szumowski J, Crawford DC. Temporal in vivo assessment of fresh osteochondral allograft transplants to the distal aspect of the femur by dGEMRIC (delayed gadolinium-enhanced MRI of cartilage) and zonal T2 mapping MRI. J Bone Joint Surg Am. 2014;96:564–72.

45. Li X, Cheng J, Lin K, et al. Quantitative MRI using T1rho and T2 in human osteoarthritic cartilage specimens: correlation with biochemical measurements and histology. Magn Reson Imaging. 2011;29:324–34.

46. Theologis AA, Schairer WW, Carballido-Gamio J, Majumdar S, Li X, Ma CB. Longitudinal analysis of T1ρ and T2 quantitative MRI of knee cartilage laminar organization following microfracture surgery. Knee. 2012;19:652–7.

47. Domayer S, Kutscha-Lissberg F, Welsch G, et al. T2 mapping in the knee after microfracture at 3.0 T: correlation of global T2 values and clinical outcome–preliminary results. Osteoarthr Cartil. 2008;16:903–8.

48. Jungmann PM, Brucker PU, Baum T, et al. Bilateral cartilage T2 mapping 9 years after mega-OATS implantation at the knee: a quantitative 3T MRI study. Osteoarthr Cartil. 2015;23:2119–28.

Part II
Core Knee Joint Preservation Cases

Chapter 6
Incidental Cartilage Defect

David R. Christian, Adam J. Beer, and Adam B. Yanke

Clinical Case Presentation

Clinical History

A 21-year-old male presents 18 months after a noncontact, twisting injury of the right knee. He has no prior history of knee injury and no symptoms prior to this event. At the time of injury, he had difficulty bearing weight and developed significant swelling within 24 h of the event. He never received a formal evaluation, but complained of inability to return to sport and high-level exercise several months after the injury. He denies experiencing any obvious instability events since the time of injury, but reports a severe lack of confidence in his injured knee. He had complaints of anterior knee pain with stairs and some occasional swelling, but no primary pain symptoms.

D. R. Christian · A. J. Beer · A. B. Yanke (✉)
Department of Orthopedic Surgery, Rush University Medical Center, Chicago, IL, USA
e-mail: Adam.yanke@rushortho.com

© Springer Nature Switzerland AG 2019   85
A. B. Yanke, B. J. Cole (eds.), *Joint Preservation of the Knee*,
https://doi.org/10.1007/978-3-030-01491-9_6

Physical Exam

The patient is 6 feet and 0 inches tall, weighs 174 pounds, and walks with a non-antalgic gait. There is no coronal plane abnormality when walking or standing. His range of motion is from −5° to 135° in his right knee, which is equal to his uninjured left knee. At the time of exam, he has a Grade I effusion and no medial or lateral joint line tenderness. Ligamentous examination reveals a 2B Lachman, negative posterior drawer, negative varus and valgus stress tests, and normal dial test.

Radiographs and Imaging

Radiographs of the right knee were obtained showing no fracture or dislocation as well as preserved joint space without evidence of tibiofemoral arthritis (Fig. 6.1). Review of

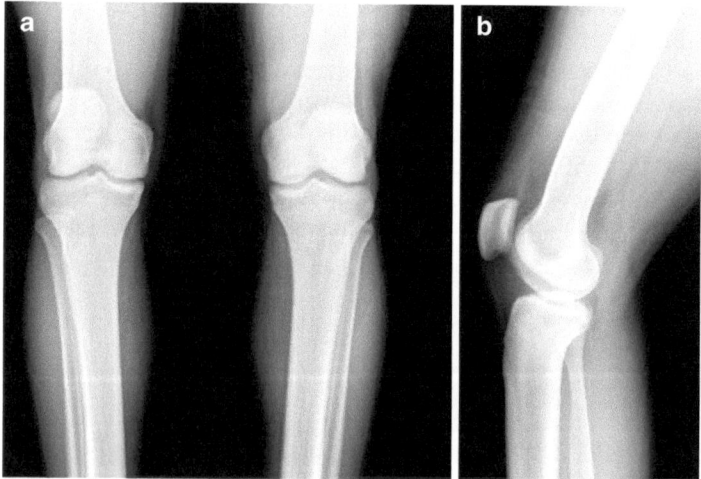

FIGURE 6.1 Preoperative radiographs. (a) Standing weight-bearing anteroposterior radiograph showing no fracture or dislocation, preserved joint space, and no evidence of tibiofemoral arthritis in either the right or left knee. (b) Lateral radiograph of the right knee showing no fracture, dislocation, or bone pathology

his right knee magnetic resonance imaging (MRI) demonstrates a complete rupture of the ACL with an intact posterior cruciate ligament (PCL), medial collateral ligament (MCL), and lateral collateral ligament (LCL). The patellofemoral and lateral compartments appear normal. There is a posterior medial meniscus tear that appears chronic in nature. There is a focal, full-thickness chondral defect of the posterior medial femoral condyle with underlying subchondral edema (Fig. 6.2).

Management

After the discussion of the risks and benefits, the patient is elected to proceed with an arthroscopically assisted ACL reconstruction utilizing a bone-patellar tendon-bone autograft. Diagnostic arthroscopy at that time revealed a small, degenerative central lateral meniscal tear, a chronic posterior medial meniscal tear, and a 20 mm × 15 mm International Cartilage

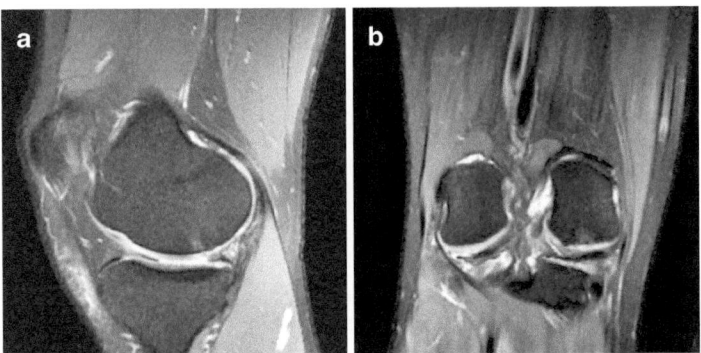

FIGURE 6.2 Preoperative magnetic resonance imaging. (a) Sagittal T2-weighted MRI image of the medial compartment in the patient's right knee depicting a full-thickness focal chondral defect of the posterior medial femoral condyle. (b) Coronal T2-weighted MRI image of the posterior aspect of the patient's knee showing a preserved lateral compartment and a full-thickness focal chondral defect of the posterior medial femoral condyle with subchondral edema

Restoration Society (ICRS) Grade III focal chondral defect of the medial femoral condyle (Fig. 6.3).

The lateral meniscal tear was mildly debrided with a shaver, and a medial meniscectomy was performed to treat the chronic medial meniscal tear. The medial femoral condyle defect was gently debrided to a stable base using a shaver to remove loose cartilage fragments. The decision was made to refrain from performing a formal cartilage restoration procedure at that time.

Literature Review and Discussion

Chondral defects of the knee are common within the general population, with one series reporting an incidence of 63% in patients undergoing arthroscopy [1]. The weight-bearing aspect of the medial femoral condyle has been identified as the most common location for such defects, although they are also often observed on the lateral femoral condyle and within the patellofemoral compartment [1]. Cartilage lesions frequently cause symptoms, including localized pain, swelling, and functional

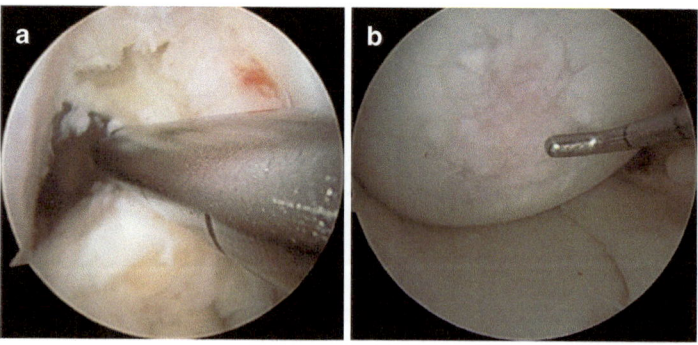

FIGURE 6.3 Surgical images. (a) Intraoperative arthroscopic image showing debridement of the ruptured ACL while protecting the PCL. (b) Intraoperative arthroscopic image showing the focal chondral defect of the posterior medial femoral condyle measuring 15 mm × 20 mm

disability, yet many defects remain asymptomatic and are only identified on advanced imaging or during arthroscopy while investigating the concurrent pathology. The association of symptomatic chondral defects with coronal malalignment, meniscus deficiency, or subchondral bone disease is often identifiable from a patient's history or imaging findings. Far less is understood, however, about the natural history of asymptomatic, incidental lesions that exist in the knee.

Whether symptomatic or asymptomatic, the decision-making process when treating any chondral defect is multifactorial and must take into consideration the defect's characteristics, such as the depth, size, location, and involvement of subchondral bone, in addition to patient-specific factors, which include varus or valgus malalignment, prior cartilage procedures, and concomitant meniscal or ligamentous pathology [2]. Depending on these factors, cartilage defects themselves may be successfully treated using a variety of methods ranging from a simple chondroplasty to more invasive cartilage restoration methods, including marrow stimulation, osteochondral grafting, and cell-based treatments. Symptomatic lesions are unlikely to improve without appropriate intervention, but when asymptomatic lesions are discovered, it is critical to weigh the risks and benefits of each treatment option.

While the outcomes of various cartilage restoration procedures for the treatment of symptomatic cartilage lesions have been reported [3–6], few studies have reported on the outcomes of asymptomatic lesions that are left untreated at the time of surgery. Shelbourne and colleagues investigated whether the presence of an untreated articular cartilage defect at the time of an ACL reconstruction would have impacted the outcome [7]. The authors compared the results of 125 ACL reconstruction patients with asymptomatic chondral defects treated with debridement to a control group of patients undergoing ACL with intact cartilage. While the final follow-up data was only available for approximately 20% of patients, they found that patients with intact cartilage had a significantly higher modified Noyes score (95.3 vs. 94.0) but demonstrated no difference in radiographic knee findings. Additionally, at least 79% of patients in both groups were able to return to sport. Despite the low follow-up percentage seen in this study, the results suggest that the presence of an asymptomatic chondral defect does not significantly impact the outcome of patients undergoing ACL reconstruction [7].

Similarly, Widuchowski and colleagues compared patients with untreated, asymptomatic Grade III and Grade IV chondral defects undergoing ACL reconstruction to patients with intact cartilage undergoing ACL reconstruction [8]. At 15-year follow-up, they reported that there was no difference between the defect and control group with the International Knee Documentation Committee (IKDC), Lysholm, and Tegner scores. Additionally, there was no difference in tibial anterior translation or reoperation rates between the two groups [8]. In agreement with the study by Shelbourne and colleagues, this study further supports that invasive cartilage restoration techniques should not be used to treat incidental chondral defects.

Chondroplasty has also been shown to provide relief in patients with symptomatic chondral defects. Hubbard compared the outcomes of patients with symptomatic defects of the medial femoral condyle who received either an arthroscopic debridement or washout and found that 80% of patients receiving a chondroplasty were pain-free at 1-year follow-up, compared to only 14% of patients in the washout group [9]. Additionally, Scillia et al. reported that 67% of National Football League players were able to return to play after arthroscopic chondroplasty, while those who also underwent a microfracture were 4.4 times less likely to return to play [10]. Messner and Maletius reported the long-term outcomes of 28 athletes with high-grade chondral damage in the weight-bearing aspect of the knee treated with arthroscopic chondroplasty [11]. Only 5 patients required further surgical intervention, and 21 patients were able return to their presurgical activity level [11]. More recently, Anderson et al. reported on a group of patients undergoing chondroplasty for symptomatic chondral defects in the absence of concurrent pathology [12]. Their cohort experienced symptomatic improvement at a mean follow-up of 31.5 months, and lower-grade lesions were correlated with greater improvement in patient-reported outcome scores [12]. Patients with patello-femoral cartilage lesions, in particular, often experience symptomatic relief after arthroscopic debridement. Federico and Reider reported outcomes of 36 patients undergoing debridement of symptomatic Grades II–IV patellar lesions for the treatment of anterior knee pain [13]. Overall, their cohort showed significant improvement in Fulkerson-Shea Patellofemoral Joint Evaluation score at final follow-up, and all but four patients stated that they benefited from the procedure [13].

When discovering an incidental chondral defect, it is important to consider the other factors associated with more invasive cartilage restoration procedures, such as wait times, costs, and postoperative rehabilitation. Autologous chondrocyte implantation (ACI) and osteochondral allograft transplantation (OCA) both require a future surgical procedure given that time is required to culture the chondrocytes in the case of ACI and acquire the allograft in the case of OCA. This exposes patients to additional general anesthesia and financial burdens associated with surgery. Microfracture and osteochondral autograft transplantation (OAT) can be performed without subsequent surgery; however, each of these procedures has its own limitations and requires significant postoperative rehabilitation. OAT requires the harvest of an osteochondral plug from a healthy region of the knee and comes with the risk of donor site morbidity, which increases with the number of plugs used [14]. Microfracture has been associated with worsening outcomes after 2-year postoperative time point and a high incidence of persistent postoperative pain [15]. Marrow stimulation can also lead to worsening pain as well as the formation of intraosseous osteophytes. Additionally, patients undergoing microfracture or OAT are instructed to be non-weight-bearing for 6 weeks, which can lead to muscular atrophy and persistent stiffness if not appropriately rehabilitated. Though not a determining factor in itself, the planned debridement approach can also avoid the uncertainty associated with what postoperative protocol the patient will be following. Arguably the worst-case scenario is a clinician deciding to perform marrow stimulation during a procedure for an incidental defect without prior discussion with the patient of the possibility as well as the changes in postoperative protocol.

Conclusion

Incidental chondral defects create a difficult clinical scenario and are commonly identified while evaluating for and treating the concurrent pathology. It is critical to determine whether the patient is experiencing any pain, swelling, or mechanical symptoms related to the identified defect. This can even involve them testing the knee before treating other associated pathologies (running in a linear fashion before performing ACL reconstruction). If symptomatic, intervention may be necessary; however, asymptomatic defects often remain asymptomatic and do not interfere with a patient's outcome. In the setting of an asymptomatic cartilage lesion while treating the concurrent pathology, the authors recommend mechanical debridement to avoid sequelae of unnecessary, more invasive intervention.

References

1. Curl WW, Krome J, Gordon ES, Rushing J, Smith BP, Poehling GG. Cartilage injuries: a review of 31,516 knee arthroscopies. Arthroscopy. 1997;13(4):456–60.
2. Oliver-Welsh L, Griffin JW, Meyer MA, Gitelis ME, Cole BJ. Deciding how best to treat cartilage defects. Orthopedics. 2016;39(6):343–50.
3. Frank RM, Lee S, Levy D, Poland S, Smith M, Scalise N, et al. Osteochondral allograft transplantation of the knee: analysis of failures at 5 years. Am J Sports Med. 2017;45(4):864–74.
4. Ebert JR, Smith A, Fallon M, Wood DJ, Ackland TR. Degree of preoperative subchondral bone edema is not associated with

pain and graft outcomes after matrix-induced autologous chondrocyte implantation. Am J Sports Med. 2014;42(11):2689–98.

5. Gobbi A, Karnatzikos G, Kumar A. Long-term results after microfracture treatment for full-thickness knee chondral lesions in athletes. Knee Surg Sports Traumatol Arthrosc. 2014;22(9):1986–96.

6. Gomoll AH, Kang RW, Chen AL, Cole BJ. Triad of cartilage restoration for unicompartmental arthritis treatment in young patients: meniscus allograft transplantation, cartilage repair and osteotomy. J Knee Surg. 2009;22(2):137–41.

7. Shelbourne KD, Jari S, Gray T. Outcome of untreated traumatic articular cartilage defects of the knee: a natural history study. J Bone Joint Surg Am. 2003;85-A(Suppl 2):8–16.

8. Widuchowski W, Widuchowski J, Koczy B, Szyluk K. Untreated asymptomatic deep cartilage lesions associated with anterior cruciate ligament injury: results at 10- and 15-year follow-up. Am J Sports Med. 2009;37(4):688–92.

9. Hubbard MJ. Articular debridement versus washout for degeneration of the medial femoral condyle. A five-year study. J Bone Joint Surg Br. 1996;78(2):217–9.

10. Scillia AJ, Aune KT, Andrachuk JS, Cain EL, Dugas JR, Fleisig GS, et al. Return to play after chondroplasty of the knee in National Football League athletes. Am J Sports Med. 2015;43(3):663–8.

11. Messner K, Maletius W. The long-term prognosis for severe damage to weight-bearing cartilage in the knee: a 14-year clinical and radiographic follow-up in 28 young athletes. Acta Orthop Scand. 1996;67(2):165–8.

12. Anderson DE, Rose MB, Wille AJ, Wiedrick J, Crawford DC. Arthroscopic mechanical chondroplasty of the knee is beneficial for treatment of focal cartilage lesions in the absence of concurrent pathology. Orthop J Sports Med. 2017;5(5):2325967117707213.

13. Federico DJ, Reider B. Results of isolated patellar debridement for patellofemoral pain in patients with normal patellar alignment. Am J Sports Med. 1997;25(5):663–9.

14. Pareek A, Reardon PJ, Maak TG, Levy BA, Stuart MJ, Krych AJ. Long-term outcomes after osteochondral autograft transfer: a systematic review at mean follow-up of 10.2 years. Arthroscopy. 2016;32(6):1174–84.

15. Mithoefer K, McAdams T, Williams RJ, Kreuz PC, Mandelbaum BR. Clinical efficacy of the microfracture technique for articular cartilage repair in the knee: an evidence-based systematic analysis. Am J Sports Med. 2009;37(10):2053–63.

Chapter 7
Small Femoral Cartilage Defect: Primary/Bone Loss

Christian Lattermann and Burak Altintas

Chief Complaint

Medial knee pain

History of Present Illness

A 28-year-old otherwise healthy male recreational basketball player presents with ongoing pain in the medial side of the knee in his right knee. He reports some soreness on and off after games or long workdays, but it started becoming outright painful during a game about 4 weeks ago. He reports pain and swelling around the joint as well as pain during weight-bearing along the medial aspect of his knee. He feels occasionally tightness and an associated loss of strength in his quadriceps at times. He denies feelings of catching, locking, or instability. The conservative treatment with ice, elevation, and anti-inflammatory therapy did not provide lasting relief.

C. Lattermann (✉)
Brigham and Women's Hospital, Harvard Medical School, Boston, MA, USA
e-mail: clattermann@bwh.harvard.edu

B. Altintas
Steadman Philippon Clinic, Vail, CO, USA

© Springer Nature Switzerland AG 2019
A. B. Yanke, B. J. Cole (eds.), *Joint Preservation of the Knee*,
https://doi.org/10.1007/978-3-030-01491-9_7

Pearls

- Insidious onset – cartilage lesions usually do not become symptomatic in a sudden fashion but first linger and then start becoming symptomatic after a specific event.
- Recurrent swelling and tightness – this is a warning sign for a chondral defect. It also affects range of motion and quadriceps function. Symptoms that linger for more than 1 year affect outcome of any chondral repair procedure. Patients with clearly documented intra-articular effusions should not undergo physical therapy until a clear diagnosis is made.
- Pain during weight-bearing – this is often more pronounced in situations of mechanical interference such as a flap or an associated meniscus tear.

Physical Examination

The patient has a normal BMI. The gait is slightly antalgic. The gross anatomic alignment of the lower extremity is neutral. The right knee has a mild effusion (recession fills with the knee in extension). There is no redness or warmth. The range of motion is symmetric from 0° to 140°. There is tenderness to palpation over the medial femoral condyle just above the joint line. Meniscal tests are negative. There is good patellofemoral tracking without crepitus, and patellofemoral glide is 2/4. The ligamentous examination shows no abnormalities when tested for Lachman test, pivot-shift test, and varus/valgus stress test. The patient has a good quadriceps activation with straight leg raise test and does not show significant atrophy of the VMO. The neurovascular examination is within normal limits.

Imaging

Imaging with standard x-rays of the knee (AP and lateral, FWB-AP, and Merchant view in 30° of flexion) is obtained to rule out acute injuries (such as the notch sign or second fracture) and chronic conditions such as osteochondritis dissecans and joint space narrowing, osteophytes, or subchondral sclerosis, indicative of osteoarthritis. In this case, the plain radiographs could not be included but did not indicate any of the above pathologies and were considered to be within normal limits. A long-leg alignment view (MTP-2 single-leg standing) shows neutral alignment. Thus, an MRI is ordered to assess articular cartilage and synovium as well as ligaments (Fig. 7.1). The 3T MRI shows a 2-cm^2-full-thickness chondral defect in the medial femoral condyle with a small subchondral edema and minimal bone loss underlying the defect. No loose body can be identified. No evidence for an osteochondritis dissecans can be found. There is no evidence of damage to the menisci or the ligaments.

Technique Description

During diagnostic arthroscopy, a full-thickness 10 mm by 20 mm chondral lesion of the medial femoral condyle within the weight-bearing zone in extension is identified (Fig. 7.2).

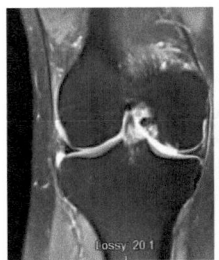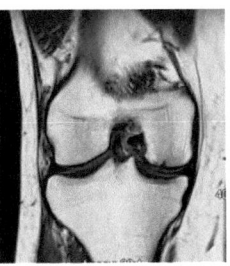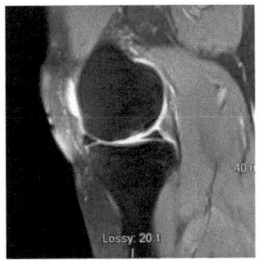

FIGURE 7.1 T1 and T2 coronal/sagittal MRI images show small chondral defect in MFC. No significant subchondral edema. The meniscus is intact

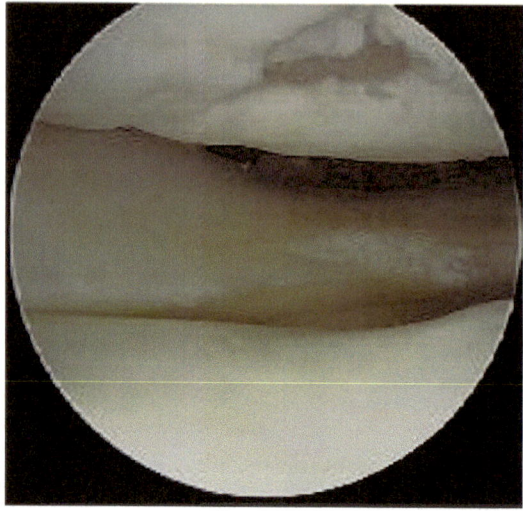

FIGURE 7.2 Grade IIIb (deep chondral lesion with intact subchondral bone). Lesion of the medial femoral condyle

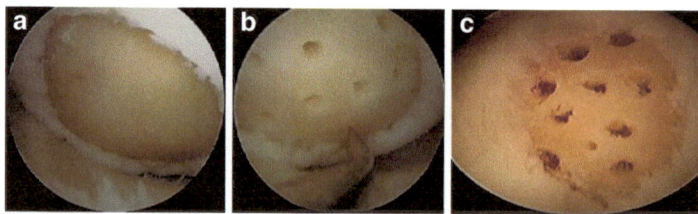

FIGURE 7.3 Microfracture technique. (**a**) Preparation of the defect with careful debridement of the calcified cartilage layer. (**b**) Careful creation of the microfracture holes using the awl (recognize the small fat globules as indicator for sufficient depth). (**c**) Blood-filled microfracture holes after deflation of the tourniquet

After confirming the absence of any ligamentous and meniscal lesions, a microfracture procedure is performed (Fig. 7.3a, b). For this, it is important to choose an adequate anteromedial portal with the help of a spinal needle to reach the lesion. The chondral defect should be debrided to expose the subchondral bone and resect any unstable chondral tissue at the margins. After the creation of a stable chondral border around the defect, the microfracture awl is inserted through the antero-medial portal under direct visualization from the proximal anterolateral viewing portal with care taken not to injure the healthy cartilage. After placing the awl close to the chondral margins of the defect, small holes of 3–5 mm depth are created. It is important to keep the awl perpendicular to the subchondral bone to avoid skiving. The distance between the holes should be approximately 3 mm. Care should be taken not to place them too close to each other to avoid fracture propagation of the subchondral bone plate. After completion of the procedure, first the tourniquet (if used) should be discontinued, and the fluid inflow should be shut off. Then the remaining fluid should be carefully suctioned under vision until the visualization of the blood outflow from the microfracture canals. Then, the arthroscope should be removed without suction (Fig. 7.3c).

Postoperative Rehabilitation Protocol

Following surgery, the patient follows the microfracture protocol described by Steadman et al. In brief, the patient is mobilized with non-weight-bearing on crutches for 6 weeks followed by gradual increase of weight-bearing in the following weeks. A continuous passive motion machine is required for 4–6 weeks and 6–8 h/day. Quadriceps-strengthening exercises are started immediately. Concomitant physiotherapy is initiated with focus on reducing the inflammation.

Pearls
• Neutral alignment – the alignment plays an important role in decision-making as a malalignment can predispose to the overloading of the joint. The alignment should be confirmed with a long-leg MTP-2 alignment film.

- Effusion – persistent effusion 4 weeks after an exacerbation with a history of "soreness" is suggestive of chondral damage. This is a reactive effusion and not an acute, post-traumatic effusion (typically after ACL, after meniscus injury, or after patella dislocation).

Approach to Treatment

The following aspects should be considered in a young active patient with acute-on-chronic onset of symptoms related to a symptomatic cartilage lesion with minimal bone loss and subchondral edema of the medial femoral condyle:

1. *Staging arthroscopy*: any patient with a potential chondral defect should be undergoing an arthroscopic evaluation. This staging arthroscopy lays the ground for the current treatment algorithm and should result in a decision to either treat the defect with a single-staged procedure, such as microfracture or an osteochondral autograft transfer, or with a two-staged procedure such as an osteochondral allograft or a cell-based procedure. It is *not advised* to plan the actual chondral repair technique without the benefit of an arthroscopic exam.
2. *Alignment*: alignment is crucial for the treatment planning. If the patient has a varus deformity with a concomitant chondral lesion on the medial side, the adequate treatment should include an osteotomy to correct the main cause.
3. *Meniscus*: the presence of a meniscal lesion plays a role in the guidance of the patient. If the lesion is reparable and good biological healing potential is present, primary repair of the meniscus should be attempted. If the meniscal lesion is unsalvageable, the only option is judicious partial resection of the tear. The patient should be counseled regarding having a higher risk of incomplete healing of the chondral lesion and developing knee osteoarthritis in the future if a meniscus lesion requires partial meniscectomy.

4. *Rehabilitation*: the patient's ability and willingness to do the required rehabilitation should not be forgotten. Especially, limited weight-bearing following microfracture should be discussed carefully and cannot be "sprung" onto the patient postoperatively. Lack of communication about the weight-bearing restrictions leads to significant confusion and noncompliance postoperatively.

Lesion Characteristics and Treatment Approach

The size of the chondral lesion and the osseous involvement are important elements in the decision-making. Arthroscopic evaluation of the defect location and size is important since the MRI may underestimate the lesion size [1]. A recent study demonstrated that commonly used intraoperative measurement tools underestimate the size of the defects, but the 3 mm probe has the highest measurement bias at all lesion locations. Thus utilization of a simple metal ruler or sliding metallic ruler tool measures the defect size more accurately [2]. This is of utmost importance since the size determines the choice of treatment.

Treatment Choices

1. Arthroscopic debridement and chondroplasty may improve the patient's symptoms despite being not curative [3]. The literature on the outcome after this technique is limited. Levy et al. showed promising results after 1 year of follow-up in 15 knees of soccer players with an average of 42 mm^2 lesion before and 112 mm^2 after debridement [4]. The use of monopolar radiofrequency as an adjuvant to mechanical chondroplasty with a shaver for the treatment of grade III chondral lesions 1.5–3 cm in diameter did not affect function outcomes when compared with mechanical

chondroplasty by the use of a shaver only after a follow-up of 19 months [5]. Another study on patients with medial femoral chondral defect of approximately 20 mm^2 and medial meniscus lesions showed superior results for bipolar radiofrequency. However, 18 of the 60 patients required revision surgeries including knee replacement surgery [6]. The 10-year follow-up showed a significant decrease in functional outcomes with 60% revision surgery rate in the debridement group versus 23.3% in the radiofrequency chondroplasty group [7]. Thus, this kind of therapy can deem reasonable for patients who are not optimal candidates for cartilage restoration such as with older age, advanced degeneration, high body mass index, or inactive patients who are unwilling to comply with the postoperative rehabilitation protocol [3].

2. Microfracture: a widely accepted treatment option for small cartilage defects of the femoral condyles without osseous involvement is the bone marrow stimulation with microfracture. In 72 patients with traumatic full-thickness chondral defects with a mean size of 2.8 cm^2, Steadman et al. showed significant improvements in Tegner and Lysholm scores with good to excellent SF-36 and WOMAC scores following the microfracture at a mean follow-up of 11 years [8]. Another study on 53 athletes with an average defect size of 4 cm^2 reported an improvement of Lysholm and IKDC scores. However, the authors also noted a decline in sport activity over time [9]. Gobbi et al. showed that patients with lesions smaller than 4 cm^2 and younger than 30 years of age showed significantly better functional outcome. Furthermore, they added that the lesion size is a more important prognostic factor than age [10]. A systematic review showed that microfracture provides effective short-term functional improvement of knee function but insufficient data are available on its long-term results [11]. A newer analysis stated that the use of microfracture for the treatment of small lesions in patients with low postoperative demands was observed to result in good clinical outcomes at short-term follow-up. However, beyond

5 years postoperatively, treatment failure after microfracture could be expected regardless of lesion size [12]. Thus modifications to the microfracture technique have emerged clinically. The available literature to support this new technology is sparse. A recent systematic review showed that the early literature on microfracture with biological adjuvants is heterogeneous reporting both equivalent and superior clinical outcomes and extremely limited in quality [13]. Future studies are needed to show the potential role of biological adjuvant therapy after

3. Osteochondral autograft transfer (OAT): this autologous transfer technique can be done "point of care" and thus does not require a second procedure. Lynch et al. showed improved clinical outcomes with a high return-to-play rate following OAT. Moreover, they suggested that OAT might be more appropriate for lesions smaller than 2 cm^2 with the known risk of failure between 2 and 4 years [14]. Another analysis is also in line with this in showing significant improvements in clinical outcome scores and good durability with successful outcomes in 75% of the patients at 12.3 years after surgery [15]. The comparison between OAT and microfracture showed no significant difference for lesions less than 3 cm^2 at midterm. However, because of variability in patient-specific factors such as age, preinjury activity level, lesion location, and size, the superiority of OAT over MFX cannot be generalized to all patient populations and therefore requires individualized patient care [16].

In summary, for a chondral lesion of 2 cm^2 size in the femoral condyle, the preferred treatment remains as either osteochondral autograft transfer (OAT) or microfracture. If there is significant involvement of subchondral bone (clearly destruction of the subchondral bone plate and extensive marrow edema), both of these techniques may reach their limit and may have to be reconsidered as primary tools to treat these lesions. Future studies will determine whether adding biologics will result in lasting superior clinical outcome.

TABLE 7.1 Different therapeutic approaches

Technique	Advantages	Disadvantages
Debridement	Easy to perform Uncomplicated postoperative rehabilitation	Not curative
Microfracture	Easy to perform Good functional outcome	Strict postoperative rehabilitation with limited weight-bearing and use of CPM
Microfracture with augmentation	Currently only experimental	The same as for microfracture Increased cost
Osteochondral transfer	Possible anatomic reconstruction of the defect	Harvest site morbidity

The advantages and disadvantages of the techniques can be depicted in Table 7.1.

References

1. Gomoll AH, Yoshioka H, Watanabe A, Dunn JC, Minas T. Preoperative measurement of cartilage defects by MRI underestimates lesion size. Cartilage. 2011;2(4):389–93. https://doi.org/10.1177/1947603510397534.
2. Flanigan DC, Carey JL, Brophy RH, et al. Interrater and intra-rater reliability of arthroscopic measurements of articular cartilage defects in the knee. J Bone Jt Surg. 2017;99(12):979–88. https://doi.org/10.2106/JBJS.16.01132.
3. Chilelli BJ, Cole BJ, Farr J, Lattermann C, Gomoll AH. The four most common types of knee cartilage damage encountered in practice: how and why orthopaedic surgeons manage them. Instr Course Lect. 2017;66:507–30. Available at: http://www.ncbi.nlm.nih.gov/pubmed/28594526.
4. Levy AS, Lohnes J, Sculley S, LeCroy M, Garrett W. Chondral delamination of the knee in soccer players. Am J Sports Med. 1996;24(5):634–9. https://doi.org/10.1177/036354659602400512.

5. Barber FA, Iwasko NG. Treatment of grade III femoral chondral lesions: mechanical chondroplasty versus monopolar radiofrequency probe. Arthroscopy. 2006;22(12):1312–7. https://doi.org/10.1016/j.arthro.2006.06.008.
6. Spahn G, Klinger HM, Mückley T, Hofmann GO. Four-year results from a randomized controlled study of knee chondroplasty with concomitant medial meniscectomy: mechanical debridement versus radiofrequency chondroplasty. Arthrosc J Arthrosc Relat Surg. 2010;26(9):S73–80. https://doi.org/10.1016/j.arthro.2010.02.030.
7. Spahn G, Hofmann GO, von Engelhardt LV. Mechanical debridement versus radiofrequency in knee chondroplasty with concomitant medial meniscectomy: 10-year results from a randomized controlled study. Knee Surg Sport Traumatol Arthrosc. 2016;24(5):1560–8. https://doi.org/10.1007/s00167-015-3810-6.
8. Steadman JR, Briggs KK, Rodrigo JJ, Kocher MS, Gill TJ, Rodkey WG. Outcomes of microfracture for traumatic chondral defects of the knee: Average 11-year follow-up. Arthroscopy. 2003;19(5):477–84. https://doi.org/10.1053/jars.2003.50112.
9. Gobbi A, Nunag P, Malinowski K. Treatment of full thickness chondral lesions of the knee with microfracture in a group of athletes. Knee Surg Sports Traumatol Arthrosc. 2005;13(3):213–21. https://doi.org/10.1007/s00167-004-0499-3.
10. Gobbi A, Karnatzikos G, Kumar A. Long-term results after microfracture treatment for full-thickness knee chondral lesions in athletes. Knee Surg Sport Traumatol Arthrosc. 2014;22(9):1986–96. https://doi.org/10.1007/s00167-013-2676-8.
11. Mithoefer K, Mcadams T, Williams RJ, Kreuz PC, Mandelbaum BR. Clinical efficacy of the microfracture technique for articular cartilage repair in the knee: an evidence-based systematic analysis. Am J Sports Med. 2009;37(10):2053–63. https://doi.org/10.1177/0363546508328414.
12. Goyal D, Keyhani S, Lee EH, Hui JH. Evidence-based status of microfracture technique: a systematic review of level I and II studies. Arthrosc J Arthrosc Relat Surg. 2013;29(9):1579–88. https://doi.org/10.1016/j.arthro.2013.05.027.
13. Arshi A, Fabricant PD, Go DE, Williams RJ, McAllister DR, Jones KJ. Can biologic augmentation improve clinical outcomes following microfracture for symptomatic cartilage defects of the knee? A systematic review. Cartilage. 2017; https://doi.org/10.1177/1947603517746722.

14. Lynch TS, Patel RM, Benedick A, Amin NH, Jones MH, Miniaci A. Systematic review of autogenous osteochondral transplant outcomes. Arthroscopy. 2015;31(4):746–54. https://doi.org/10.1016/j.arthro.2014.11.018.
15. Assenmacher AT, Pareek A, Reardon PJ, Macalena JA, Stuart MJ, Krych AJ. Long-term outcomes after osteochondral allograft: a systematic review at long-term follow-up of 12.3 years. Arthroscopy. 2016;32(10):2160–8. https://doi.org/10.1016/j.arthro.2016.04.020.
16. Pareek A, Reardon PJ, Macalena JA, et al. Osteochondral autograft transfer versus microfracture in the knee: a meta-analysis of prospective comparative studies at midterm. Arthroscopy. 2016;32(10):2118–30. https://doi.org/10.1016/j.arthro.2016.05.038.

Chapter 8
Large Cartilage Defects: Primary/Bone Loss

Luis Eduardo Tirico and William Bugbee

Primary Bone Loss

Case Presentation

An athletic 17-year-old male high school soccer player presents with a 4-year history of intermittent anteromedial pain in the right knee when performing sports. The patient has been diagnosed with osteochondritis dissecans 3 years prior but did not receive any specific treatment. The current episode occurred in the last 6 months and did not resolve with rest and avoidance of sports. New onset of mechanical symptoms and swelling has also been observed.

On physical examination, the patient stands 6 ft. and 1 in. tall, weighs 172 lb., and walks with a slight external rotation on the right limb, with neutral alignment in both limbs. A trace effusion on the right knee was noted along with maintained

L. E. Tirico
Knee Surgery Department, Orthopedic and Traumatology Institute, University of São Paulo Medical School, São Paulo, Brazil
e-mail: luis.tirico@hc.fm.usp.br

W. Bugbee (✉)
Joint Preservation and Cartilage Repair Service, Medical Direction of Orthopaedic Research, Division of Orthopaedic Surgery, Scripps Clinic, La Jolla, CA, USA
e-mail: bugbee.william@scrippshealth.org

© Springer Nature Switzerland AG 2019
A. B. Yanke, B. J. Cole (eds.), *Joint Preservation of the Knee*,
https://doi.org/10.1007/978-3-030-01491-9_8

107

range of motion at −5–135 degrees. Pain was noted in the medial compartment with flexion and internal rotation of the knee from 60 to 20 degrees of flexion. Mild tenderness to palpation of the medial femoral condyle is present. No ligament instability is noticed, and the meniscal tests were negative.

Digital weight-bearing AP and lateral and tunnel view radiographs of the patient showed a radiolucent rounded lesion on the lateral aspect of the medial femoral condyle involving approximately 40% of the weight-bearing area. Magnetic resonance imaging was performed, and an osteochondral lesion was seen on the weight-bearing surface of the medial femoral condyle measuring approximately 20 × 30 mm (Figs. 8.1 and 8.2). A fluid-filled break in the articular surface was present, and there was fluid at the interface of the fragment with the host bone. Edema was present in the bed of the defect (Fig. 8.3).

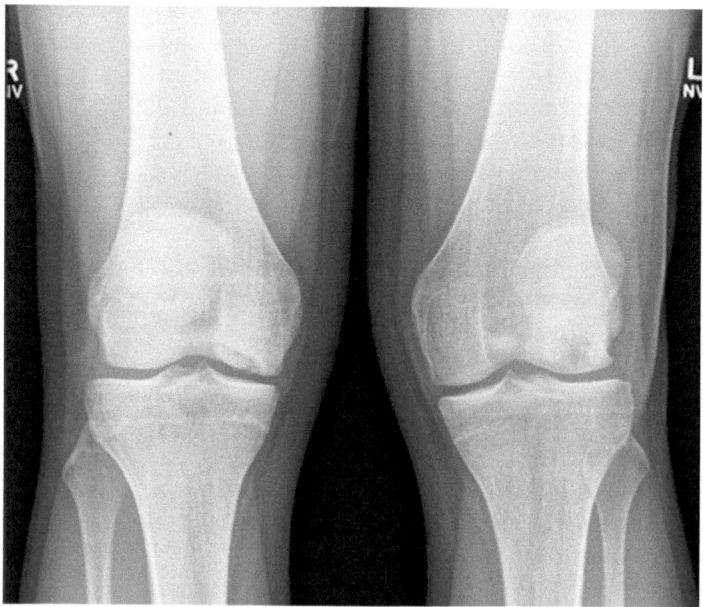

FIGURE 8.1 A preoperative weight-bearing radiograph demonstrating a radiolucent rounded lesion of the medial femoral condyle

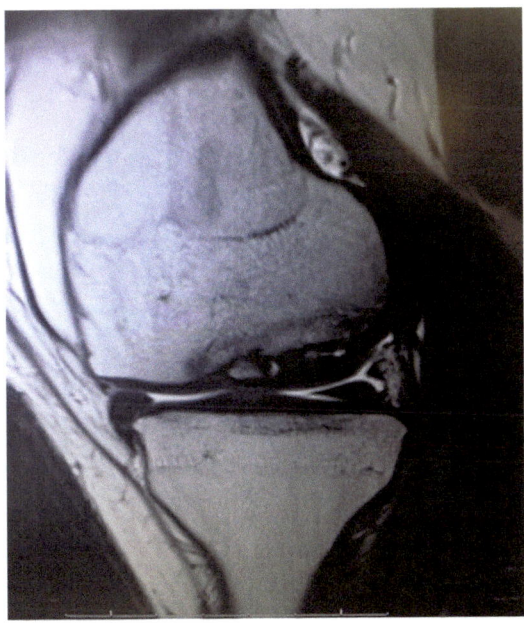

FIGURE 8.2 Sagittal T1 magnetic resonance image showing an osteo-chondritis dissecans lesion in the medial femoral condyle

The patient's history and imaging findings are consistent with the diagnosis of osteochondritis dissecans (OCD) of the knee. While the presence of external rotation of the limb is not commonly seen (Wilson's sign), anterior knee pain on knee range of motion in flexion and internal rotation (Wilson's test) is usually found in symptomatic cases. The presence of effusion is usually correlated with an osteochondral lesion on the knee. On digital radiographs, OCD in the classic position of the medial femoral condyle is best seen on the AP view. A disruption of the subchondral bone plate best seen on the lateral view is often present, particularly with large, unstable lesions. Completing the investigation with an MRI study is usually necessary for a thorough visualization of the lesion and therapeutic planning. Nonoperative treatment of OCD is usually the first line of treatment, and it has been

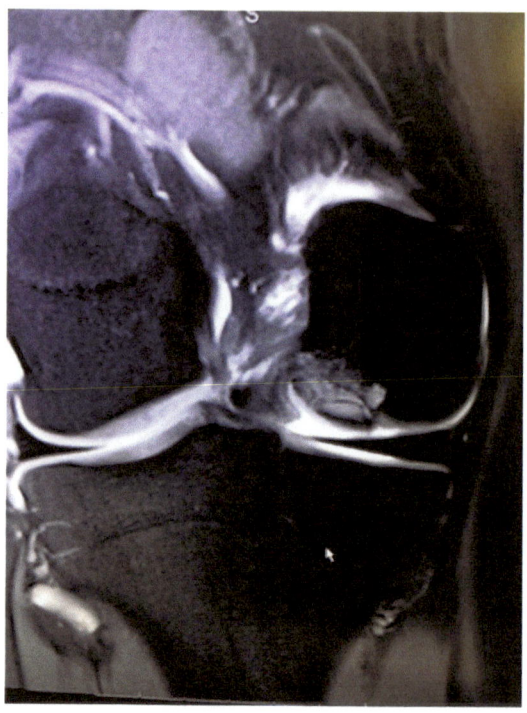

FIGURE 8.3 Coronal T2 magnetic resonance image of the lesion showing fluid at the interface of the fragment with the host bone suggesting lack of stability. Edema is present in the bed of the defect

reported to be successful in 50–94% of patients with open physes and stable lesions [4, 9]. When the physes are closed or the lesion is unstable or detached, surgical treatment is usually indicated. In this case we chose to use fresh osteochondral allograft (OCA) because of the size of the lesion, fragmentation of the bony fragment, and the fibrous and cystic maturity of the interface of the bone and its bed. Furthermore the use of fresh osteochondral allografts provides the option to restore both the osseous and chondral components at the same time with mature hyaline cartilage and a structured osseous component. As the majority of OCD lesions are located in the femoral condyles, dowel technique OCA is best indicated for this type of repair.

Management

The surgical procedure is performed with the patient in a supine position with a tourniquet on the proximal ipsilateral thigh. A leg or foot holder is extremely helpful to position and maintain the knee in between 70° and 120° of flexion. A standard midline incision is made and elevated subcutaneously, and an anteromedial 5 cm arthrotomy was executed. The joint is entered by incising the fat pad and retinaculum without disrupting the anterior horn of the meniscus or damaging the articular surface. Once the joint capsule and synovium have been incised and retractors carefully placed, the knee is brought to a degree of flexion that presents the lesion into the arthrotomy site (Fig. 8.4).

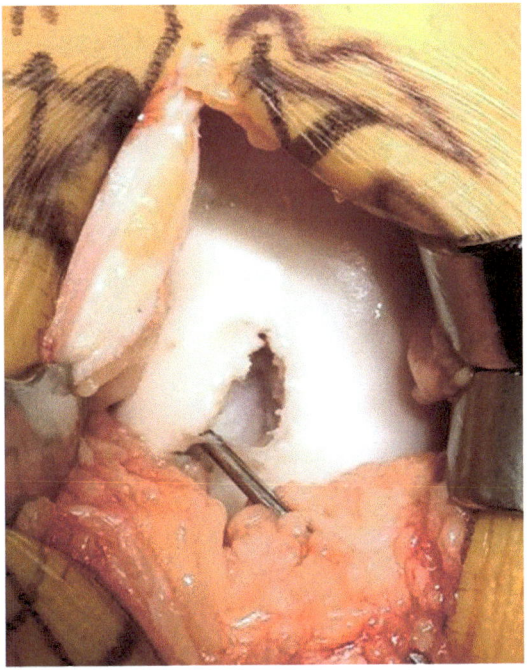

FIGURE 8.4 Arthrotomy showing an osteochondral defect in the medial femoral condyle. A nerve hook is elevating the osteochondral lesion showing instability of the fragment

Extending the arthrotomy proximal or distal may be necessary to mobilize the extensor mechanism. Care is taken for the positioning of the retractor within the notch, to protect the cruciate ligaments and articular cartilage. The unstable fragment is excised sharply and measured (Fig. 8.5). The lesion is then inspected and palpated with a probe, to determine the extent, margins, and maximum size (Fig. 8.6).

Dowel surgical technique is our preferred choice for the treatment of femoral condyle lesions whenever feasible, and a commercial set of instruments is used for this type of OCA transplantation (Fig. 8.7).

A guide wire is driven through the sizing dowel into the center of the lesion, perpendicular to the curvature of the articular surface. The cartilage surface is scored, and a special reamer is used to remove the remaining articular cartilage

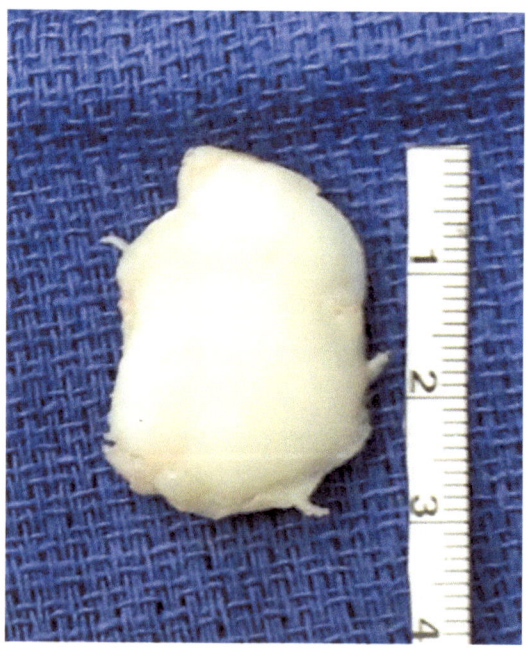

FIGURE 8.5 Large osteochondral defect removed from the knee. Fragment was not suited for fixation

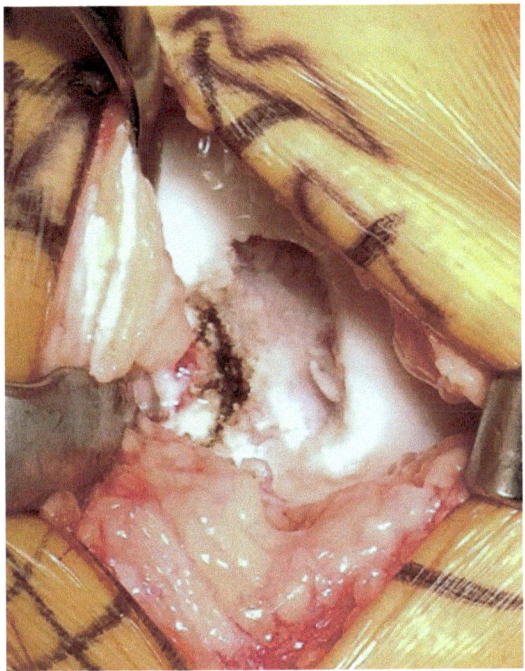

FIGURE 8.6 Osteochondral defect on the lateral portion of the medial femoral condyle showing a sclerotic subchondral bed. The lesion is uncontained into the femoral notch, a typical finding

and 3–4 mm of the subchondral bone. In deeper lesions, the pathologic bone is removed until there is a healthy, bleeding bone. Generally, the preparation depth does not exceed 5–8 mm. Bone grafting is performed to fill any deeper or more extensive osseous defects or cysts or to modify the fit of the graft if there is a depth mismatch between the recipient socket and allograft plug. At this point the guide pin is removed (Fig. 8.8), and depth measurements are made and recorded in the four quadrants of the prepared recipient site.

The corresponding anatomic location of the recipient site is identified on the graft (Fig. 8.9). The graft is placed into a graft holder (or, alternately, held with bone-holding forceps).

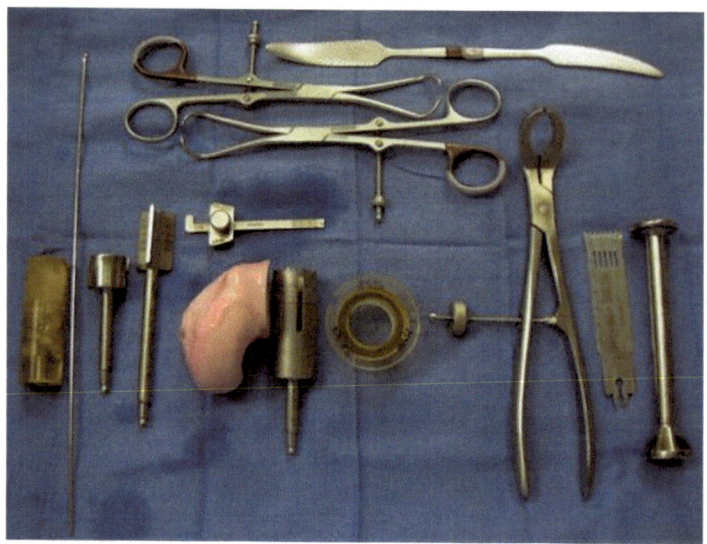

FIGURE 8.7 A set of instruments used for the osteochondral allograft dowel technique transplantation

A graft-harvesting guide is placed in the appropriate position, again perpendicular to the articular surface, exactly matching the orientation used to create the recipient site. The appropriate size-matched coring saw is used to core out the graft (Fig. 8.10). The graft is cut from the donor condyle and removed as a long plug (Fig. 8.11). Depth measurements, which were taken from the recipient, are transferred to the graft, and the excess bone is trimmed with a saw (Fig. 8.12). The graft is irrigated copiously with a high-pressure lavage to remove all marrow elements.

The graft is then inserted by hand in the appropriate rotation and is gently pressed into place manually. To fully seat the graft, the joint can be carefully brought through a range of motion, allowing the opposing articular surface to seat the graft. Finally, a very gentle tamping is performed to fully seat the graft. Once the graft is seated, a determination is made

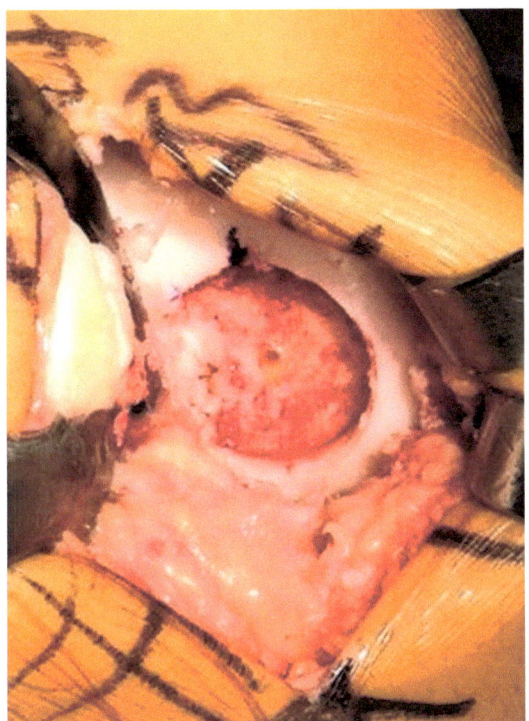

Figure 8.8 Recipient socked with the bleeding subchondral bone

whether additional fixation is required (Fig. 8.13). Typically, press-fit fixation is used with no additional type of fixation. The knee is then brought through a complete range of motion in order to confirm that the graft is stable and that there is no catching or soft-tissue obstruction noted.

Outcome

Postoperatively, full range of motion is implemented and tolerated immediately after surgery. Patient was allowed 25% weight-bearing for 4–6 weeks after surgery. Progressive

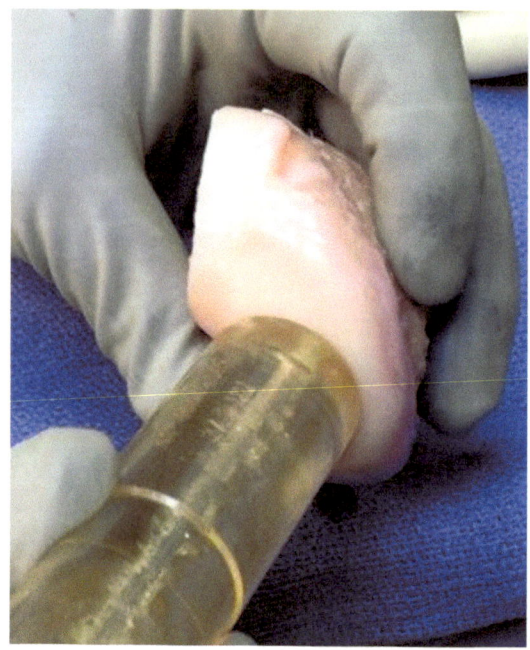

FIGURE 8.9 Anatomical location and size matching on the donor condyle

weight-bearing is then implemented and tolerated. The patient is allowed to return to recreational and sports activities by 4–6 months, once complete functional recovery and radiographic healing are demonstrated (Fig. 8.14a–d).

Literature Review

Osteochondritis dissecans affects approximately 15–30 per 100,000 patients, and it is most prevalent in adolescents and young adults. Conservative treatment is usually indicated as the initial treatment, and an improved response is usually seen within 6 months of treatment in cases that tend to evolve to the healing of the lesion. Juvenile patients and medial OCD have a better chance of healing with conservative treatment

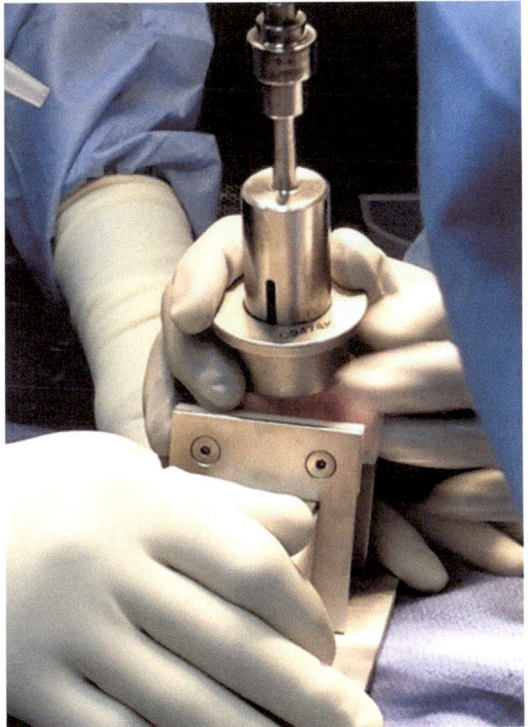

FIGURE 8.10 Graft positioned in the graft holder and the appropriate saw used to core out the graft

than adult patients and lateral lesions [2]. Surgical procedure is indicated for unstable lesions or symptomatic patients that failed conservative treatment and varies between minimally invasive procedures, such as drilling, fixation, debridement, and fragment excision, and restorative procedures such as microfracture, autologous osteochondral transplantation (OAT), autologous chondrocyte implantation (ACI), OCA, and stem cell transplantation [6]. Good outcomes in surgical treatment of OCD with surface procedures such as microfracture, ACI, and stem cell transplantation have been described [1, 3]. However, a lesion that is deeper than 8–10 mm requires a surgical technique that will restore the subchondral bone. In

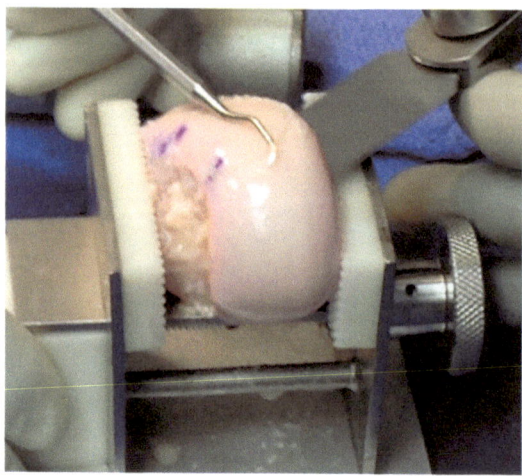

FIGURE 8.11 Saw blade is used to cut the graft from the donor femoral condyle as a long plug that will be trimmed after matching the depth with the socket in the recipient condyle. An instrument is used to secure the graft into the bone until the cut is finalized

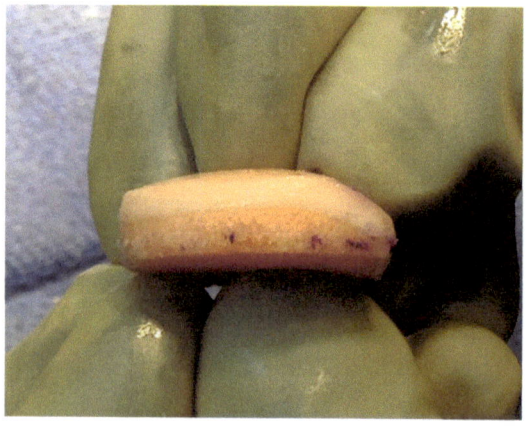

FIGURE 8.12 Final adjustment on the depth of the graft showing the minimum amount of bone necessary to restore the subchondral bone at the recipient socket

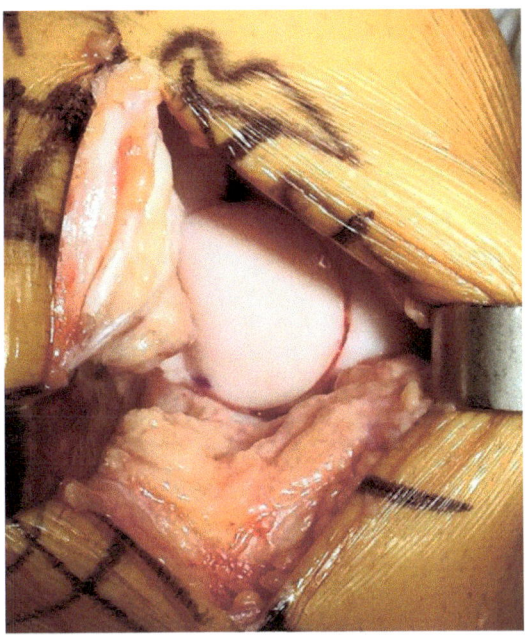

FIGURE 8.13 Final view of the graft implanted restoring the defect on the medial femoral condyle. The graft should be positioned flush to the articular surface

this scenario, OAT can be used for lesions smaller than 1.5 cm^2, whereas ACI sandwich technique and OCA are better indicated for larger lesions [7, 8]. Outcomes with OCA for OCD have been described by Sadr et al. [8] evaluating outcomes in 149 knees with a mean follow-up of 6.3 years. Clinical scores improved significantly from preoperative to latest follow-up ($p < 0.001$), and failure rate was 8% (12/149), with a mean time to failure of 6.1 ± 1.3 years. Graft survivorship was 95% at 5 years and 93% at 10 years, showing that OCA is effective for the treatment of OCD lesions with durable long-term results. Return to sport in patients who underwent OCA transplantation for OCD in the knee was also studied by

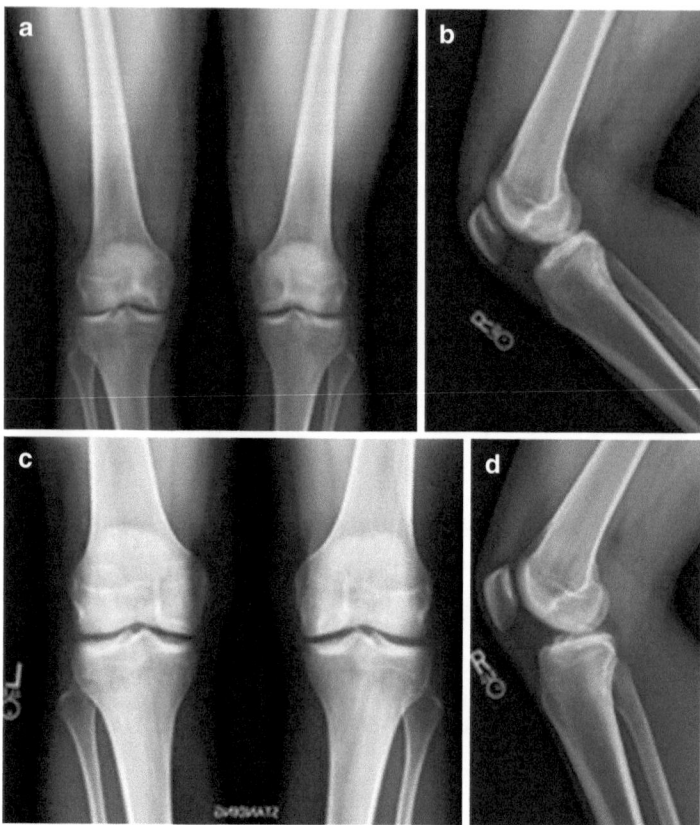

FIGURE 8.14 (**a**) Preoperative AP radiographs. (**b**) Preoperative lateral radiographs. (**c**) One-year postoperative AP radiographs. (**d**) One-year postoperative lateral radiographs

Nielsen et al. [5] Among the 149 knees treated for OCD in active sporting individuals, return to sport and recreation was 75%%. Among the 25% (37/149 who did not return to sport or activity), reasons included both knee-related problems and lifestyle characteristics.

Clinical Pearls/Pitfalls

- OCA may be used for primary cartilage repair of large osteochondral lesions or as a salvage procedure following a failed previous cartilage repair. COA can anatomically restore large or complex lesions of any anatomic surface and is particularly useful in dealing with disorders of the subchondral bone.
- OCA has the advantage of restoring both the osseous and chondral components caused by OCD lesion.
- The guide wire for OCA dowel technique must be placed perpendicular to the articular surface when preparing the host area. This is of paramount importance particularly in cases of classic OCD on the lateral wall of the medial femoral condyle, once the center of the lesion is usually situated oblique to the weight-bearing central area of the condyle.
- Depth of resection of the area to be grafted must be kept to a minimum, until healthy subchondral bone is found.
- Pulsatile lavage of the osseous surface is used to remove marrow elements in order to decrease immunogenicity of the graft.
- Medial condyle lesions are usually long and narrow, and two grafts might be needed in cases of larger lesions. When using two grafts, they can be placed adjacent to one another ("snowman") or overlapping a small part in its interface ("MasterCard").
- When using more than one plug, the direction of the plugs must be convergent to one another, in order to restore the curved articular surface of the femoral condyle.
- For simple dowel plugs, adjuncting fixation is rarely necessary.
- Rehabilitation is simple and usually rapid as bone healing reliably occurs and the articular surface of the graft is mature hyaline cartilage and can accept full loading.

References

1. Bentley G, Biant LC, Vijayan S, Macmull S, Skinner JA, Carrington RW. Minimum ten-year results of a prospective randomised study of autologous chondrocyte implantation versus mosaicplasty for symptomatic articular cartilage lesions of the knee. J Bone Joint Surg Br. 2012;94(4):504–9.
2. Hefti F, Beguiristain J, Krauspe R, et al. Osteochondritis dissecans: a multicenter study of the European Pediatric Orthopedic Society. J Pediatr Orthop B. 1999;8(4):231–45.
3. Knutsen G, Drogset JO, Engebretsen L, et al. A randomized trial comparing autologous chondrocyte implantation with microfracture. Findings at five years. J Bone Joint Surg Am. 2007;89(10):2105–12.
4. Krause M, Hapfelmeier A, Moller M, Amling M, Bohndorf K, Meenen NM. Healing predictors of stable juvenile osteochondritis dissecans knee lesions after 6 and 12 months of nonoperative treatment. Am J Sports Med. 2013;41(10):2384–91.
5. Nielsen ES, McCauley JC, Pulido PA, Bugbee WD. Return to sport and recreational activity after osteochondral allograft transplantation in the knee. Am J Sports Med. 2017;45:1608–14. https://doi.org/10.1177/0363546517694857.
6. Pascual-Garrido C, Moran CJ, Green DW, Cole BJ. Osteochondritis dissecans of the knee in children and adolescents. Curr Opin Pediatr. 2013;25(1):46–51.
7. Peterson L, Minas T, Brittberg M, Lindahl A. Treatment of osteochondritis dissecans of the knee with autologous chondrocyte transplantation: results at two to ten years. J Bone Joint Surg Am. 2003;85-A Suppl 2:17–24.
8. Sadr KN, Pulido PA, McCauley JC, Bugbee WD. Osteochondral allograft transplantation in patients with osteochondritis dissecans of the knee. Am J Sports Med. 2016;44(11):2870–5.
9. Wall EJ, Vourazeris J, Myer GD, et al. The healing potential of stable juvenile osteochondritis dissecans knee lesions. J Bone Joint Surg Am. 2008;90(12):2655–64.

Chapter 9
Osteochondritis Dissecans of the Knee

Michael L. Redondo, Adam J. Beer, and Adam B. Yanke

Case Presentation

History

The patient is a 15-year-old female tennis player with a 3-month history of right anteromedial knee pain and mechanical symptoms while playing tennis and walking. The patient reports her knee locks approximately twice per day when she is not playing tennis. The patient endorses pain when her knee is locked. She reports symptoms of instability though difficult to predict. She denies swelling and has no prior surgical history for this knee.

Physical Examination

On physical examination, the patient is 5 feet and 6 inches tall weighing 138 pounds with a body mass index of 22.1. The patient displayed normal gait with no atrophy or asymmetry in either limb. She had mild to moderate tenderness to palpation along the medial joint line and the medial femoral condyle

M. L. Redondo · A. J. Beer · A. B. Yanke (✉)
Department of Orthopedic Surgery, Rush University Medical
Center, Chicago, IL, USA
e-mail: adam.yanke@rushortho.com

© Springer Nature Switzerland AG 2019   123
A. B. Yanke, B. J. Cole (eds.), *Joint Preservation of the Knee*,
https://doi.org/10.1007/978-3-030-01491-9_9

(MFC). No effusion was appreciated in the right knee joint, and the patient's active range of motion was −5° to 135°. Wilson's sign, which is when patients hold the affected leg in relative external rotation to avoid contact between the tibial spine and an MFC lesion, was equivocal.

Diagnostic Imaging

Standard four-view X-rays were obtained and revealed open growth plates with a lucency at the lateral aspect of the MFC (Fig. 9.1a). Subchondral sclerosis was present deep to the lesion. There was no evidence of a loose body or joint space narrowing that was observed. Magnetic resonance imaging (MRI) revealed a 2 cm osteochondritis dissecans defect at the lateral aspect of the MFC (Fig. 9.1b). The fragment was not displaced, but fluid was noted deep to the defect with adjacent bone marrow signal on T2. Her anterior cruciate

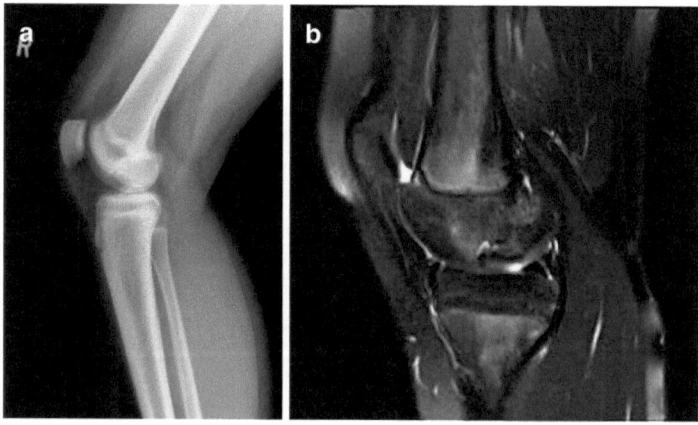

FIGURE 9.1 (a) Lateral view radiograph of the right knee of a 15-year-old female demonstrating an osteochondral dissecans lesion of the medial femoral condyle. (b) Sagittal T2-weighted image of the right knee of a 15-year-old male demonstrating osteochondral dissecans lesion of the medial femoral condyle with evidence of an unstable lesion

ligament (ACL), posterior cruciate ligament (PCL), menisci, lateral femoral condyle (LFC), patella, and trochlea are all intact.

Management

The patient was offered a period of non-weight-bearing given their physeal status. However, due to the signs of an unstable lesion based on both history and imaging, the patient and family elected to proceed with arthroscopic evaluation and treatment. The treatment plan was to evaluate the joint arthroscopically and perform arthroscopic reduction with internal fixation versus debridement. The patient was counseled on the potential for hardware removal and future surgery if the fragment was not able to be fixed.

Surgical Technique

In this case, the patient was positioned with an ACL leg holder and with the foot of the table lowered to allow for hyperflexion if necessary for fixation. Diagnostic arthroscopy was performed through a standard inferolateral portal. No loose bodies or cartilage wear was identified in the patellofemoral or lateral tibiofemoral compartment. The patient's medial tibiofemoral joint demonstrated the expected OCD lesion on the MFC, which was measured to be approximately 12 mm × 16 mm (Fig. 9.2). Importantly, the lesion was ballotable with a probe. This is crucial to not only confirm the unstable aspect of the lesion but to also help define the edges of the fragment. In this case the most obvious peripheral fissures were central (toward the notch) and at the proximal and distal aspect of this. Using a bankart elevator, these two areas were extended to develop a medial hinge (Fig. 9.3). This allowed visualization of the sclerotic base under the fragment. An angled curette was used to debride the overlying subchondral bone to develop a bleeding surface and remove the underlying cortical bone (Fig. 9.4).

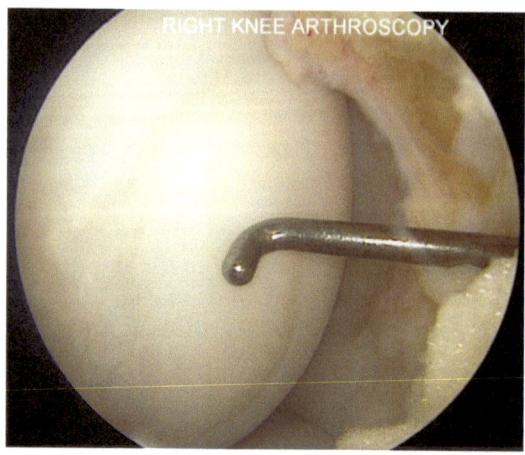

FIGURE 9.2 Intraoperative arthroscopic photograph of an osteochondritis dissecans lesion of the medial femoral condyle in a
15-year-old female measuring to be approximately 12 mm × 16 mm

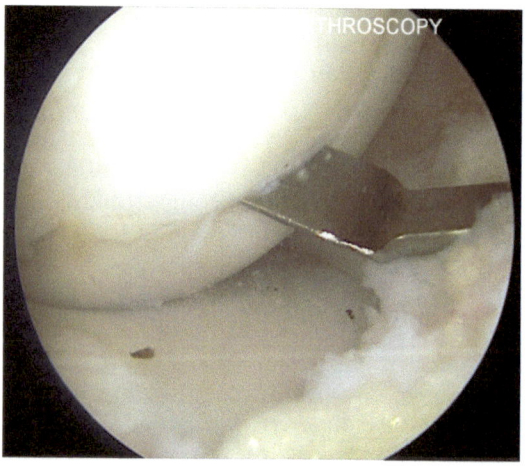

FIGURE 9.3 Intraoperative arthroscopic photograph of the distal
aspect of the osteochondritis dissecans lesion being unroofed using
an elevator

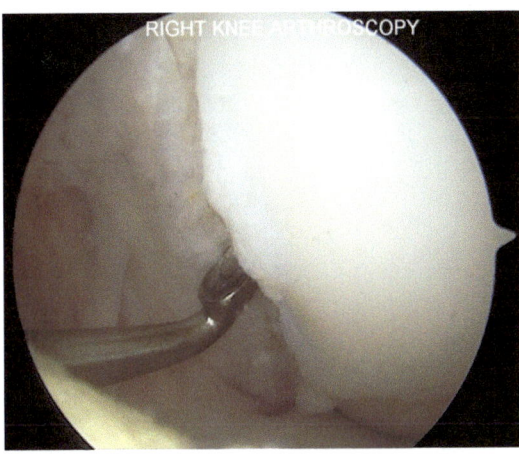

FIGURE 9.4 Intraoperative arthroscopic photograph of an angled curette being used to debride the underlying sclerotic base of the osteochondritis dissecans lesion

In order to create marrow stimulation at the base of the defect, a 45° PowerPick (Arthrex, Naples, Florida) was utilized to drill the base of the lesion (Fig. 9.5). After completion of this process, visual confirmation should demonstrate bleeding from the base of the defect. Through percutaneous stab incisions, the fragment was reduced using two cannulated wires that were intentionally placed to mirror the placement of our headless cannulated screws. With two wires in place, the cannulated drill was used from the Acutrak standard headless variable compression screws to drill through the fragment and the defect base (Fig. 9.6). To complete the fixation, two 16 mm standard size headless screws were recessed 2–3 mm relative to the articular surface (Fig. 9.7). After fixation, we probed the repair site to confirm the stability and quality of the fixation.

Postoperatively, the patient was counseled to refrain from weight-bearing activities and to begin range of motion movements immediately by way of a continuous passive motion (CPM) device. Two weeks postoperatively, the patient began

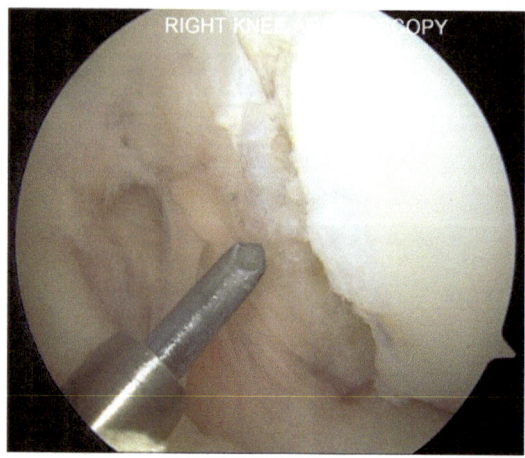

FIGURE 9.5 Intraoperative arthroscopic photograph of a PowerPick (Arthrex, Naples, Florida) being used to drill marrow access channels into the subchondral bone at the base of the osteochondritis dissecans lesion

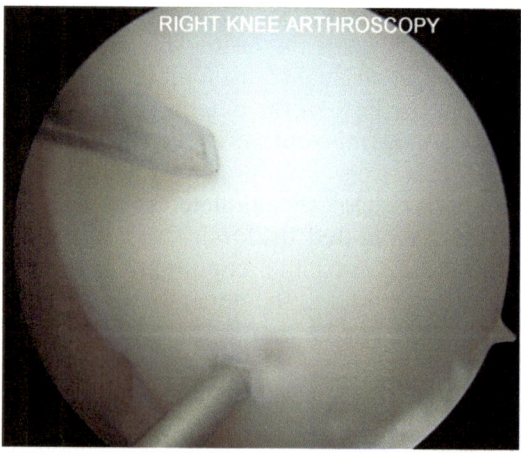

FIGURE 9.6 Intraoperative arthroscopic photograph of the right knee demonstrating placement of a guide pin into an osteochondritis dissecans lesion of the medial femoral condyle

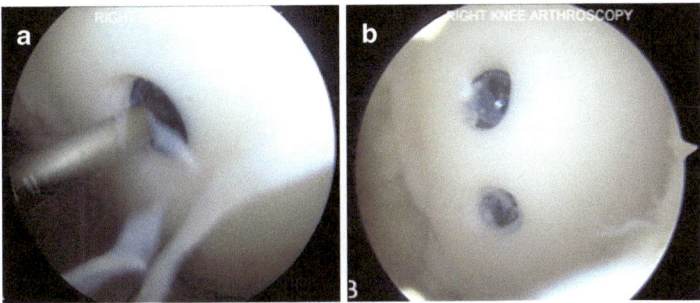

FIGURE 9.7 (**a**) Intraoperative arthroscopic photograph of the right knee demonstrating placement of a headless screw into an osteochondritis dissecans lesion of the medial femoral. (**b**) Intraoperative arthroscopic photograph of the right knee demonstrating two headless screws recessed 2–3 mm relative to the articular surface after fixation of an osteochondritis dissecans lesion of the medial femoral condyle

6 full weeks of physical therapy with protective bracing and ambulation restrictions. At 6 weeks the patient was allowed to discontinue the brace, CPM, and weight-bearing restrictions. Prior to fixation, it was discussed that screw removal occurs routinely at 3 months from surgery and full activity can resume 2 weeks after removal assuming stability was confirmed.

Outcome

Three months following arthroscopic reduction and internal fixation, the patient reported that she was not experiencing any pain or swelling. Surveillance diagnostic plain radiographs revealed the hardware with appropriate alignment and no interval radiolucency or migration (Fig. 9.8). At the time of hardware removal, the lesion was well secured, and the patient was able to return to all activities per the protocol listed above (Fig. 9.9).

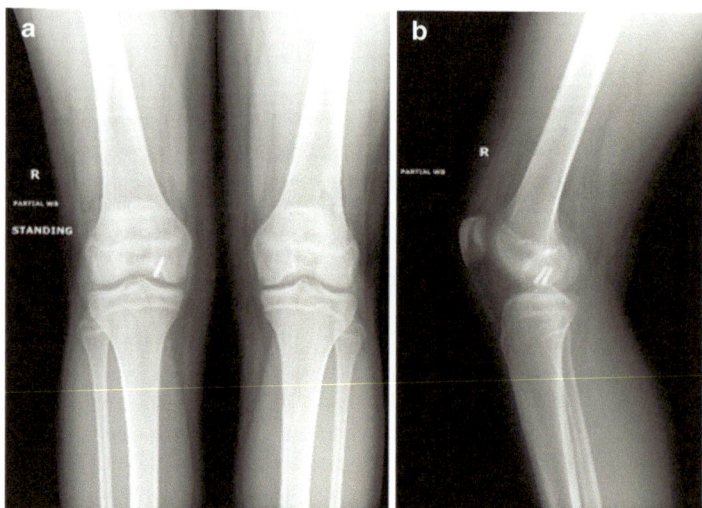

FIGURE 9.8 Standing anteroposterior (**a**) and lateral (**b**) surveillance diagnostic plain radiographs displaying appropriate hardware alignment, no interval radiolucency, or migration

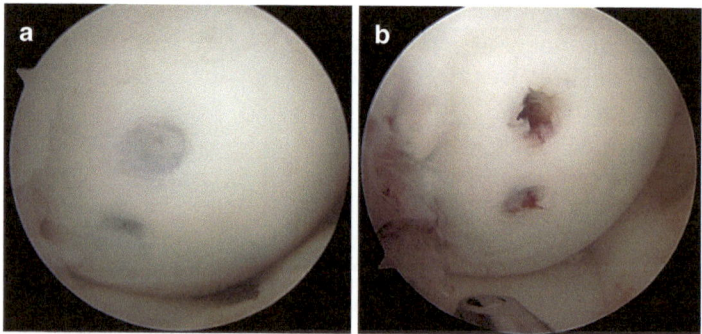

FIGURE 9.9 An arthroscopic image at the time of hardware removal of a well secured lesion prior to screw removal (**a**) and after screw removal (**b**)

Literature Review

Prevalence and Risk Factors

Though the exact prevalence is unknown, the reported prevalence of OCD is between 15 and 29 incidences per 100,000 patients [1–4]. The peak incidence of OCD has been reported at age 15, and the highest incidence for developing the lesions is reported to be between ages 12 and 19 [2, 5]. Several risk factors have been associated with OCD (Table 9.1). Individuals who are male, active sports participants, or of African-American ethnicity are at an increased risk. Interestingly, the male sex has been reported to increase the risk of OCD development approximately fourfold, yet the incidence of OCD young females is on the rise, which is thought to be due to increasing numbers of females who participate in sports [5]. Anatomic risk factors, such as having a discoid lateral meniscus or prominent tibial spine, have also been identified [6–8].

Though OCD lesions may occur in the ankle, elbow, shoulder, wrist, and hip, the vast majority of OCD lesions involve the knee [7]. Within the knee, the MFC (70–80%) accounts for the majority of OCD lesions, followed by the LFC (15–20%), and the patella (5–10%) [4, 7, 9]. In a large multicenter study that examined OCD in the medial compartment of the knee, Hefti et al. [10] reported that 51% of OCD in the MFC is on the lateral aspect of the condyle. Bilateral OCD lesions have been reported in approximately 10% of cases [9, 11].

TABLE 9.1 Risk factors for development of OCD lesions of the knee

Risk factors
Male sex
Age (12–19 years of age)
Active sports participant
African-American ethnicity
Discoid lateral meniscus

Despite being a common knee pathology, the etiology of OCD has not been fully elucidated. However, once identified, at least four stages of the disease have been established. Classification systems have been based upon radiographs, MRI, and, most importantly, arthroscopic findings (Table 9.2). Additionally, De Smet et al. [14] have defined four T2-weighted MRI criteria correlated with successful non-operative treatment of OCD. Irrespective of which staging classification system is used, it is pivotal to determine the lesion's stability, as this is widely considered to be the most prominent determining factor when choosing treatment modality.

Clinical Considerations

The clinical presentation of OCD is variable and largely dependent on the pathology's staging, size, and stability. In the early stages of the disease, OCD lesions can be asymptomatic and are often found incidentally on imaging for unrelated injuries. The initial symptoms of the condition are variable, nonspecific, and poorly localizable. Similarly, asymptomatic lesions should not be treated with surgery. As the disease advances, patients are more likely to develop joint effusions, instability, or painful mechanical symptoms, such as catching and locking from an unstable lesion or a resulting loose body.

OCD also displays nonspecific findings on physical examination. Localized tenderness to palpation is a fairly consistent (40–70%) finding [7, 15]. Anterior condylar pain is a common finding in MFC lesions resulting in Wilson's sign, as well as an avoidance gait [16, 17]. Range of motion is generally intact until the more advanced stages of the disease. Passive extension may be impacted by pain, mechanical symptoms induced by a loose body, and quadriceps atrophy in chronic lesions [4, 15, 18]. Finally, due to OCD's nonspecific physical examination, a high index of suspicion is recommended to exclude other structural causes of referred knee pain, such as ligamentous deficiency, meniscal involvement, and associated hip pathology.

TABLE 9.2 Describes the Dipaola and ICRS classifications for staging OCD lesions on MRI and arthroscopy, respectively

Dipaola et al. [12]	Stage	MRI findings
	I	Intact cartilage with signal changes
	II	High-signal breach of cartilage
	III	A thin, high-signal rim extending behind the osteochondral fragment, indicating synovial fluid around the fragment
	IV	Mixed- or low-signal loose body in the center of the lesion or within the joint
ICRS [13]	Stage	Arthroscopic findings
	I	Stable lesions with continuous but softened area of intact cartilage
	II	Partial discontinuity but stable when probed
	III	Complete discontinuity but not yet dislocated
	IV	Dislocated fragment or a loose body within the bed
De Smet	**T2-weighted MRI criteria associated with success of non-operative management of OCD**	
	A line of high-signal intensity at least 5 mm in length between the OCD lesion and underlying bone	
	An area of increased homogeneous signal	
	At least 5 mm in diameter, beneath the lesion, a focal defect of 5 mm, or more in the articular surface	
	A high-signal line traversing the subchondral plate into the lesion	

Confirmatory imaging is often necessitated due to OCD's nonspecific presentation and examination. Radiographs are essential for characterization of the lesion location, assessment of skeletal maturity, and exclusion of other bony pathologies. Plain radiographs of the knee should include standard weight-bearing anteroposterior and lateral views. Posteroanterior and merchant views at 45° of flexion can be considered for suspected MFC or patellar lesions, respectively [15]. OCD, especially in later-stage cases, may appear on plain radiographs as well as circumscribed osseous fragments separated from the underlying subchondral bone by a radiolucent line [7, 18]. Contralateral knee radiographs are suggested in order to provide comparisons for assessing the presence of asymmetric physeal status, joint space narrowing, and ossification irregularities.

MRI has a superior sensitivity and specificity compared to plain radiographs, making MRI useful for the identification and diagnosis of OCD [16]. Not only can MRI reliably differentiate OCD from other pathologies or abnormal ossification, it also allows for detailed characterization of lesion size, location, depth, and associated loose bodies. In particular, T2 MRI is worthwhile for identifying osseous edema, articular cartilage surface instability or incongruity, and subchondral separation [16]. Diagnostic imaging, like MRI, is an essential component of preoperative planning, yet arthroscopy remains the gold standard for staging OCD lesions.

The patient's history, examination, and results on diagnostic imaging are all paramount in diagnosing OCD of the knee. The main goals of OCD management are to promote healing of the osteochondral unit and mitigate the progression of osteoarthritis via restoration of joint congruity. The senior author's OCD management algorithm (Fig. 9.10) is largely based upon lesion stability but considers physeal

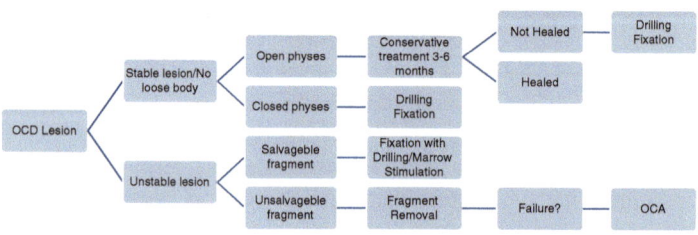

FIGURE 9.10 Chart demonstrating a decision tree for the senior author's treatment approach to a patient with osteochondritis dissecans

status, fragment salvageability, and lesion size for a patient-focused approach.

When weighing options for the course of treatment, physeal status is a unique consideration. OCD can be divided into juvenile OCD (JOCD), which occurs in the setting of an open epiphyseal plate, or adult OCD (AOCD), which develops after the physis has closed. Though AOCD may develop de novo, most AOCD is hypothesized to be the result of unresolved or previously asymptomatic JOCD. The prognosis and management of AOCD and JOCD differ. JOCD lesions with intact articular cartilage surfaces retain the potential to heal and respond effectively to non-operative, conservative management [1, 7, 18]. In contrast, AOCD lesions are more likely to be unstable and generally require surgical intervention.

Non-operative Management

Non-operative or conservative management of OCD is typically recommended for stable lesions, especially stable JOCD [15]. Experts have described several factors associated with the failure of non-operative treatment [18], but lesion staging and stability remain the ultimate deciding factors in management and prognosis. Regardless of physeal status, stable lesions are more likely to heal when taking a non-operative approach. Unstable AOCD lesions almost certainly require surgical intervention [16].

The rationale for non-operative treatment is to reduce the loading on the injured aspect of the knee in an effort to promote spontaneous healing. This is generally implemented by incorporating pain management through activity modification. Activity modification, the mainstay of non-operative management, includes restricting weight-bearing, participation in sports, and participation in other high-impact activities [15, 18]. Essentially, the clinician can restrict to activities that do not cause symptoms. For some patients this can range from no high-level sports to complete non-weight-bearing during activities of daily living. Finally, immobilization by bracing or casting is highly recommended against [19].

The senior author recommends non-operative management of OCD primarily for stable lesions in skeletally immature patients. The likelihood that a JOCD lesion will heal spontaneously is estimated to be 50–94% at 6–18 months [2, 16, 18]. In a large, multicenter, 452-patient trial, those with open epiphyseal plates responded significantly better to conservative management than skeletally mature patients [10]. At the mean follow-up of 33 years, Linden reported that stable JOCD treated non-operatively did not increase the rate of degenerative joint changes, regardless of the type of conservative management used [20]. However, other studies have reported that patients diagnosed with JOCD have up to a 50% chance of developing radiographic evidence of osteoarthritis at an older age [19]. OCD that presented after physeal closure, as in AOCD, however, was more likely to display premature osteoarthritis [19, 20].

Surgical Intervention

As previously mentioned, surgical options for patients who fail conservative management for OCD include palliative (fragment excision), reparative (fixation or subchondral drilling), and restorative techniques (marrow stimulation, ACI, OAT, and OCA) [7]. The widely agreed-upon indications for operative treatment are detached or unstable lesions and/or patients who have failed conservative management with a closed or nearly closed (6–12 months away) physis [1, 3]. Due to the large breadth of current surgical management options, no singular standard of care exists. Treatment is typically patient-specific and based upon the patient's demand and goals, as well as physeal status, lesion size, lesion stability, and lesion grade. Furthermore, the aforementioned arthroscopic grading scheme remains pivotal to surgical decision-making.

Despite the absence of clear guidelines for when surgical intervention is indicated, the outcomes for surgical intervention are generally positive. Recently, Trinh et al. [3] published a systematic review examining 30 studies (levels I-IV) and evaluating a total of 862 knees. The mean postoperative follow-up was 77 months, and the minimum follow-up was 24 months. Overall, outcomes were significantly better when treating JOCD surgically as compared to AOCD. Nearly all the included studies demonstrated significant clinical and radiographic improvements in surgically treated JOCD at short-, mid-, and long-term follow-up [3]. Interestingly, patients who underwent isolated fragment excision experienced worse outcomes than those who underwent other surgical techniques. Furthermore, in a study that examined 20 patients with a prior OCD excision, 6 patients had significantly poor outcomes, and 5 failures were reported at a mean follow-up of 9 years [21]. Additionally, equally disappointing outcomes were seen with regardless of the subject's skeletal maturity [21].

A review of 25 recent articles demonstrated that the most common technique used to repair stable lesions is transarticular drilling [22]. A separate study reported that the most important prognostic factor for OCD subchondral drilling is age, as up to 100% of JOCD patients experienced radiographically visible healing within 6 weeks to 2 years postoperatively [19]. Similar results have also been reported in retrograde drilling, which is the authors preference and preserves the articular surface. In comparison, AOCD lesions repaired with OCD drilling display less radiographic healing and poorer symptomatic outcomes. This is likely due to a higher prevalence of more advanced-stage, unstable lesions with decreased rates of spontaneous healing (5%–50%) [1, 23].

Restorative procedures focus on replacing or regenerating damaged articular cartilage with either hyaline or hyaline-like fibrocartilage repairs. For the treatment of OCD, the senior author considers these techniques if fixation is not possible due to the size and level of fragmentation or if the patient has failed a prior reparative procedure. The cartilage restoration method is dependent on factors such as lesion size, quality of subchondral bone, and the goals and demand of the patient.

Initial treatment of fragment excision should be followed by a period of non-operative management. If the patient continues to have no joint space narrowing on surveillance radiographs, swelling, or pain, the lesion should be left without further treatment. If symptoms develop, then treatments that can be considered include marrow stimulation, osteochondral autograft transplant, or osteochondral allograft transplant. OAT may be considered as a first-line treatment for small (<2 cm^2) OCD lesions when the subchondral bone quality would not support marrow stimulation or if the patient's habits of physical activity are of higher demand [1, 24]. Gudas et al. [25] reported on 50 children with OCD lesions of the knee randomized to receive microfracture or OAT. Both groups had excellent short-term outcomes, yet patients who underwent microfracture displayed significant deterioration in International Cartilage Repair Society (ICRS) scores with 41% continuing to failure. Importantly, only 14% of patients in the microfracture group returned to their preinjury level at 4.2 years after surgery versus 81% in the OAT group [25]. These studies highlight the shortcomings of isolated marrow stimulation for OCD lesions, and this is rarely recommended.

The approach to treating large OCD lesions (>2 cm^2) may also be delineated by the quality of subchondral bone below the defect and the activity demands of the patient. ACI is a two-stage, cellular-based autograft technique. It is ideal for symptomatic, unipolar, well-contained chondral defects that are larger than 2 cm^2 in the absence of significant bone loss [15, 24]. Reported ACI outcomes are favorable, as studies have detailed significant improvements in patient-reported pain and function. Many authors have reviewed efficacy of treating OCD with ACI and have found good or excellent results in 73–86% of patients [26, 27]. Peterson et al. reported on 58 patients who underwent ACI for their knee OCD and found that 91% of patients had good or excellent results at 2–10 years after surgery [27]. Among patients with JOCD who were treated with ACI prior to physeal closing, 91% achieved good to excellent outcomes, compared with 77% in those treated after skeletal maturity had been reached, which suggests that early treatment is optimal [27].

Conversely, OCA is indicated for larger OCD lesions with or without subchondral bone loss, as well as in patients who have failed other restorative techniques. OCA allows for the simultaneous restoration of the osteochondral defect with a single graft. OCA should be viewed as a strong therapeutic option especially for patients with high physical demand and lesions greater than 2 cm^2 [7]. Potential OCA disadvantages include limited graft availability, decreased cell viability, immunogenicity, and disease transmission [28]. It has been reported that OCA provides good to excellent clinical outcomes with long-term follow-up, as patient-reported outcomes have demonstrated improvement in upward of 90% of cases [7, 29]. It should be considered that most OCD treatment that utilized cell-based transplantations occurs in Europe where OCA is not available. It is the authors preferred treatment to approach symptomatic OCD defects post-excision with OCA in the vast majority of patients.

Conclusion

OCD is a common and well-known condition, yet much remains to be understood about it. OCD of the knee requires a timely diagnosis to prevent progression of the lesion and degeneration of the joint. In stable JOCD, non-operative management is highly effective. Indications for surgical treatment are based on lesion stability, physeal status, and failure of prior treatments. Reestablishment of the joint congruity, fragment stabilization, and early range of motion are primary goals for preservation of the osteochondral fragment. The question of whether or not to treat the condition surgically by way of a cartilage restoration procedure (marrow stimulation, ACI, OAT, and OCA) depends on the size of the lesion, quality of the subchondral bone, and demand of the patient, though most patients are appropriately treated with OCA. The overall goal for the treatment of adult OCD lesions is to relieve pain, decrease mechanical symptoms, and prevent development of secondary osteoarthritis.

References

1. Pascual-Garrido C, McNickle AG, Cole BJ. Surgical treatment options for osteochondritis dissecans of the knee. Sports Health. 2009;1:326–34.
2. Yang JS, Bogunovic L, Wright RW. Nonoperative treatment of osteochondritis dissecans of the knee. Clin Sports Med. 2014;33:295–304.
3. Trinh TQ, Harris JD, Flanigan DC. Surgical management of juvenile osteochondritis dissecans of the knee. Knee Surg Sports Traumatol Arthrosc Off J ESSKA. 2012;20:2419–29.
4. Kocher MS, Tucker R, Ganley TJ, Flynn JM. Management of osteochondritis dissecans of the knee: current concepts review. Am J Sports Med. 2006;34:1181–91.
5. Kessler JI, Nikizad H, Shea KG, Jacobs JC, Bebchuk JD, Weiss JM. The demographics and epidemiology of osteochondritis dissecans of the knee in children and adolescents. Am J Sports Med. 2014;42:320–6.
6. Jacobs JC, Archibald-Seiffer N, Grimm NL, Carey JL, Shea KG. A review of arthroscopic classification systems for osteochondritis dissecans of the knee. Clin Sports Med. 2014;33:189–97.
7. Erickson BJ, Chalmers PN, Yanke AB, Cole BJ. Surgical management of osteochondritis dissecans of the knee. Curr Rev Musculoskelet Med. 2013;6:102–14.
8. Cavaignac E, Perroncel G, Thépaut M, Vial J, Accadbled F, De Gauzy JS. Relationship between tibial spine size and the occurrence of osteochondritis dissecans: an argument in favour of the impingement theory. Knee Surg Sports Traumatol Arthrosc Off J ESSKA. 2017;25:2442–6.
9. Kon E, Vannini F, Buda R, et al. How to treat osteochondritis dissecans of the knee: surgical techniques and new trends: AAOS exhibit selection. J Bone Joint Surg Am. 2012;94:e1(1–8).
10. Hefti F, Beguiristain J, Krauspe R, et al. Osteochondritis dissecans: a multicenter study of the European pediatric orthopedic society. J Pediatr Orthop B. 1999;8:231–45.
11. Gomoll AH, Flik KR, Hayden JK, Cole BJ, Bush-Joseph CA, Bach BR. Internal fixation of unstable Cahill Type-2C osteochondritis dissecans lesions of the knee in adolescent patients. Orthopedics. 2007;30:487–90.
12. Dipaola JD, Nelson DW, Colville MR. Characterizing osteochondral lesions by magnetic resonance imaging. Arthroscopy. 1991;7:101–4.

13. Brittberg M, Winalski CS. Evaluation of cartilage injuries and repair. J Bone Joint Surg Am. 2003;85-A Suppl 2:58–69.
14. De Smet AA, Ilahi OA, Graf BK. Untreated osteochondritis dissecans of the femoral condyles: prediction of patient outcome using radiographic and MR findings. Skelet Radiol. 1997;26:463–7.
15. Pascual-Garrido C, Moran CJ, Green DW, Cole BJ. Osteochondritis dissecans of the knee in children and adolescents. Curr Opin Pediatr. 2013;25:46–51.
16. Edmonds EW, Polousky J. A review of knowledge in osteochondritis dissecans: 123 years of minimal evolution from König to the ROCK study group. Clin Orthop Relat Res. 2013;471:1118–26.
17. Shea KG, Jacobs JC, Carey JL, Anderson AF, Oxford JT. Osteochondritis dissecans knee histology studies have variable findings and theories of etiology. Clin Orthop Relat Res. 2013;471:1127–36.
18. Cruz AI, Shea KG, Ganley TJ. Pediatric knee osteochondritis Dissecans lesions. Orthop Clin North Am. 2016;47:763–75.
19. Bruns J, Werner M, Habermann C. Osteochondritis Dissecans: etiology, pathology, and imaging with a special focus on the knee joint. Cartilage. 2018;9:346–62. https://doi.org/10.1177/1947603517715736.
20. Linden B. The incidence of osteochondritis dissecans in the condyles of the femur. Acta Orthop Scand. 1976;47:664–7.
21. Anderson AF, Pagnani MJ. Osteochondritis dissecans of the femoral condyles. Long-term results of excision of the fragment. Am J Sports Med. 1997;25:830–4.
22. Abouassaly M, Peterson D, Salci L, et al. Surgical management of osteochondritis dissecans of the knee in the paediatric population: a systematic review addressing surgical techniques. Knee Surg Sports Traumatol Arthrosc Off J ESSKA. 2014;22:1216–24.
23. Winthrop Z, Pinkowsky G, Hennrikus W. Surgical treatment for osteochondritis dissecans of the knee. Curr Rev Muscoskelet Med. 2015;8:467–75.
24. Richter DL, Schenck RC Jr, Wascher DC, Treme G. Knee articular cartilage repair and restoration techniques: a review of the literature. Sports Health. 2016;8:153–60.
25. Gudas R, Kalesinskas RJ, Kimtys V, et al. A prospective randomized clinical study of mosaic osteochondral autologous transplantation versus microfracture for the treatment of osteochondral defects in the knee joint in young athletes. Arthroscopy. 2005;21:1066–75.

26. Bartlett W, Gooding CR, Carrington RW, Skinner JA, Briggs TW, Bentley G. Autologous chondrocyte implantation at the knee using a bilayer collagen membrane with bone graft. A preliminary report. J Bone Joint Surg Br. 2005;87:330–2.

27. Peterson L, Minas T, Brittberg M, Lindahl A. Treatment of osteochondritis dissecans of the knee with autologous chondrocyte transplantation: results at two to ten years. J Bone Joint Surg Am. 2003;85-A Suppl 2:17–24.

28. Pascual-Garrido C, Friel NA, Kirk SS, et al. Midterm results of surgical treatment for adult osteochondritis dissecans of the knee. Am J Sports Med. 2009;37(Suppl 1):125S–30S.

29. Sadr KN, Pulido PA, McCauley JC, Bugbee WD. Osteochondral allograft transplantation in patients with osteochondritis dissecans of the knee. Am J Sports Med. 2016;44:2870–5.

Chapter 10
Post-meniscectomy Syndrome

Trevor R. Gulbrandsen, Katie Freeman, and Seth L. Sherman

Clinic Presentation: Medial Post-meniscectomy Syndrome

Patient is a 15-year-old female who presents with 6 months of worsening left knee medial-based pain and activity-related swelling. Initially at age 12, the patient sustained a bucket-handle medial meniscus tear that was treated with hybrid all-inside and inside-out medial meniscus repair. The repair failed, and she subsequently underwent subtotal medial meniscectomy 1 year following index arthroscopy. The patient did well following this procedure with resolution of her pain and mechanical symptoms. She was able to resume

The original version of this chapter was revised. A correction to this chapter is available at https://doi.org/10.1007/978-3-030-01491-9_19

T. R. Gulbrandsen
Department of Orthopaedic Surgery, University of Iowa Hospitals and Clinics, Iowa City, IA, USA

K. Freeman
Department of Orthopedic Surgery and Rehabilitation, University of Nebraska Medical Center, Omaha, NE, USA

S. L. Sherman (✉)
Department of Orthopaedic Surgery, University of Missouri, Columbia, MO, USA

Missouri Orthopaedic Institute, Columbia, MO, USA

© Springer Nature Switzerland AG 2019
A. B. Yanke, B. J. Cole (eds.), *Joint Preservation of the Knee*,
https://doi.org/10.1007/978-3-030-01491-9_10

sporting activity until the past 6 months when she noted worsening medial pain (VAS 6–8) and activity-related swelling. At present, she rates her knee 50% of normal. She has symptoms at night and with ADL and had to discontinue competitive gymnastics because of her symptoms. The patient has tried and failed considerable conservative treatment including NSAIDs, Tylenol, compression sleeves and unloader bracing, activity modification, and extensive "core-to-floor" physical therapy.

On physical exam, her BMI is 22. She stands with bilateral neutral alignment and walks with a slow non-antalgic gait. Double limb squat is symmetric but painful on the left. She has good quadriceps tone, mild effusion, focal tenderness over the medial compartment, negative McMurray, and stable ligaments.

Weight-bearing AP, PA flexion, and lateral and Merchant views demonstrate no joint space narrowing (Fig. 10.1). The patient is skeletally mature. Mechanical axis view demonstrates neutral alignment. Magnetic resonance imaging (MRI) demonstrates medial meniscal deficiency with foci of subchondral bone signal within the medial femoral condyle. There is no focal cartilage defect noted on MRI (Fig. 10.2).

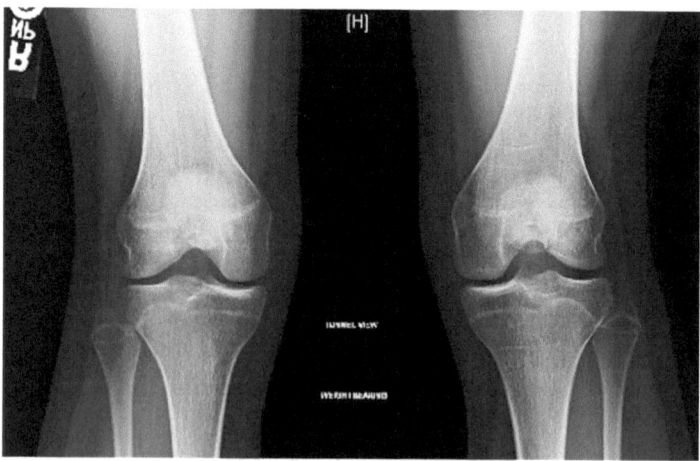

FIGURE 10.1 Preoperative weight-bearing Rosenberg radiograph

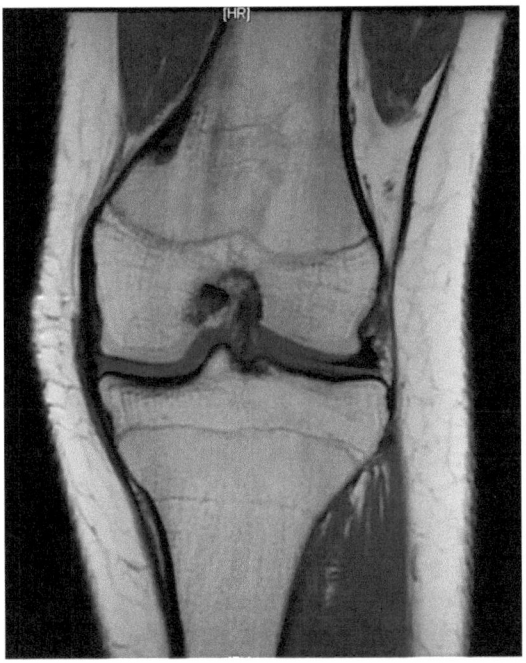

FIGURE 10.2 T1-weighted coronal MRI showing medial meniscal deficiency

Diagnosis/Assessment

This patient's clinical examination and imaging studies are consistent with medial post-meniscectomy syndrome. She is likely experiencing overload secondary to meniscus deficiency manifest as biologic effusions and pain in the medial compartment. Despite optimization of dynamic flexibility and strength, the patient has persistent symptoms that are affecting her ability to sleep, her daily life, and her quality of life. At this point, surgical intervention is warranted. Her problem list is isolated to medial meniscus deficiency with neutral alignment, ligamentous stability, and no focal cartilage defects. The patient is indicated for salvage intervention, which would be an isolated medial meniscus allograft transplantation.

Management

Examination under anesthesia demonstrated no abnormalities and was followed by diagnostic arthroscopy. The patellofemoral and lateral compartments remained pristine. Synovectomy and lysis of adhesions were performed to remove scar tissue from prior injury and surgery. Arthroscopy confirmed medial meniscal deficiency (Fig. 10.3). When possible, a 2–3 mm rim of healthy remaining tissue was maintained for repair to the native structures. Ideally punctate bleeding should be noticed so the repair is not performed to the white zone. The MFC had Grade I-early Grade II changes and the MTP had Grade I softening. There was no indication for cartilage treatment and no contraindications to moving forward with medial MAT.

The deep MCL was trephinated with a spinal needle to improve access to the medial compartment. A power rasp was utilized to perform a reverse notchplasty beneath the femoral PCL insertion. A FlipCutter guide was utilized to create a 9.5 mm wide × 10 mm deep socket in the anatomic posterior root insertion of the medial meniscus, and a shuttle suture was passed. An accessory high anteromedial portal was established with the knee in deep flexion. A k-wire was placed into the anterior root insertion, and an outside-in reamer was utilized in an antegrade fashion which was used

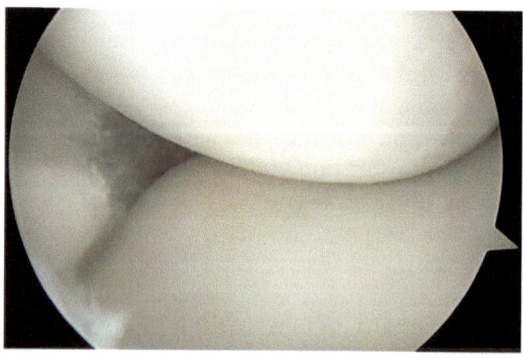

FIGURE 10.3 Evidence of meniscal deficiency in the medial compartment

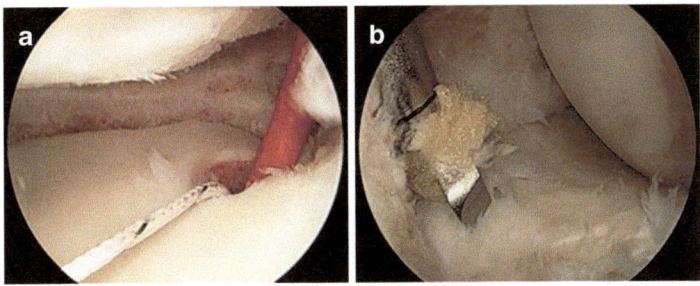

FIGURE 10.4 (**a**) Posterior meniscal tunnel using ACL guide to pass shuttle stitch (left). (**b**) Low-profile reaming of anterior meniscal tunnel (right)

to create a 9.5 mm wide × 10 mm deep socket just anterior and medial to the ACL insertion. An ACL guide was used to pass a shuttle suture from the anterior tibial socket to the anteromedial cortex of the tibia. An inside-out technique was used to pass shuttle sutures at the junction of the middle meniscus with the anterior and posterior horns, respectively. A passport cannula was placed, and all shuttle sutures were retrieved through the medial portal (Fig. 10.4).

The medial meniscus allograft was prepared using TightRope ABS (attachable button system) for suspensory cortical fixation of both anterior and posterior bone plugs. The bone plugs were 9 mm wide by 3 mm in depth. Labral tape horizontal mattress sutures were passed at the junction of the mid-body of the meniscus with the anterior and posterior horns, respectively.

The MAT was shuttled into the joint. The posterior bone plug was seated first and fixed with the suspensory cortical sutures for provisional fixation. Posterior all-inside sutures and several inside-out sutures were then passed to help secure the meniscus to the rim posteriorly and in the mid-body of the meniscus. The anterior bone plug was then well seated and provisionally fixed (Fig. 10.5).

There was minimal graft mismatch which was reduced by recessing both bone plugs slightly deeper into the sockets so that the meniscus had precise fit. The knee was placed in extension, and the sutures were retrieved through a small medial-

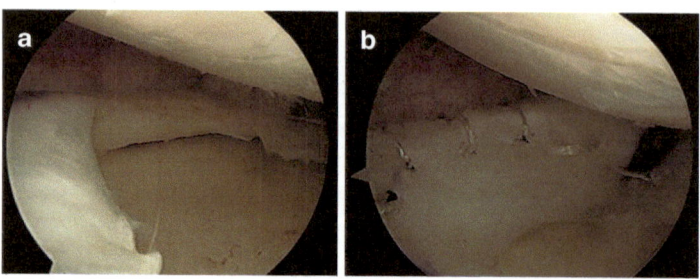

FIGURE 10.5 (**a**) MAT placement. (**b**) MAT with inside out suture placement

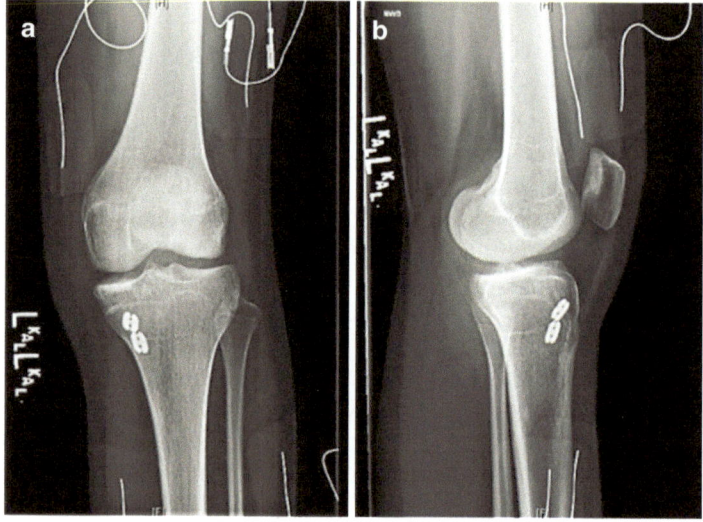

FIGURE 10.6 AP (**a**) and lateral (**b**) views of the left knee showing postoperative medial MAT suspensory cortical fixation

based incision. The labral tapes were secured to the tibia using PushLock anchors to restore meniscotibial attachments, and the inside-out sutures were tied. Direct visualization showed the meniscus was nicely approximated to the rim with excellent fixation. Outside-in PDS sutures were placed anteriorly and tied over the capsule. The knee was taken through a range of motion demonstrating stability of the medial MAT. Postoperative radiographs were obtained (Fig. 10.6).

Outcome

The patient had an uneventful course after the medial MAT. On follow-up at 3 months, the patient had achieved full ROM, normalized her gait, and had minimal pain that was relieved with NSAIDs. At 6 months postoperative, she continued to report minimal pain but had significant improvement of her subjective assessment scores, including Knee Injury and Osteoarthritis Scores (KOOS) of 95.59 for daily living, 91.67 for pain, 70 for sports and recreation, and 87.5 for symptoms. Her Lysholm Knee Scoring Scale was 78, as well as a 10 on her Marx score and a 7 on the Tegner Activity Scale.

Clinical Presentation: Lateral Post-meniscectomy Syndrome

This female patient presented to our clinic at age 12 with symptoms of diffuse knee pain, swelling, and inability to fully extend the knee for 1 year following a football injury. She was diagnosed with a chronic locked bucket-handle tear of her lateral meniscus and indicated for arthroscopic surgery. Unfortunately, the meniscus was not reducible, and she was treated with subtotal lateral meniscectomy. Her cartilage surfaces were pristine at this time. She had slight asymmetric valgus and was strictly monitored for signs/symptoms of post-meniscectomy syndrome. She was treated with lateral unloader brace, NSAIDs, and home exercise program. While she was initially improved after index arthroscopy, serial follow-up over several months demonstrated progressive valgus deformity and onset of lateral-based pain and activity-related swelling even with ADLs.

On physical exam, she has a BMI of 24. She walks with a non-antalgic gait and has symmetric double limb squat with pain on the left. She has asymmetric valgus, left greater than right. Her knee has a trace effusion and tenderness over the lateral joint line with a negative McMurray. Ligaments are stable and ROM is normal. Distal neurovascular intact.

Weight-bearing AP, PA flexion, and lateral, Merchant, and bilateral standing mechanical axis view radiographs demonstrated asymmetric valgus without lateral joint space narrowing (Fig. 10.7). Magnetic resonance imaging (MRI) revealed a trace effusion, evidence of mild fibrillation of her cartilage surface in her lateral compartment with femoral subchondral edema and early sclerosis. Lateral meniscus deficiency was noted (Fig. 10.8).

Diagnosis/Assessment

This case highlights the rapid progression of lateral knee joint breakdown that follows subtotal lateral meniscectomy in the valgus active female. In general, MAT is indicated for symptomatic meniscal deficiency and is not recommended as a

FIGURE 10.7 AP weight-bearing alignment view showing left knee valgus malalignment with right knee varus malalignment

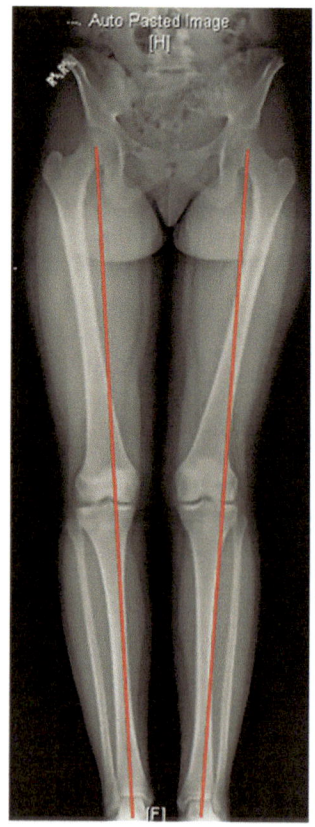

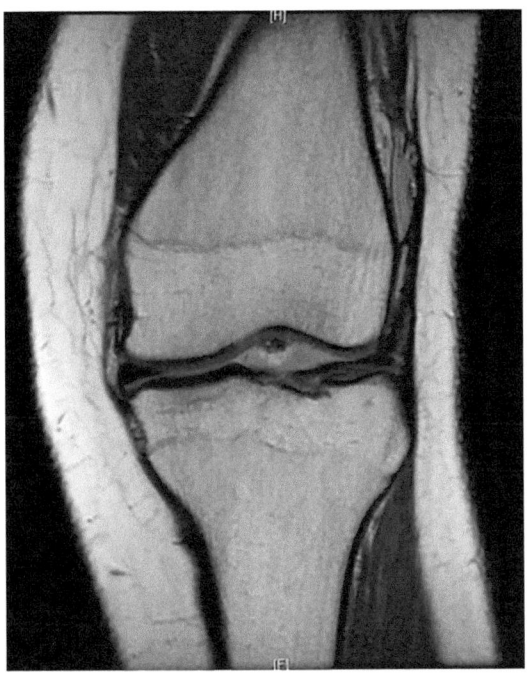

FIGURE 10.8 Initial T1-weighted coronal MRI of the left knee showing lateral meniscal deficiency

prophylactic procedure. However, the valgus active female with meniscal deficiency is a rare exception to this overall rule. As can be seen in this case vignette, the patient had only transient symptomatic relief before return of painful swelling several months after arthroscopy. Even in this short time, her valgus had worsened, and she began to develop chondral surface changes and subchondral edema in the lateral compartment. This is a scenario with a poor natural history and one in which aggressive surgical treatment is strongly considered. In her case, her problem list includes asymmetric valgus and lateral meniscus deficiency. Her ligaments are stable, and she has no obvious focal, full-thickness cartilage defects. She is indicated for either combined realignment osteotomy and lateral MAT versus staged intervention or osteotomy followed by lateral MAT/cartilage restoration at a later date.

The lateral compartment is convex, and the lateral meniscus covers more of the surface than the medial meniscus. As such, the lateral side is more sensitive to changes relating to partial or subtotal meniscectomy. There is significant increase in contact pressure, decreased contact area, and often rapid progression of cartilage wear following meniscectomy. This is amplified in the setting of valgus alignment and hastened by attempts at increased high-demand activity in young female athletes. Given the natural history of this condition, surgeons should have a low threshold for action to avoid onset of lateral-based arthritis at a young age.

In general, surgeons prefer the use of bone plug MAT on the medial side and trough-type MAT on the lateral side, given the close proximity of the lateral meniscus root insertions. Both techniques have demonstrated acceptable clinical outcomes for MAT, and technique is based largely on surgeon preference. In our hands, we prefer lateral MAT with small bone plugs placed in anatomic sockets and secured with suspensory cortical fixation. Despite the small bone bridge between the root insertions, mechanical testing has demonstrated root insertion strength near native meniscus without tunnel convergence. Advantages of this technique include all-arthroscopic visualization throughout the entire procedure, maintenance of bone stock, ability to handle graft mismatch in real time, and no need to "flip" the meniscus into a tight compartment, among others.

Management

After careful discussion with the patient and family, decision was made to proceed with staged intervention. The first stage would include arthroscopic evaluation of her cartilage surfaces followed by distal femoral varus producing osteotomy. Second stage would include lateral MAT plus cartilage restoration if indicated. At arthroscopy, progression of Grade I-II cartilage changes over the lateral femoral condyle and lateral tibial plateau was noted. Medial and patellofemoral compartments remained pristine. Arthroscopic lysis of adhesions was performed.

Standard lateral-based approach was taken for distal femoral osteotomy. Using fluoroscopic guidance, a guidewire was placed parallel to the joint line at the level of the epicondyles. The osteotomy guide was then placed over this guidewire, and two pins were placed in line with the planned osteotomy and confirmed with fluoroscopy. Blunt retractors were placed subperiosteally posteriorly around the femur to protect the neurovascular structures. The osteotomy was performed with a saw and completed with osteotomes. Osteotomy wedges were used to open to the desired correction, which was 7.5°, as measured from preoperative templating. The plate was secured with 4.5 mm cortical screws proximally and 6.5 mm cancellous screws distally. The osteotomy site was packed with a combination of Beta-tricalcium phosphate wedges soaked in BMAC (bone marrow aspirate concentrate).

The patient recovered uneventfully from her DFO. Alignment radiographs were obtained (Fig. 10.9). She elected to proceed with lateral MAT 5 months after osteotomy. There was progression to Grade II chondral disease on the lateral femoral condyle and lateral tibial plateau but no focal, full-thickness cartilage lesions and no indication for cartilage restoration which was not performed. The lateral meniscus remnant was debrided down to a healthy peripheral 2–3 mm rim when present. A FlipCutter was used to prepare a 9.5 mm × 10 mm socket at the posterior root insertion of the lateral meniscus. A shuttle suture was passed. The FlipCutter was again utilized to create a 9.5 mm × 10 mm deep socket at the anterior root insertion adjacent to but avoiding the ACL. Shuttle sutures were passed. Inside-out zone-specific cannula was used to pass a shuttle stitch just anterior to the popliteal hiatus. This was retrieved through an accessory posterolateral incision (Fig. 10.10).

The lateral MAT was prepared on the back table. Bone plugs 9 mm wide and 3 mm deep were secured with Fiberloop sutures through the bone/soft tissue junction on both ends. Fiberwire suture was placed in the meniscus at the level of the popliteal hiatus to assist in graft passage.

A passport cannula was placed and sutures retrieved through the cannula which was subsequently removed. The MAT was shuttled into the joint and the root sutures secured

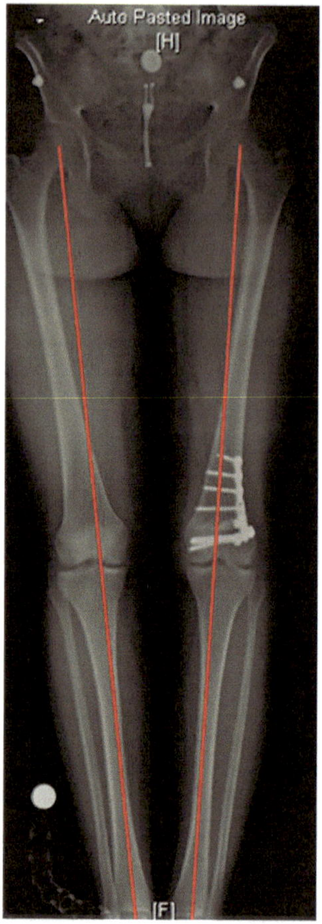

FIGURE 10.9 Post DFO AP
alignment showing left knee valgus correction

with cortical buttons. Hybrid all-inside, inside-out, and outside-
in meniscus repair technique was performed (Fig. 10.11).

Outcome

The patient did well in her early postoperative lateral MAT
recovery (Fig. 10.12). By 6 months post-MAT, she completed
physical therapy. At this time she had continual improvement
in her subjective assessment scores including Knee Injury and
Osteoarthritis Outcome Scores (KOOS) of 95.59 for daily
living, 86.11 for pain, 60 for sports and recreation, and 96.88

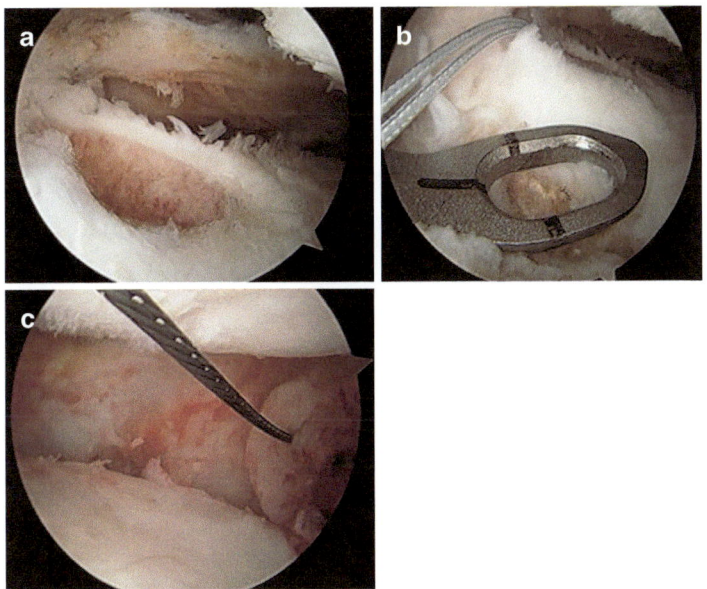

FIGURE 10.10 (**a**) 9.5 mm × 10 mm deep socket at the anterior root insertion adjacent to the ACL. (**b**) Drill guide. (**c**) Placement of Fiberwire suture to assist in graft passage

for symptoms. Her Lysholm Knee Scoring Scale was 78. She reported no pain or swelling. By 1 year posterolateral MAT, she had completely normalized her ADLs and could participate in low-impact athletic activities. At 18 months she experienced symptomatic distal femoral hardware and underwent removal of hardware with postoperative symptomatic improvement. At 2 years posterolateral MAT, the patient had normalized her ADLs and was able to fully participate in low-impact activities without significant limitations.

Literature Review

Despite the above clinical vignette, post-meniscectomy syndrome is less commonly encountered following medial meniscectomy as compared to lateral meniscectomy. The medial compartment is concave, and the medial meniscus covers less

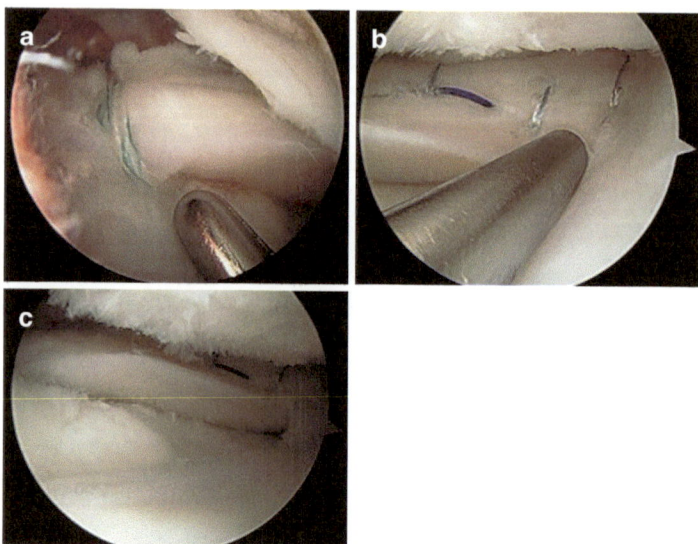

FIGURE 10.11 (**a**) Placement of MAT. (**b**) Hybrid all-inside, inside-out, and outside-in meniscus repair technique shown on final lateral MAT placement. (**c**) Final lateral MAT placement

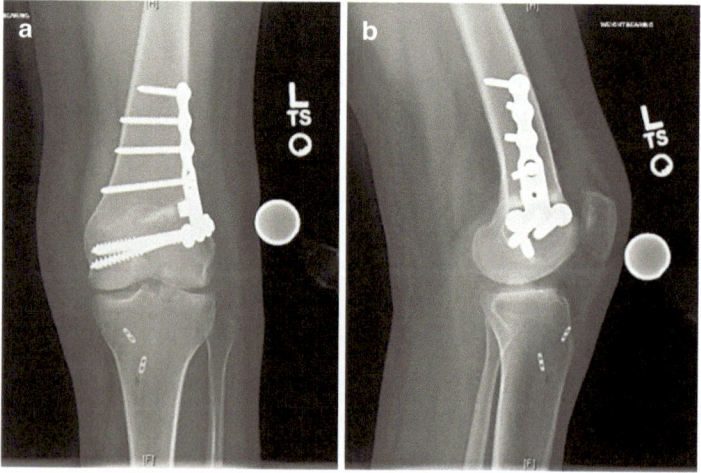

FIGURE 10.12 AP (**a**) and lateral (**b**) views of the left knee showing postoperative changes with DFO and lateral MAT suspensory cortical fixation placement

of the surface area of the medial tibial plateau. Therefore, meniscectomy has less detrimental effect on the contact areas and contact pressures in the medial compartment and is less likely to lead to early and symptomatic post-meniscectomy syndrome. Additionally, these characteristics also make it less likely for there to be cartilage breakdown in the medial compartment and less need for concomitant cartilage restoration procedure at the time of MAT as compared to the lateral side. More often the case, medial meniscus deficiency is associated with failure of ACL reconstruction, and medial MAT is often performed as a combined procedure alongside revision ACL surgery with the indication of improving functional stability.

There are several surgical techniques that may be utilized for medial MAT including fixation that is soft tissue only, with bone plugs, or with an osseous trough. Guidance in choosing between these techniques can be obtained through the literature but is not conclusive. Ultimately, all techniques have good reported outcomes, and due to procedural complexity, the technique the surgeon is most facile with should be utilized. Considerations to take into account are the increased distance in medial meniscal insertional footprint compared to the lateral side and run in an oblique orientation in the axial plane. As such, anatomic trough techniques require loss of significant bone stock and also require violation of at least a portion of the native ACL. Additionally, combined ACL reconstruction/medial MAT can be more challenging using the trough technique. However, the native donor root relationship is preserved with the trough technique which is not the case when utilizing bone plugs. When compared to soft tissue-only MAT which is technically the easiest, clinical outcomes are similar but may result in increased graft extrusion.

Several studies have shown favorable outcomes of the medial MAT using bone plugs. Ha et al. performed a 2-year follow-up study on medial MAT using the bone plug technique. They reported significant improvement of the mean IKDC scores (from 60.3 to 85.4 ($P < 0.05$) and mean Lysholm scores (from 68.2 preoperatively to 89.7 postoperatively ($P < 0.05$)). Additionally, they reported that 100%, 83.3%, and 94.4% of patients had healing at the anterior root, the posterior root, and the meniscal rim on MRI, respectively. Second-look arthroscopy further supported these findings [1].

Verdonk et al. performed a study on 39 medial MAT and 61 lateral MAT with a mean follow-up of 7.2 years. Using the modified Hospital for Special Surgery (HSS) function and pain scoring system, they reported a significant improvement in regard to both pain and function from preoperative to the time of final follow-up. Additionally, they reported that the cumulative survival rates for the lateral and medial allografts were 69.8% and 74.2% at 10 years [2].

Furthermore, LaPrade and colleagues performed a prospective 2-year follow-up study that showed significant subjective improvements associated with lateral and medial MAT. In this study, 19 patients underwent medial MAT with baseline Cincinnati scores of 52.3. In post-MAT, these scores improved to 73.2 ($P < 0.001$). This groups IKDC subjective scores preoperatively averaged at 51.2 and improved to 68.2 ($P < 0.001$) postoperatively. Furthermore, this study included 21 patients who underwent lateral MAT. This group had baseline Cincinnati scores of 57.8. There were 15 patients with follow-up scores averaging 77.9 ($P < 0.001$). All 21 patients who underwent lateral meniscal improved from baseline scores of 57.6 to an average of 76.6 ($P < 0.001$) [3].

Several studies have demonstrated success with the bone-in-slot technique. McCormick et al. [4] reported upon MAT survival in 172 patients at a mean follow-up of 59 months with a minimum 2-year follow-up. Only eight patients (4.7%) went on to require revision MAT or total knee replacement at final follow-up. Additionally, Kaplan-Meier survival analysis showed no significant difference between medial MAT or lateral MAT. Additionally, Saltzmann et al. [5] reported on the survivorship of the same MAT technique when performed concomitantly with ACL reconstruction. These authors reported overall survival of 40 patients (33 medial MAT, 7 lateral MAT) at a mean 5-year follow-up which was 80%, and there was no significant increase in joint space narrowing from preoperative radiographs.

Return to sport following meniscus transplant remains controversial. Chalmers et al. studied the results of the bone trough MAT in high school and high-level athletes who had meniscal deficiency and symptomatic post-meniscectomy syndrome. Thirteen athletes were followed post-MAT for a mean of 3.3 years (range 1.9–5.7), and their ability to return to their preinjury level of play was analyzed. More than three-quarters (77%) of the athletes who underwent MAT had significant improvements and were able to return to their desired level of play, while the remaining athletes (23%) required further surgery including one revision MAT, one partial meniscectomy, and one meniscal repair [6].

There is still controversy regarding the treatment of post-meniscectomy syndrome. In general, MAT is indicated for patients with symptomatic meniscal deficiency who have failed conservative treatment and have symptoms with activities of daily living. Being able to return to sport following MAT should be considered icing on the cake. Although patients with meniscal deficiency often advance to radiographic osteoarthritis, clinical symptoms do not accurately correlate with these findings [7, 8]. Additionally, there is no clear evidence that meniscal allograft transplantation decreases the radiographic advancement of osteoarthritis [9]. Therefore, MAT is currently not indicated for asymptomatic patients. These patients should be closely followed over time for subjective and objective signs and symptoms of meniscal deficiency. A specific clinical scenario that should be followed closely is the valgus active female status post-functional lateral meniscectomy. In this case, the patient may develop rapid progression of lateral-based osteoarthritis. Overall, the main goal of MAT is to provide relief of symptoms and improve quality of life. The technique used to perform MAT varies and ultimately should be left to the treating physician based on comfort level. Although there may still be an increased risk of progression toward osteoarthritis, there is growing evidence that MAT provides clinical improvements with potential for chondroprotection [10].

Clinical Pearls

- Patients with functional or subtotal meniscectomy must be counseled effectively and followed at regular intervals for signs/symptoms of meniscus deficiency.
- Symptoms include compartment-based pain, swelling, and mechanical symptoms.
- Signs include progressive limb deformity, joint space narrowing, and chondral or subchondral changes on serial advanced imaging studies.
- Morphological differences between medial and lateral compartments predict differences in clinical onset of post-meniscectomy syndrome.
- The medial compartment is more tolerant to meniscectomy changes as it concaves and is more conforming. The lateral compartment is convex and less tolerant to meniscectomy.
- Malalignment increases the risk of post-meniscectomy syndrome, particularly in the case of the valgus active female following subtotal meniscectomy.
- While prophylactic MAT is generally not indicated, the natural history of lateral meniscal deficiency is poor, and early surgery should be considered, particularly in the setting of valgus malalignment.
- There is no MAT technique that has demonstrated clinical superiority. In general, surgeons in the USA utilize bone plug MAT medially and trough MAT laterally.
- Managing patient expectation is *CRITICAL*. This is a salvage intervention intended to improve quality of life. Sporting goals are secondary and may not be achievable or allowed. This surgery will not last forever, and it is likely the patient will require other procedures throughout their lifetime.

References

1. Ha JK, Sung JH, Shim JC, Seo JG, Kim JG. Medial meniscus allograft transplantation using a modified bone plug technique: clinical, radiologic, and arthroscopic results. Arthroscopy. 2011;27:944–50.
2. Verdonk PC, Demurie A, Almqvist KF, Veys EM, Verbruggen G, Verdonk R. Transplantation of viable meniscal allograft. Survivorship analysis and clinical outcome of one hundred cases. J Bone Joint Surg Am. 2005;87(4):715–24.
3. LaPrade RF, Wills NJ, Spiridonov SI, Perkinson S. A prospective outcomes study of meniscal allograft transplantation. Am J Sports Med. 2010;38(9):1804–12.
4. McCormick F, Harris JD, Abrams GD, Hussey KE, Wilson H, Frank R, Gupta AK, Bach BR Jr, Cole BJ. Survival and reoperation rates after meniscal allograft transplantation: analysis of failures for 172 consecutive transplants at a minimum 2-year follow-up. Am J Sports Med. 2014;42(4):892–7.
5. Saltzman BM, Meyer MA, Weber AE, Poland SG, Yanke AB, Cole BJ. Prospective clinical and radiographic outcomes after concomitant anterior cruciate ligament reconstruction and meniscal allograft transplantation at a mean 5-year follow-up. Am J Sports Med. 2017;45(3):550–62.
6. Chalmers PN, Karas V, Sherman SL, Cole BJ. Return to high-level sport after meniscal allograft transplantation. Arthroscopy. 2013;29:539–44.
7. Andersson-Molina H, Karlsson H, Rockborn P. Arthroscopic partial and total meniscectomy: a long-term follow-up study with matched controls. Arthroscopy. 2002;18(2):183–9.
8. McNicholas MJ, Rowley DI, McGurty D, et al. Total meniscectomy in adolescence: a thirty-year follow-up. J Bone Joint Surg Br. 2000;82(2):217–21.
9. Elattar M, Dhollander A, Verdonk R, Almqvist KF, Verdonk P. Twenty-six years of meniscal allograft transplantation: is it still experimental? A meta-analysis of 44 trials. Knee Surg Sports Traumatol Arthrosc. 2011;19(2):147–57.
10. Verdonk PC, Verstraete KL, Almqvist KF, De Cuyper K, Veys EM, Verbruggen G, Verdonk R. Meniscal allograft transplantation: long-term clinical results with radiological and magnetic resonance imaging correlations. Knee Surg Sports Traumatol Arthrosc. 2006;14(8):694–706.

Chapter 11
Chondral Defects
of the Patella: Diagnosis
and Management

Andreas H. Gomoll and Brian J. Chilelli

Case Presentation

The patient is a 33-year-old female who presented with
chronic right anterior knee pain. She endorses significant
crepitus in the right knee. She reports the pain is located
directly behind the patella, worse with weight-bearing, especially going up and down stairs. In particular, she complains
of night pain that is exacerbated after prolonged use. She
endorses significant swelling associated with the pain. She
also reports difficulty with rising from a seated position
after prolonged sitting. She rates her symptoms as 7/10. She
has tried ice, TENS unit, physical therapy, corticosteroid
injection, and viscosupplementation. The patient reports
injections improved her symptoms, but not significantly. The
patient also comes today for discussion and evaluation of
her MRI on the right knee. She is interested in discussing
surgery.

A. H. Gomoll
Department of Orthopedic Surgery,
Hospital for Special Surgery, New York, NY, USA

B. J. Chilelli (✉)
Northwestern Medicine, Regional Medical Group Orthopaedics,
Warrenville, IL, USA
e-mail: brian.chilelli@nm.org

© Springer Nature Switzerland AG 2019   163
A. B. Yanke, B. J. Cole (eds.), *Joint Preservation of the Knee*,
https://doi.org/10.1007/978-3-030-01491-9_11

Physical Exam

Evaluation of the right lower extremity reveals skin that is warm, dry, and intact. There is a mild intra-articular effusion in the left knee. She has significant pain and audible patellofemoral crepitus with single leg squat on the right side. She is tender to palpation on the right knee overlying the patellar tendon, but otherwise non-tender to palpation. She is stable to varus and valgus stress at 0 and 30°. She is ligamentously intact and has a mild J sign.

Diagnostic Imaging

Merchant view radiograph of the patellofemoral joint revealed a preserved joint space without subluxation or significant tilt (Fig. 11.1b). Magnetic resonance imaging demonstrated right knee full-thickness chondral loss on the proximal aspect of the patella with subchondral cyst formation (Fig. 11.1a). The trochlea is completely spared,

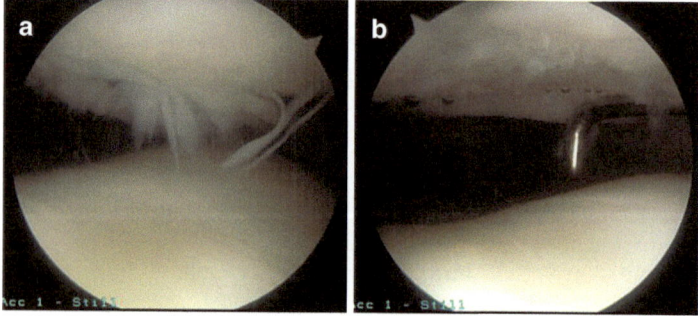

FIGURE 11.1 (**a**) Sagittal MRI PD FS sequence demonstrating a chondral defect of the mid- to proximal patella with mild associated subchondral edema and a small cyst; (**b**) Merchant view of the patellofemoral joint demonstrating preserved joint space without subluxation or significant tilt

with no element of dysplasia. The ACL, PCL, LCL, and MCL are intact.

Management

Conservative and operative management were discussed with the patient. Due to exhausting all conservative options, her history, and MRI, the patient elected to proceed with staging arthroscopy and biopsy for matrix-associated autologous chondrocyte implantation (MACI).

On diagnostic arthroscopy, the patient had a grade 3 to grade 4 cartilage lesion in the patella that was 25 × 20 mm in size (Fig. 11.2a). The patellar lesion was central and distal. The trochlear cartilage was intact. The remainder of her knee was normal. After visualization, the patella lesion was debrided using a 4.0 mm shaver for full visualization (Fig. 11.2b). The chondroplasty completed until the formation of a stable rim and no element of any loose flap-type component.

The patient reported significant relief after chondroplasty. However, her anterior left knee pain, symptoms, and physical exam findings reverted 4 months after arthroscopy. After discussion, the patient elected to proceed with the MACI and TTO.

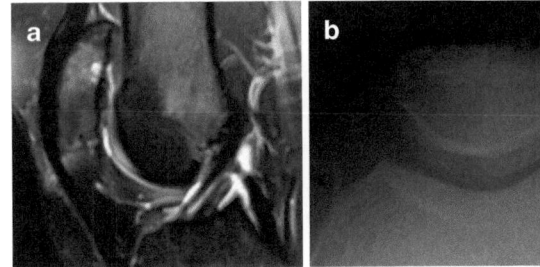

FIGURE 11.2 A staging arthroscopy image through the lateral portal of an isolated patella cartilage defect prior (**a**) and after (**b**) debridement of the lesion

Surgical Technique

The patient was positioned supine with all osseous promi-
nences padded. Anesthesia was induced without any difficulty, and antibiotics were given within 30 min of skin
incision. The operative extremity was prepped and draped in
the normal sterile fashion using chlorhexidine, and a tourniquet was placed. A timeout was performed that confirmed
the side, site, and type of surgery to be correct. A longitudinal
skin incision was made along the length of the patella at the
midline and then developed down to the lateral retinaculum
where Bovie electrocautery was used to perform an arthrotomy. The arthrotomy was completed up to the inferior edge
of the vastus lateralis and down to the origin of the patellar
tendon. After completing this, the patella was everted to
expose the articular cartilage. No damage on the trochlea was
found; however, the patient did have a large grade 3 to grade
4 patellar defect, which was 20 × 25 mm and located central
and distal (Fig. 11.3a). The defect was fully debrided using a
ring curet, an 11-blade knife, and saline down to the bony bed
(Fig. 11.3b). The calcified cartilage layer was removed. After
full preparation, we then moved our attention to the tibial
tubercle.

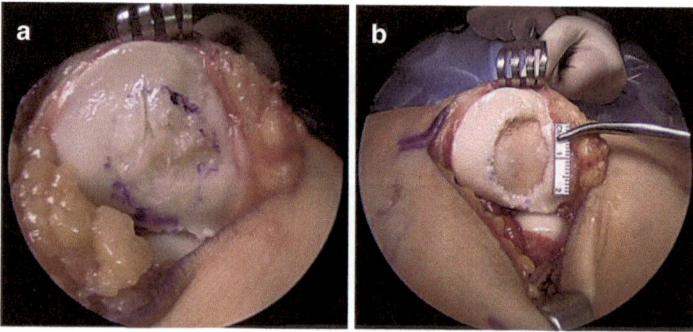

Figure 11.3 (a) Intraoperative image of an everted patella to
expose the large grade 3 to grade 4 articular cartilage defect. (b) The
same patellar defect after full debridement down to the bone bed

The tibial tubercle osteotomy was made through a separate 7 cm incision at the tibial tubercle and distal. Medial and lateral flaps were made to the anterior compartment fascia which was incised using Bovie electrocautery. After elevating the musculature, full visualization of the lateral aspect of the tibia was achieved. An Arthrex guide set to 90° was used to make an anterior to posterior cut just through the anterior cortex. A lateral to medial cut was made using an ACL saw blade and tapering distally. After release with osteotomes proximally, a tricortical bone graft was performed in a wedge that was 1 cm at its maximum height in order to anteriorize the bone. Two 4.5 screws were used in a standard AO technique. The screws were countersunk to place fixation from lateral to medial. After completion, the area was copiously irrigated, and we turned our attention back to the MACI portion of the case.

The Chondro-Gide membrane patch (Geistlich Pharma AG, Switzerland) was cut and injected and soaked with one vial of cultured cells. After this was complete, thrombin-soaked sponges were placed in the base of the defect with the tourniquet down to reduce bleeding. Any additional punctate bleeding was stopped adequately using fibrin glue. The tourniquet was then reinflated, and the joint was copiously irrigated. The patch was sewn in place using 6-0 Vicryl. After 50% of the patch was sewn in place, fibrin glue was placed peripherally, and the remaining vial of the ACI cells was injected underneath the patch. The remainder of the patch was secured with 6-0 Vicryl and the fibrin glue (Fig. 11.4). After adequate seal was confirmed, the patellofemoral joint was reduced. The arthrotomy was closed with #1 Vicryl, the subcutaneous skin with a 2-0 Monocryl, and the skin with running 3-0 Prolene. The fasciotomy was closed with #1 Vicryl, and the subcutaneous skin with a 2-0 Monocryl followed by a running 3-0 Prolene. The wound was dressed with Steri-Strips, gauze, Kerlix, Ace wrap, Recovery Plus ice unit, and brace locked in extension.

Postoperatively, the patient was counseled to be restricted to partial heel-based weight-bearing activities and full extension bracing and to begin range of motion movements immediately by way of a continuous passive motion (CPM) device. Two weeks postoperatively, the patient began 6 full weeks of

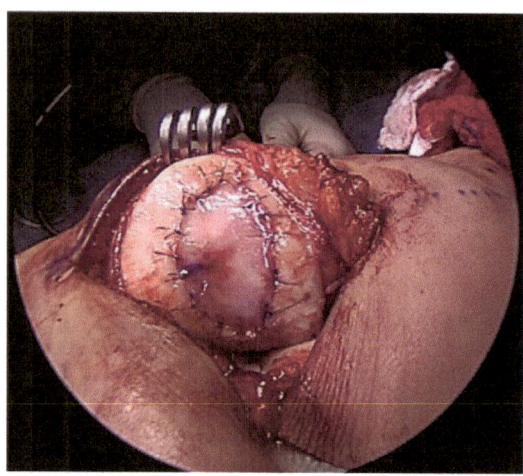

FIGURE 11.4 An intraoperative image of an isolated patella cartilage defect repaired with matrix-associated autologous chondrocyte implantation using the Chondro-Gide membrane patch

physical therapy with protective bracing and continued weight-bearing restrictions. At 6 weeks the patient was counseled to continue physical therapy and allowed to advance to weight-bearing as tolerated.

Outcome

Six months following MACI and TTO, the patient reported improving anterior knee pain, mild clicking in the front of the knee, and mild difficulty in squatting. The patient endorses improved stiffness and no effusion. On physical examination, range of motion was 0/0/125. No effusion or tenderness to palpation was identified. Mild patellofemoral crepitus remained.

History and Clinical Evaluation

When patients with patella cartilage injuries are symptomatic, they will typically present with anterior knee pain that is exacerbated by activity. The most common activities include bending, kneeling, squatting, running, jumping, and using stairs; all of which involve loading a flexed knee. Posterior knee pain can occur but most people will describe pain deep to the patella or may point to an area just below the patella. Swelling will occasionally arise and patients may experience catching or locking as a result of an unstable cartilage flap. A thorough history is obtained and includes questions about patellar instability (acute or chronic). In patients with known patellar instability, is important to distinguish between transient pain as a result of a specific unstable event and pain as a result of a chondral defect that has occurred secondary to instability.

Physical examination starts with assessing a patient's gait and inspecting for lower extremity malalignment. The Q angle (anterior superior iliac spine to the central patella to the tibial tubercle) can be measured, and an elevated value (>14 in males and >17 in females) may be associated with patellar maltracking or instability [1]. For this test, the patella needs to be located in the groove. A laterally subluxed patella will result in a falsely low Q angle. Palpation of the joint is performed to determine if an effusion is present and to assess for patellar translation and apprehension. Motion is observed while paying close attention to patellar tracking and mobility throughout the entire range of motion. The patient should be evaluated for generalized ligamentous laxity as well as lower extremity malalignment or malrotation.

Imaging

Radiographs are obtained and include standing anteroposterior, lateral, merchant, and 45° flexion posteroanterior views. These images are analyzed for fractures, loose bodies, joint space narrowing, osteophytes, patella alta, patellar subluxation, and patellar tilt. MRI is useful to detect chondral or osteochondral defects and to further characterize them. Determining the size of the lesion is helpful for prognostic purposes and to aid in surgical decision-making, but MRI has been shown to underestimate lesion size by as much as 60% [2]. In addition to evaluating lesion characteristics, MRI can be used to determine tibial tubercle-trochlear groove (TT-TG) distance, presence of trochlear dysplasia, patellar height, subchondral edema, and associated ligamentous injuries. A recent MRI comparative study concluded that a flat and shallow trochlea, trochlea dysplasia, and patella alta are associated with the development of patellar cartilage defects [3]. The tibial tubercle-posterior cruciate ligament (TT-PCL) distance has been found to be an effective alternative method for determining the position of the tibial tubercle [4]. This measurement is not influenced by the rotation of the knee or shape of the trochlea, and values greater than or equal to 24 are considered abnormal. Computed tomography (CT) or CT arthrogram may be particularly useful when evaluating for subchondral bone deficiency.

Treatment Options

Nonoperative Treatment

The initial approach to managing most patients with patellar cartilage defects should focus on conservative measures. Nonetheless, patients with mechanical symptoms as a result of an unstable chondral flap or osteochondral fragment may be considered for early surgical intervention. The mainstays of nonoperative treatment include activity modification, anti-inflammatory medications, physical therapy, bracing, and injections (cortisone or hyaluronic acid). Physical therapy focuses on quadriceps strengthening to improve patellofemoral biomechanics. However, newer studies confirm the importance of a more comprehensive approach to physical therapy which includes core strengthening, hip abductor and external rotator strengthening, and iliotibial (IT) band stretching [5–8]. Nonoperative treatment should be attempted for 6 weeks to 6 months prior to determining whether or not it has been successful.

Surgical Treatment

Surgical treatment is reserved for the subset of patients who fail nonoperative management or for individuals who have displaced chondral or osteochondral fragments resulting in mechanical symptoms. Incidental cartilage lesions of the patella found at the time of ACL reconstruction or meniscus surgery should not be treated with cartilage repair since it is unclear whether or not that lesion is or will be symptomatic. Surgical options for known symptomatic full-thickness defects include arthroscopic chondroplasty, open reduction internal fixation (ORIF) of the chondral/osteochondral fragments, marrow stimulation, osteochondral autograft transfer (OAT), osteochondral allograft transplantation (OCA), autologous chondrocyte implantation (ACI), and particulated juvenile articular cartilage (PJAC). The goal of surgery is to restore the chondral surface anatomy with tissue that exhibits biomechanical properties as closely as possible to native articular cartilage. Additional procedures such as lateral release/lengthening, MPFL reconstructions, tibial and femoral rotational osteotomies, and tibial tubercle osteotomies can be combined with cartilage restoration surgery. Patellofemoral arthroplasty is used as a salvage procedure for failed cartilage procedures or for patients who are not candidates for cartilage restoration. Surgical decision-making depends on defect characteristics such as size, location, and status of the subchondral bone. Other associated conditions include instability and malalignment. Patient factors also play a vital role in the decision-making process. Compliant patients with realistic expectations who comprehend the postoperative rehabilitation process are ideal candidates. Relative contraindications include smokers, patients with increased BMI, non-compliant patients, and radiographic evidence of joint space narrowing (Kellgren Lawrence grades III–IV).

Marrow Stimulation

Marrow stimulation can be considered for small (<2 cm²) full-thickness chondral defects of the patella. This technique is most commonly performed through an arthroscopic approach, which can be technically challenging to orient the instruments perpendicular to the defect. Alternatively, an open arthrotomy can be performed allowing for eversion of the patella. Unfortunately, there is a paucity of outcome studies looking at isolated patellar chondral defects treated with microfracture. Instead, several studies combine femoral condyle and patellofemoral data. Most of these studies report good outcomes at short term for small lesions in low-demand patients but acknowledge that deterioration of clinical outcomes should be expected after 2–5 years [9–11]. Kreuz et al. [12] reported outcomes based on location of the defect following microfracture in 70 patients. There were 32 femoral condyle, 11 tibia, 16 trochlear, and 11 patella defects. Good results were documented at 6 months and 18 months, but deterioration in outcome scores and MRI defect filling occurred at 36 months. In addition, the trochlea and patella groups experienced greater deterioration compared to the femoral condyle group. The authors concluded that young patients (<40 years) with femoral condyle lesions are associated with a better prognosis.

Osteochondral Autograft Transfer

Osteochondral autograft transfer is used to treat small (<2 cm²) full-thickness chondral or osteochondral defects of the patella. It restores the articular surface with native hyaline cartilage and can be used to address concomitant abnormal subchondral bone and/or deficiency. However, it can be difficult to match the complex morphology of the patella utilizing donor femoral condyle cylinders that often have a different hyaline cartilage thickness and structural properties than that of the native patella [13, 14]. In a retrospective study, 33 patients were followed for an average of 19.3 months after undergoing osteochondral autograft transfer mosaicplasty to treat patellofemoral cartilage defects [15]. The mean age was 31 and the average lesion size was 2.4 cm². The results were good in 24 cases and fair in 9 cases. The mean Lysholm knee score prior to surgery was 51.9 and increased to 85.5 at final follow-up. In another series, Nho et al. [16] reported on 22 patients treated with OAT for patella defects with an average size of 1.65 cm². Significant improvements were documented at a mean follow-up of 28.7 months with improved IKDC (47.2–74.4), ADL (60.1–84.7), and SF-36 (64.0–79.4). Similarly, Astur et al. [17] found statistically significant improvements in Lysholm, Kujala, Fulkerson, and SF-36 scores following OAT to treat symptomatic patellar defects. In this study there were 33 patients followed for 2 years with all defects measuring less than 2.5 cm². Results reported by Bentley et al. [18] were less encouraging with a high failure rate associated with mosaicplasty for patellar cartilage lesions. All five of the patients who underwent surgery failed at a mean follow-up of 1.7 years. As a result the authors considered mosaicplasty of the patella to be contraindicated.

Osteochondral Allograft Transplantation

Osteochondral allograft transplantation is ideal for large defects (>2–4 cm²) of the patella and can be used to address associated subchondral bone pathology. Similar to OAT, matching the complex architecture of the patella can be technically challenging. In a recent case series, 28 knees in 27 patients with a mean age of 33.7 were treated with OCA for isolated full-thickness patellar chondral defects [18]. This series represented a challenging patient population since 26 of 28 knees (92.9%) had previous procedures (mean, 3.2 procedures) and the mean allograft area was 10.1 cm². Survivorship at 5 and 10-years was 78.1% and at 15 years was 55.8%. Failures were documented in 8 of the 28 knees (28.6%) but among the 20 knees with grafts in situ, 89% of patients were extremely satisfied or satisfied with the results. The authors concluded that the outcomes in their study were inferior to published outcomes following OCA for femoral condyle defects. Similarly, a systematic review of 19 studies discovered a trend toward inferior results following OCA to treat patellofemoral lesions compared to treated tibial and femoral condyle lesions [19]. Torga Spak et al. [20] reported a high reoperation rate (86%, 12/14) in their series of 14 fresh patellofemoral allografts (11 patients), but 10 of the 11 patients in the study stated that they would repeat the procedure. At last follow-up, 8 grafts were still in place, 4 for more than 10 years, 2 for more than 5 years, and 2 for more than 2 years. Of the non-surviving grafts, three survived more than 10 years.

Autologous Chondrocyte Implantation

Autologous chondrocyte implantation is used to treat medium to large (>2–4 cm²) chondral defects of the patella. This technique makes it easier to match the native surface architecture of the patella compared to OAT and OCA. In a prospective study, 25 knees in 23 patients were treated with ACI and anteromedialization of the tibial tubercle for isolated patellar articular cartilage lesions [21]. The mean age was 31.0 with a mean defect size of 6.4 cm². At an average follow-up of 7.6 years, significant improvements were observed in the IKDC score (42.5–75.7), modified Cincinnati Knee Rating System score (3.0–7.0), Lysholm score (40.2–79.3), and SF-12 score. The majority of patients (83%, 19/23) rated their surgery as good or excellent. Another prospective study involved 39 patellofemoral defects (14 patella, 18 trochlea, 7 bipolar) in 38 patients treated with ACI with a mean follow-up of 37 months [22]. The lesions were large (5.4 cm² patella, 4.3 cm² trochlea, 8.8 cm² bipolar) and tibial tubercle anteromedialization was performed as indicated in 28 patients. At final outcome significant improvements were observed in all outcome measure including modified Cincinnati, Lysholm, and VAS scores. Second-look arthroscopy in 22 patients revealed repair tissue that scored a median of 11 of 12 points using the International Cartilage Repair Society cartilage repair assessment. There were 3 failures, and 25 patients underwent subsequent surgery, including 14 to remove hardware from a prior osteotomy. In a recent long-term prospective series, Kon et al. [23] reported on 32 patients treated with matrix-assisted autologous chondrocyte transplantation (MACT) for full-thickness chondral lesions of the patellofemoral joint. The final follow-up was at 10 years and included the same cohort of patients who were evaluated at 2 and 5 years. The average defect size was 4.45 cm^2 and included 20 patellar lesions, 8 trochlear lesions, and 4 patients with multiple patellofemoral lesions. All scores (IKDC, EuroQol visual analog scale, and Tegner) showed a statistically significant improvement at 2-, 5-, and 10-year follow-up with respect to the preoperative level. In addition, there was no worsening observed at last follow-up compared to 5-year follow-up. The authors concluded that the long-term results were reassuring since their previous study showed that the short-term improvement was not maintained at midterm follow-up with worsening of results from 2 to 5 years after MACT [24]. Gomoll et al. [25] performed a large multicenter study consisting of 110 patients treated with ACI for cartilage defects of the patella with an average follow-up of 90 months. The average age was 33 and patellar defect size was 5.4 cm^2. Significant outcome score improvements were documented as a group (IKDC 40–69, modified Cincinnati 3.2–6.2, WOMAC 50.4–28.6). Of importance, 86% of patients rated their knee as good or excellent at final follow-up, and 92% stated they would undergo the procedure again. In another study, Von Keudell et al. [26] presented 30 consecutive patients with isolated chondral lesions of the patella treated with ACI. At an average follow-up of 7.3 years, knee function was rated as good to excellent in 83% (25/30) of patients, fair in 13% (4/30) of patients, and poor in 3% (1/30) of patients. Significant improvements in all outcome scores were seen. The average lesion size was 4.7 cm^2 and 19 of 30 patients underwent concomitant tibial tubercle osteotomy. There were three failures, all of which were workers' compensation (WC) cases and had an average age of 42 years compared to the non-WC age of 28 years.

Particulated Juvenile Articular Cartilage

Particulated juvenile articular cartilage (PJAC) is an emerging technique to treat patellofemoral chondral defects of any size. An advantage of this technique includes the improved ability to recreate the complex patellofemoral surface anatomy, similarly seen with ACI. In addition, it is readily available and therefore can be useful for treating patellofemoral defects when concomitant osteochondral allograft transplantation is performed for femoral condyle lesions. While this technique brings promise to cartilage repair surgery, there are few outcome studies to date, especially involving isolated patella lesions. Tompkins et al. [27] followed 13 patients with 15 patellar defects (2 bilateral lesions) treated with PJAC (Tompkins 2013). At an average follow-up of 28.8 months, the majority (11 of 15, 73%) of knees were found to have normal or near normal cartilage repair based on MRI evaluation with a mean fill of the defect of 89%. Favorable outcome scores (IKDC, VAS, KOOS, Tegner, and Kujala) were documented at final follow-up. Three patients required reoperation for symptomatic grafts, and two patients required knee manipulation under anesthesia.

Concurrent Procedures (Osteotomy, Soft Tissue Stabilization)

Tibial tubercle osteotomy (TTO) can be performed in isolation or in combination with other procedures to treat patellar instability and patellofemoral cartilage lesions. The most common technique, as described by Fulkerson [28], involves anteromedialization of the tibial tubercle. Lateral patella and trochlea lesions have the greatest potential to benefit since biomechanical studies demonstrate decreased lateral patellofemoral contact pressures following this procedure while medial, proximal, and diffuse lesions are less likely to have a favorable result [29, 30]. Concomitant osteotomy and cartilage repair have gained popularity as a result of encouraging results reported in recent studies when combining these procedures. A systematic review consisting of 11 studies observed significantly greater improvements in multiple clinical outcomes in subjects undergoing ACI combined with osteotomy compared to ACI alone [31]. Gillogly et al. [21] achieved good to excellent results in 83% of patients (19 of 23) at a mean of 7.6 years following ACI and TTO. In a cohort of 62 patients, Pascual-Garrido et al. [32] discovered a tendency toward better outcomes in patients undergoing ACI combined with anteromedialization compared to dislocated ACI. On the contrary, no significant difference was observed in patients treated with and without TTO at the time of patellofemoral ACI in a recent, large, multicenter study [25]. The authors concluded that most of the defects in their patient population were pan-patellar, which would be expected to result in less of a response following TTO than patients in other studies that had more lateral defects. However, they stressed that TTO is indicated to normalize an abnormal biomechanical environment. Additional procedures such as medial patellofemoral ligament (MPFL) reconstruction should be considered when treating patellar chondral defects associated with recurrent patellar instability. Siebold et al. [33] treated ten patients with a combination of MPFL reconstruction and ACI. All patients had a history of two or more patella dislocations and full-thickness cartilage lesions of the patella measuring on average 7.2 cm^2. All patients reported a stable patella with no instability at a mean follow-up of 2 years. Improved subjective and objective scores were achieved in all patients, and complete fill of the defect was noted in 80% of lesions based on postoperative MRI.

Conclusion

Treatment of patellar chondral defects is challenging as a result of the complex biomechanical environment of the patellofemoral joint. Lesion characteristics and patient factors should be carefully considered when developing a surgical plan. Associated conditions such as malalignment and instability can be addressed with concomitant procedures when indicated. Small chondral lesions (<2 cm^2) can be successfully treated with OAT and PJAC, while larger lesions (>2–4 cm^2) are better treated with ACI or OCA. There is conflicting evidence to recommend for or against marrow stimulation. Subchondral bone loss (>6–10 mm) is best addressed with OAT or OCA.

References

1. Mihalko WM, Boachie-Adjei Y, Spang JT, et al. Controversies and techniques in the surgical management of patellofemoral arthritis. Instr Course Lect. 2008;57:365–80.
2. Gomoll AH, Yoshioka H, Watanabe A, et al. Preoperative measurement of cartilage defects by MRI underestimates lesion size. Cartilage. 2011;2(4):389–93.
3. Mehl J, Feucht MJ, Bode G, et al. Association between patellar cartilage defects and patellofemoral geometry: a matched-pair MRI comparison of patients with and without isolated patellar cartilage defects. Knee Surg Sports Traumatol Arthrosc. 2016;24:838–46.
4. Seitlinger G, Scheurecker G, Hogler R, Labey L, Innocenti B, Hofmann S. Tibial tubercle-posterior cruciate ligament distance: a new measurement to define the position of the tibial tubercle in patients with patellar dislocation. Am J Sports Med. 2012;40(5):1119–25.
5. Chevidikunnan MF, Saif AA, Gaowgzeh RA, et al. Effectiveness of core muscle strengthening for improving pain and dynamic balance among female patients with patellofemoral pain syndrome. J Phys Ther Sci. 2016;28:1518–23.
6. Santos TR, Oliveira BA, Ocarino JM, et al. Effectiveness of hip muscle strengthening in patellofemoral pain syndrome patients: a systematic review. Phys Ther. 2015;19:167–76.

7. Alba-Martín P, Gallego-Izquierdo T, Plaza-Manzano G, et al. Effectiveness of therapeutic physical exercise in the treatment of patellofemoral pain syndrome: a systematic review. J Phys Ther Sci. 2015;27:2387–90.
8. Peng HT, Song CY. Predictors of treatment response to strengthening and stretching exercises for patellofemoral pain: an examination of patellar alignment. Knee. 2015;22:494–8.
9. Goyal D, Keyhani S, Lee EH, Hui JH. Evidence-based status of microfracture technique: a systematic review of level I and II studies. Arthroscopy. 2013;29(9):1579–88.
10. Gobbi A, Karnatzikos G, Kumar A. Long-term results after microfracture treatment for full-thickness knee chondral lesions in athletes. Knee Surg Traumatol Arthrosc. 2014;22:1986–96.
11. Mithoefer K, McAdams T, Williams RJ, et al. Clinical efficacy of the microfracture technique for articular cartilage repair in the knee: An evidence-based systematic analysis. Am J Sports Med. 2009;37:2053–63.
12. Kreuz PC, Steinwachs MR, Erggelet C, et al. Results after microfracture of full-thickness chondral defects in different compartments in the knee. Osteoarthr Cartil. 2006;14:1119–25.
13. Gomoll AH, Minas T, Farr J, et al. Treatment of chondral defects in the patellofemoral joint. J Knee Surg. 2006;19(4):285–95.
14. Bentley G, Biant LC, Carrington RW, et al. A prospective, randomized comparison of autologous chondrocyte implantation versus mosaic- plasty for osteochondral defects in the knee. J Bone Joint Surg (Br). 2003;85(2):223–30.
15. Emre TY, Atbasi Z, Demircioglu DT, et al. Autologous osteochondral transplantation (mosaicplasty) in articular cartilage defects of the patellofemoral joint: retrospective analysis of 33 cases. Musculoskelet Surg. 2016.
16. Nho SJ, Foo LF, Green DM, Shindle MK, Warren RF, Wickiewicz TL, Potter HG, Williams RJ. Evaluation of patellar resurfacing with press-fit osteochondral autograft plugs. Am J Sports Med. 2008;36(6):1101–9.
17. Astur DC, Arliani GG, Binz M, et al. Autologous osteochondral transplantation for treating patellar chondral injuries. J Bone Joint Surg. 2014;96:816–23.
18. Gracitelli GC, Meric G, Pulido PA, Gorz S, De Young AJ, Bugbee WD. Fresh osteochondral allograft transplantation for isolated patellar cartilage injury. Am J Sports Med. 2015;43(4):879–84.
19. Chahal J, Gross AE, Gross C, et al. Outcomes of osteochondral allograft transplantation in the knee: systematic review. Arthroscopy. 2013;29(3):575–88.

20. Torga Spak R, Teitge RA. Fresh osteochondral allografts for patellofemoral arthritis: long-term followup. Clin Orthop Relat Res. 2006;444:193–200.
21. Gillogly SD, Arnold RM. Autologous chondrocyte implantation and anteromedialization for isolated patellar articular cartilage lesions: 5-to11-year follow-up. Am J Sports Med. 2014;42(4):912–20.
22. Farr J. Autologous chondrocyte implantation improves patellofemoral cartilage treatment outcomes. Clin Orthop Relat Res. 2007;463:187–94.
23. Kon E, Filardo G, Gobbi A, et al. Long-term results after hyaluronan-based MACT for the treatment of cartilage lesions of the patellofemoral joint. Am J Sports Med. 2016;44(3):602–8.
24. Gobbi A, Kon E, Berruto M, et al. Patellofemoral full-thickness chondral defects treated with second-generation autologous chondrocyte implantation: results at 5 years' follow-up. Am J Sports Med. 2009;37(6):1083–92.
25. Gomoll AH, Gillogly SD, Cole BJ, et al. Autologous chondrocyte implantation in the patella: a multicenter experience. Am J Sports Med. 2014;42(5):1074–81.
26. Von Keudell A, Han R, Bryant T, et al. Autologous chondrocyte implantation to isolated patella cartilage defects: two- to 15-year follow-up. Cartilage. 2016;8(2):146–54.
27. Tompkins M, Hamann JC, Diduch DR, Bonner KF, Hart JM, Gwathmey FW, Milewski MD, Gaskin CM. Preliminary results of a novel single-stage cartilage restoration technique: particulated juvenile articular cartilage allograft for chondral defects of the patella. Arthroscopy. 2013;29(10):1661–70.
28. Fulkerson J, Becker G, Meaney J, Miranda M, Folcik M. Anteromedial tibial tubercle transfer without bone graft. Am J Sports Med. 1990;18(5):490–7.
29. Beck PR, Thomas AL, Farr J, Lewis PB, Cole BJ. Trochlear contact pressures after anteromedialization of the tibial tubercle. Am J Sports Med. 2005;33:1710–5.
30. Stephen JM, Lumpaopong P, Dodds AL, Williams A, Amis AA. The effect of tibial tuberosity medialization and lateralization on patellofemoral joint kinematics, contact mechanics, and stability. Am J Sports Med. 2015;43(1):186–94.
31. Trinh TQ, Harris JD, Siston RA, et al. Improved outcomes with combined autologous chondrocyte implantation and patellofe- moral osteotomy versus isolated autologous chondrocyte implanta- tion. Arthroscopy. 2013;29(3):566–74.

32. Pascual-Garrido C, Slabaugh MA, L'Heureux DR, et al. Recommendations and treatment outcomes for patellofemoral articular cartilage defects with autologous chondrocyte implantation: pro- spective evaluation at average 4-year follow-up. Am J Sports Med. 2009;37(Suppl 1):33S–41S.
33. Siebold R, Karidakis G, Fernandez F. Clinical outcome after medial ptellofemoral ligament reonstruction and autologous chondrocyte implantation following recurrent patella dislocation. Knee Surg Traumatol Arthrosc. 2014;22:2477–83.

Chapter 12
Bipolar Articular Chondral Lesions of the Knee

Brian Waterman, Annabelle Davey, Michael L. Redondo, and Brian J. Cole

Introduction

Also known as "kissing lesions," bipolar chondral defects are less common than isolated chondral lesions in the non-arthritic knee. In published literature, bipolar lesions are often inappropriately classified as having either widespread osteoarthritis (OA) [1] or multiple isolated lesions [2], so it is difficult to ascertain the exact prevalence, with rates reported at 9–18%. In a multicenter study of 1020 patients undergoing knee arthroscopy specifically for the treatment of a symptomatic cartilage lesion (61% male; mean age, 37.6 years), 95 cases (9.3%) of bipolar chondral lesions were identified [3]. Of these 95 cases, 27 (28%) were patellofemoral, 57 (60%) involved the medial tibiofemoral articulation, and 11 (12%) affected lateral compartment [3]. In a different study of 1000 patients

B. Waterman
Wake Forest School of Medicine, Winton-Salem, NC, USA

A. Davey
University of Vermont, College of Medicine, Burlington, VT, USA

M. L. Redondo · B. J. Cole (✉)
Department of Orthopedic Surgery,
Rush University Medical Center, Chicago, IL, USA
e-mail: brian.cole@rushortho.com

© Springer Nature Switzerland AG 2019
A. B. Yanke, B. J. Cole (eds.), *Joint Preservation of the Knee*,
https://doi.org/10.1007/978-3-030-01491-9_12

183

undergoing knee arthroscopy (59% male; mean age, 47 years), 57% of arthroscopies revealed chondral or osteochondral lesions, with bipolar lesions found in 103 patients (10%) [4]. Patients with bipolar lesions are more likely to have a degenerative or indolent onset rather than traumatic etiology [3]. Additionally, patients are likely to present with a greater degree of dysfunction [3]. Solheim et al. reported that while mean Lysholm score was not significantly affected by lesion location, number of lesions, or total area of lesions, mean Lysholm score was significantly lower for patients with bipolar lesions than for patients with isolated lesions [4].

Despite a significant prevalence in younger and physically active patients, bipolar lesions are often a relative contraindication for multiple surgical cartilage restoration or resurfacing procedures [5]. However, under treatment may contribute to heightened risk of revision reoperation or secondary arthroplasty with further degenerative progression [6]. Due to this disconnect, chondral restoration procedures are being increasingly explored. These treatments are often accompanied by adjunctive procedures to address associated pathology, correct underlying coronal or rotational malalignment, and off-load treated chondral defects. Spahn et al. reported that malalignment was significantly associated with the occurrence of bipolar lesions of the medial tibiofemoral joint (87.8%), lateral tibiofemoral joint (57.2%), and patellofemoral articulation (15.8%) [3]. Additionally, malalignment may contribute to faster rate of arthritic progression [7, 8]. Furthermore, meniscal procedures are commonly performed concomitantly in patients with tibiofemoral lesions. Spahn et al. reported a significantly higher incidence of concomitant meniscal tear in the medial tibiofemoral lesion group (57.1%) than in the patellofemoral lesion group (16.9%) [3]. Notably, combined meniscus allograft transplantation (MAT) and chondral restoration [osteochondral allograft transplantation (OCA), autologous chondrocyte implantation (ACI)] for biologic knee reconstruction has shown promise at midterm follow-up [9, 10]. However, in a study with long-term follow-up, failure occurred in four out of seven knees with bipolar lesions treated with combined MAT and ACI [11]. Additionally, ligament repair is a common concomitant procedure in the treatment of bipolar chondral lesions. This is due to the relatively high incidence of ligament injury and bipolar lesions. Previous rupture or chronic insufficiency of the ACL has been reported to increase the likelihood of developing bipolar lesions and secondary arthritis [12, 13]. Additionally, both PCL and MPFL injury are associated with chondral lesions [14, 15].

Despite the prevalence of bipolar lesions in patients with knee dysfunction, there is a lack of published literature and high-level evidence focusing specifically on treatments for bipolar lesions. The following cases present patients with bipolar chondral lesions treated with different cartilage restoration or resurfacing procedures.

Clinical Case Presentation

Case 1

A 36-year-old female with a BMI of 21.3 kg/m^2 presented initially with anterior left knee pain. She had experienced a patellar dislocation 20 years prior while playing soccer, which was initially treated conservatively with closed reduction at the time of injury and physical therapy. After approximately 15 years, the patient developed persistent anterior knee pain, episodic subluxations, and intermittent effusion exacerbated by stair-climbing, kneeling, and running. She was subsequently treated with further physical therapy, McConnell taping, and a patellofemoral stabilizer brace, which improved stability but did not reduce activity-related pain. Upon further presentation, she exhibited a pathologic J sign with audible crepitations during an active range of motion arc of 0–140°, and no evidence of generalized ligamentous instability. She also demonstrated positive patellar apprehension, lateral tilt, and patellofemoral grind test. Plain and advanced radiographic imaging revealed no frank evidence of arthritis, slight patella alta, and a focal chondral defect in the apex of the patella (Figs. 12.1 and 12.2). At the time of diagnostic staging arthroscopy, bipolar lesions of the lateral patella (28 mm × 20 mm) and lateral trochlea (10 mm × 12 mm) were observed, and chondroplasty was performed. Rotational malalignment was not an issue.

Due to limited improvement, the patient underwent particulated juvenile allograft cartilage transplantation (DeNovo NT, Zimmer Biomet, Warsaw, IN) to the patella, microfracture of the trochlea, and tibial tubercle osteotomy with anteromedialization at 5 months following the initial arthroscopy. The anteromedialization was performed with 10–12 mm of correction. For the patella, a subvastus arthrotomy was performed and extended distally to allow eversion of the patella for defect

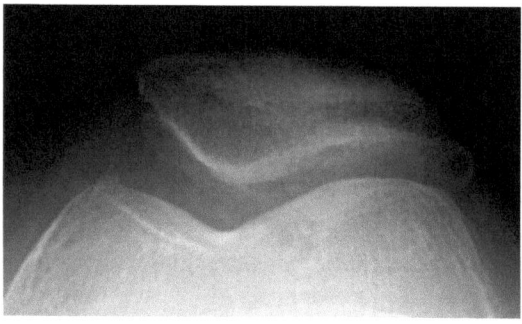

Figure 12.1 Sunrise view of plain axial radiographs displaying patellar malalignment

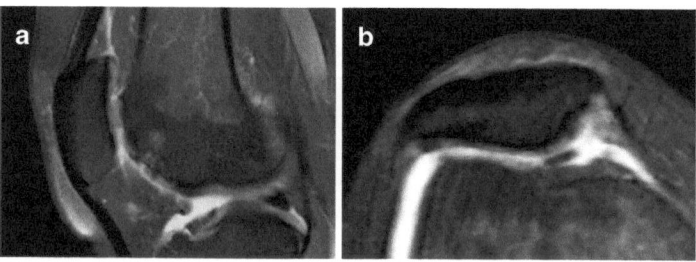

Figure 12.2 Axial and sagittal T2-weighted MRI displaying bipolar patellofemoral chondral defects

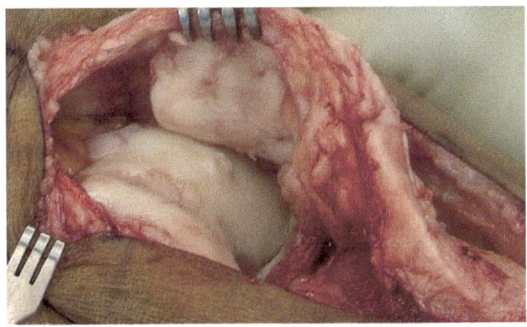

FIGURE 12.3 An intraoperative photo displaying the patella everted through a subvastus arthrotomy exposing a bipolar patellofemoral defect

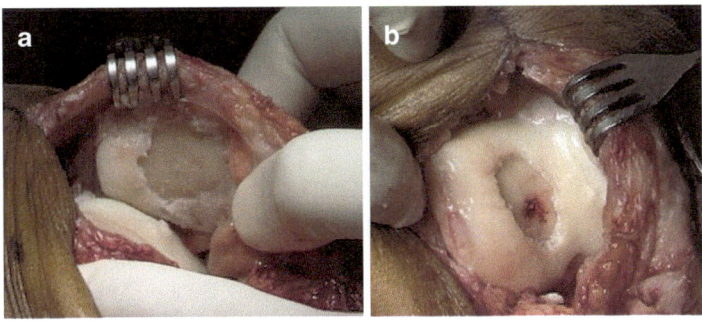

FIGURE 12.4 An intraoperative photos displaying left knee bipolar defects after preparation via curettage (**a**) Patellar Defect (**b**) Trochlear Defect

exposure (Fig. 12.3). Vertical walls were created, and a pineapple bur was used to create subchondral vents to improve the adherence of the de novo allograft material. Minced particulate allograft cartilage was placed in the defect to approximate a 50% lesion fill and then secured with fibrin glue. On the trochlear side, the lesion had progressed in size to an uncontained lesion, and the subchondral plate demonstrated a sclerotic base with intralesional osteophyte formation. Accordingly, gentle curettage was performed to restore the normal contour of the subchondral bone (Fig. 12.4), and nanofracture was performed using a 1.5-mm-powered drill. Finally, a titrated lateral lengthening procedure was performed to address tilt and achieve congruity. Postoperatively, the patient was given a cryotherapy unit and continuous passive motion device to facilitate edema control and prevent excessive scar formation. Partial weight-bearing was permitted with the brace locked in full extension for ambulation with crutches.

At 6-week follow-up, physical examination revealed notable quadriceps atrophy, with passive range of potion from 0° to 90°. Continued brace wear with crutches was encouraged, and physical therapy was initiated. At 3-month follow-up, the patient was instructed to progress to further strengthening and core-based exercises outside of the brace.

At 6 months, the patient reported generally doing well. The patient did not have significant difficulty with ambulation or stairs. The patient affirms that she has not done any running yet. The patient has full passive range of motion and rates her pain level at 1–2/10, compared to 5/10 at best prior to surgery. She did not require any additional formal physical therapy.

Particulated juvenile allograft cartilage (PJAC) transplantation remains a fairly new technique, and the available case series and indications are still evolving. Unipolar lesion treated with PJAC has demonstrated modest success in series by Tompkins et al., Bucketwalter et al., and Farr et al., although these series are limited to only 25 patients with short-term follow-up. Recent Level V evidence again suggests that bipolar lesions are a contraindication to juvenile transplantation due to shear of lesions against each other destabilizing the transplanted material [16]. Notably, the patient in this case underwent tibial tubercle osteotomy to off-load the bipolar lesions and diminish shear stress, which can also be facilitated through additional use of an overlying type I/III collagen patch.

Case 2

A 28-year-old male former college basketball player with a BMI of 27.6 presented with sharp lateral left knee pain aggravated by walking, standing, bending, and twisting, swelling, and painful mechanical symptoms. The patient had a history of left knee lateral meniscal tear 12 years prior and underwent two lateral meniscectomies on separate occasions. He previously received prior hyaluronic acid injections in the left knee and had failed a prolonged course of physical therapy and activity modification. Plain radiography revealed KL grades II to III with lateral joint space narrowing (Fig. 12.5). No other osseous abnormality including fracture or dislocation was observed.

Based on recent arthroscopic images, the patient was indicated for combined osteochondral allograft transplantation to the lateral femoral condyle, microfracture to the lateral tibial plateau, and lateral meniscal allograft transplantation. Standard diagnostic arthroscopy was performed to reveal normal medial compartment, no ligamentous damage and normal patellofemoral articulation. Inspection of the lateral compartment revealed meniscal insufficiency with bipolar lesions of the lateral femoral condyle and the lateral tibial plateau measuring 25 mm × 25 mm and 12 mm × 12 mm, respectively (Fig. 12.6). In order to prepare for the lateral meniscal allograft transplant, a complete meniscectomy was performed, with care to preserve the peripheral meniscal rim

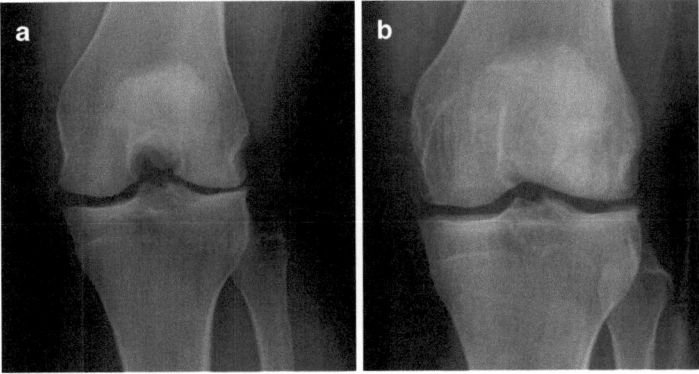

Figure 12.5 Preoperative imaging of (a) standing posterior-anterior Rosenberg radiograph and (b) standard anterior-posterior radiograph displaying lateral joint space narrowing of the left knee

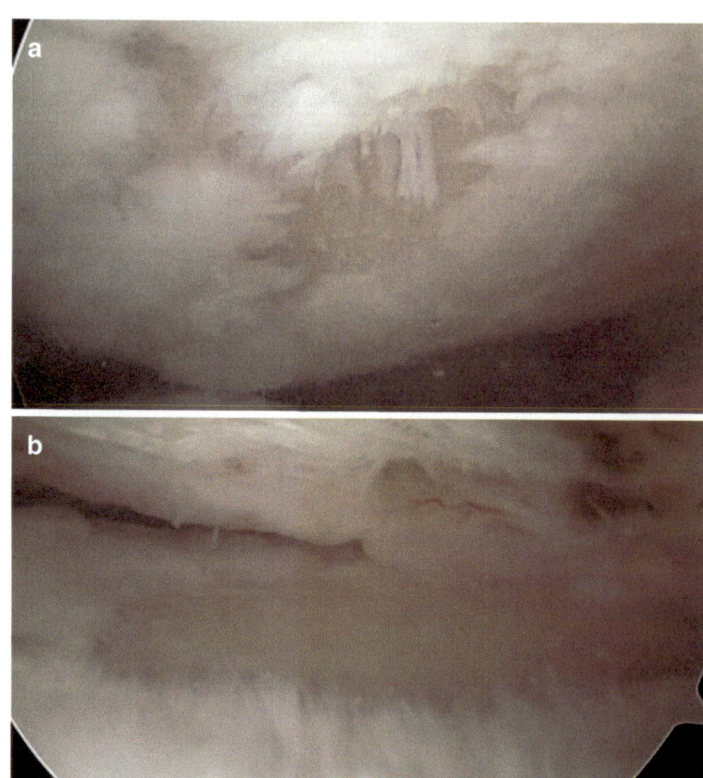

FIGURE 12.6 Arthroscopic images through the lateral portal of (**a**) a grade IV lateral femoral condyle defect and (**b**) a grade IV lateral tibial plateau cartilage defect of the left knee

for fixation. A posterolateral accessory approach was performed, with an incision 1/3 above and 2/3 below the joint line, and the lateral head of the gastrocnemius was elevated to expose the posterior capsule. A 10 mm × 8 cm slot was made through a cannulated guide and transpatellar portal, and a pituitary rongeur and box rasp were used to contour the recipient site. The meniscus was thawed and prepared to match the recipient slot, while maintaining the native anterior and posterior horn attachments on the bone block. The graft was subsequently manually inserted through an extended anterior incision while carefully pulling on traction sutures placed at the junction of the anterior two-thirds of the meniscus and exiting lateral to the popliteal fossa. Inside-out suture repair was then performed in a vertical mattress pattern on the superior and inferior surface of the meniscus and additional all-inside device posteriorly. Finally, a 7 × 23 mm biocomposite screw was placed for interference fixation lateral to the bone block. After fixation, the arthrotomy incision was then extended further proximally to expose and debride the tibial plateau defect to stable margins. Marrow stimulation was performed with both curettage and microfracture awl fenestration (Fig. 12.7). On the corresponding femoral condylar lesion, central guide pin placement and reaming were performed to achieve a depth of 7 mm and diameter of 25 mm. The fresh osteochondral allograft was sized and prepared for a line-to-line fit and gently impacted into place. Flush margins with the surrounding intact articular cartilage were obtained, and final arthroscopic images confirmed

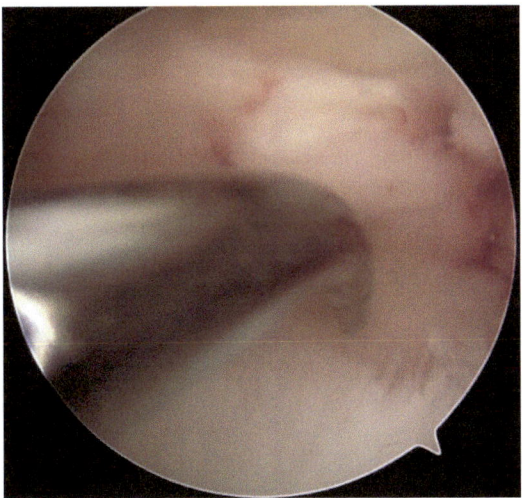

FIGURE 12.7 An arthroscopic image displaying marrow stimulation of a grade IV lateral tibial plateau defect

secure fixation of both the meniscal and osteochondral allograft (Figs. 12.8 and 12.9).

At 6-week follow-up, the patient was able to achieve full extension and flexion to 90°. He demonstrated minimal

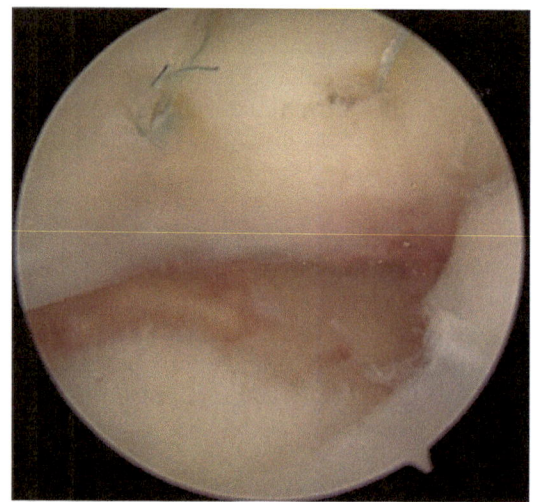

FIGURE 12.8 An arthroscopic image displaying confirm secure fixation of a lateral meniscus allograft transplantation of the left knee

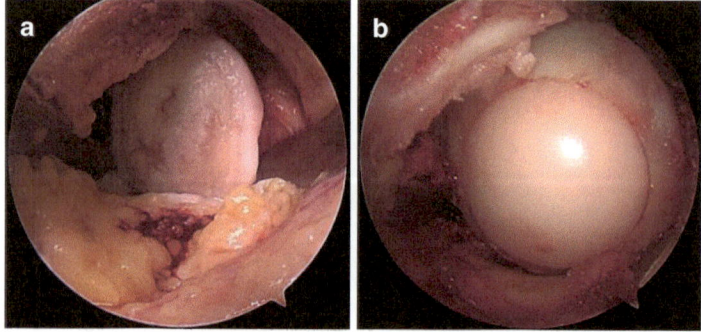

FIGURE 12.9 (**a**) An arthroscopic image displaying a lateral femoral condyle defect prior to preparation. (**b**) An arthroscopic image displaying secure fixation of an osteochondral allograft transplantation on the lateral femoral condyle

tenderness and was instructed to gradually progress weight-bearing to full at 8 weeks while increasing his range of motion as tolerated. At 6-month follow-up, physical examination revealed trace effusion, no lateral joint line tenderness, and range of motion from 0° to 115° flexion. Surveillance MRI revealed a stable meniscus, incorporation of the osteochondral allograft, and resolution of underlying marrow edema in the tibia. At this point, the patient was cleared for running and jumping, and he returned at 1-year follow-up with continuing improvement and full resumption of all pre-injury activities despite mild degenerative changes in the lateral compartment on routine radiographs.

There is a paucity of literature on treatment of bipolar lesions with osteochondral allograft transplantation. Most existing series suggest that treatment of bipolar lesions has worse outcomes than the treatment of isolated lesions. Ghazavi et al., Chu et al., and Fischer et al. reported bipolar lesions as a contraindication for osteochondral allograft transplantation in 1997 and 1999 and 2006, respectively [17–19]. Additionally, a high reoperation rate (50%) was observed for patients undergoing bipolar osteochondral allograft transplantation in more contemporary series [20]. However, this study did note that patients who did not undergo reoperation had significant clinical improvement.

Comprehensive treatment of patellofemoral lesions requires optimization of axial or coronal plane malalignment and dynamic patellar instability in order to ensure reproducible outcomes. Importantly, this patient had previously undergone tibial tubercle osteotomy with MPFL reconstruction to both off-load symptomatic defects and decrease shear stress or eccentric loading patterns. The combination of these procedures may serve to both prevent recurrence of patellar instability and enhance likelihood of symptomatic relief with revision osteochondral allograft transplantation.

Meniscal allograft transplantation is fairly common in conjunction with treatment of tibiofemoral lesions, especially bipolar lesions, because it has been shown to effectively provide symptomatic relief and improve joint contact forces and dynamic loading patterns [21]. However, it also has a significantly higher failure rate in patients with bipolar lesions [21]. There is limited data to suggest the success of microfracture alongside other hybrid treatments of bipolar lesions. However, multiple lesions have been reported to do worse with microfracture than isolated defects at both midterm and long-term follow-up [22, 23]. Additionally, microfracture is contraindicated by larger lesion size (>2-cm²), degenerative etiology, and untreated malalignment – all factors commonly associated with bipolar lesions. This suggests that bipolar lesions are a relative contraindication to microfracture, although further research is necessary to delineate its role, particularly on the tibial surface where limited options exist.

Other Treatments

There are many emerging options for treatment of chondral lesions, but more research is needed to determine if they will be effective for bipolar lesions. Bone marrow aspirate concentrate (BMAC) has shown promise in the treatment of focal chondral defects and in early stage OA [24], and platelet-rich plasma (PRP) has shown promise for treatment of overall degenerative changes in the knee [25]. However, more research is necessary to determine if BMAC and PRP are appropriate and effective treatments for bipolar lesions. Additionally, procedures using scaffolds for new cartilage to grow, in conjunction with either BMAC or PRP, have shown promising results for treatment of focal chondral lesions [26, 27]. Gobbi and Whyte reported superior outcomes of an HA scaffold supplemented with BMAC as compared to microfracture at 5-year follow-up for the treatment of large lesions and multiple lesions, although the study does not specify if this included any bipolar lesions [26]. Siclari et al. included 10 patients with bipolar lesions in their larger study cohort of patients undergoing treatment of one lesion with a PGA-HA scaffold and PRP injection [27]. There was significant improvement in KOOS score at 5-year follow-up of the total cohort, but subgroup analysis did not include the presence of bipolar lesions and did not address the outcomes of the original 10 bipolar lesion patients [27]. More research is necessary to determine the effectiveness of these procedures for treatment of bipolar lesions. Additionally, while novel hybrid techniques show promise for the treatment of chondral lesions, to the best of the authors' knowledge, there does not exist any literature examining these techniques in patients with bipolar lesions.

Bipolar lesions cause a high degree of dysfunction in patients and are often difficult to treat. This is complicated by the relative dearth of literature detailing evidence-based treatment strategies of bipolar lesions. Further research is warranted to determine the most appropriate and effective treatment for this complicated pathology.

References

1. Widuchowski W, Widuchowski J, Trzaska T. Articular cartilage defects: study of 25,124 knee arthroscopies. Knee. 2007;14(3):177–82.
2. Curl WW, Krome J, Gordon ES, Rushing J, Smith BP, Poehling GG. Cartilage injuries: a review of 31,516 knee arthroscopies. Arthroscopy. 1997;13(4):456–60.
3. Spahn G, Fritz J, Albrecht D, Hofmann GO, Niemeyer P. Characteristics and associated factors of Klee cartilage lesions: preliminary baseline-data of more than 1000 patients from the German cartilage registry (KnorpelRegister DGOU). Arch Orthop Trauma Surg. 2016;136(6):805–10.
4. Solheim E, Krokeide AM, Melteig P, Larsen A, Strand T, Brittberg M. Symptoms and function in patients with articular cartilage lesions in 1,000 knee arthroscopies. Knee Surg Sports Traumatol Arthrosc. 2016;24(5):1610–6.
5. Versier G, Dubrana F. Treatment of knee cartilage defect in 2010. Orthop Traumatol Surg Res: OTSR. 2011;97(8 Suppl):S140–53.
6. Lonner JH, Hershman S, Mont M, Lotke PA. Total knee arthroplasty in patients 40 years of age and younger with osteoarthritis. Clin Orthop Relat Res. 2000;380:85–90.
7. Cahue S, Dunlop D, Hayes K, Song J, Torres L, Sharma L. Varus-valgus alignment in the progression of patellofemoral osteoarthritis. Arthritis Rheum. 2004;50(7):2184–90.

8. Sharma L, Song J, Dunlop D, et al. Varus and valgus alignment and incident and progressive knee osteoarthritis. Ann Rheum Dis. 2010;69(11):1940–5.

9. Bhosale AM, Myint P, Roberts S, et al. Combined autologous chondrocyte implantation and allogenic meniscus transplantation: a biological knee replacement. Knee. 2007;14(5):361–8.

10. Harris JD, Hussey K, Saltzman BM, et al. Cartilage repair with or without meniscal transplantation and osteotomy for lateral compartment chondral defects of the knee: case series with minimum 2-year follow-up. Orthop J Sports Med. 2014;2(10):2325967114551528.

11. Ogura T, Bryant T, Minas T. Biological knee reconstruction with concomitant autologous chondrocyte implantation and meniscal allograft transplantation: mid- to long-term outcomes. Orthop J Sports Med. 2016;4(10):2325967116668490.

12. Cantin O, Lustig S, Rongieras F, et al. Outcome of cartilage at 12years of follow-up after anterior cruciate ligament reconstruction. Orthop Traumatol Surg Res: OTSR. 2016;102(7):857–61.

13. Chalmers PN, Mall NA, Moric M, et al. Does ACL reconstruction alter natural history?: a systematic literature review of long-term outcomes. J Bone Joint Surg Am. 2014;96(4):292–300.

14. Ringler MD, Shotts EE, Collins MS, Howe BM. Intra-articular pathology associated with isolated posterior cruciate ligament injury on MRI. Skelet Radiol. 2016;45(12):1695–703.

15. Zhang GY, Zheng L, Shi H, Ji BJ, Feng Y, Ding HY. Injury patterns of medial patellofemoral ligament after acute lateral patellar dislocation in children: correlation analysis with anatomical variants and articular cartilage lesion of the patella. Eur Radiol. 2017;27(3):1322–30.

16. Riboh JC, Cole BJ, Farr J. Particulated articular cartilage for symptomatic chondral defects of the knee. Curr Rev Musculoskelet Med. 2015;8(4):429–35.

17. Chu CR, Convery FR, Akeson WH, Meyers M, Amiel D. Articular cartilage transplantation. Clinical results in the knee. Clin Orthop Relat Res. 1999;360:159–68.

18. Fischer M, Koller U, Krismer M. The use of fresh allografts in osteochondrosis dissecans of the lateral femoral condyle. Oper Orthop Traumatol. 2006;18(3):245–58.

19. Ghazavi MT, Pritzker KP, Davis AM, Gross AE. Fresh osteochondral allografts for post-traumatic osteochondral defects of the knee. J Bone Joint Surg Br. 1997;79(6):1008–13.

20. Meric G, Gracitelli GC, Gortz S, De Young AJ, Bugbee WD. Fresh osteochondral allograft transplantation for bipolar reciprocal osteochondral lesions of the knee. Am J Sports Med. 2015;43(3):709–14.
21. Lee BS, Bin SI, Kim JM, Kim WK, Choi JW. Survivorship after meniscal allograft transplantation according to articular cartilage status. Am J Sports Med. 2017;45(5):1095–101.
22. Gobbi A, Karnatzikos G, Kumar A. Long-term results after microfracture treatment for full-thickness knee chondral lesions in athletes. Knee Surg Sports Traumatol Arthrosc. 2014;22(9):1986–96.
23. Gobbi A, Nunag P, Malinowski K. Treatment of full thickness chondral lesions of the knee with microfracture in a group of athletes. Knee Surg Sports Traumatol Arthrosc. 2005;13(3):213–21.
24. Chahla J, Dean CS, Moatshe G, Pascual-Garrido C, Serra Cruz R, LaPrade RF. Concentrated bone marrow aspirate for the treatment of chondral injuries and osteoarthritis of the knee: a systematic review of outcomes. Orthop J Sports Med. 2016;4(1):2325967115625481.
25. Kon E, Buda R, Filardo G, et al. Platelet-rich plasma: intra-articular knee injections produced favorable results on degenerative cartilage lesions. Knee Surg Sports Traumatol Arthrosc. 2010;18(4):472–9.
26. Gobbi A, Whyte GP. One-stage cartilage repair using a hyaluronic acid-based scaffold with activated bone marrow-derived mesenchymal stem cells compared with microfracture: five-year follow-up. Am J Sports Med. 2016;44(11):2846–54.
27. Siclari A, Mascaro G, Kaps C, Boux E. A 5-year follow-up after cartilage repair in the knee using a platelet-rich plasma-immersed polymer-based implant. Open Orthop J. 2014;8:346–54.

Part III
Complex Knee Joint Preservation Cases

Chapter 13
Revision Cartilage Treatment

Andrew J. Riff and Andreas H. Gomoll

Case Presentation

A 40-year-old man initially presented to our office in 2010 with a 9 month history of right medial-sided knee pain and locking symptoms that abated with manual manipulation. At that time, physical examination revealed a mild varus alignment, and MRI revealed a large, chronic-appearing osteochondritis dissecans lesion involving the medial femoral condyle (MFC) measuring roughly 3 cm × 3 cm. Three months after an initial arthroscopy for chondrocyte harvest and loose body removal, he underwent valgus-producing high tibial osteotomy (HTO) and autologous chondrocyte implantation (ACI) sandwich technique of the MFC using autologous distal femoral cancellous bone graft (Fig. 13.1a–c).

Following the HTO and ACI sandwich procedure, the patient did well for a 7 year interval with the ability to participate in hiking, running, and cycling. However, he represented in 2017 with 2 months of increased pain after he missed a step

A. J. Riff (✉)
IU Health Physicians Orthopedics & Sports Medicine, Indianapolis, IN, USA
e-mail: ariff@iuhealth.org

A. H. Gomoll
Department of Orthopedic Surgery, Hospital for Special Surgery, New York, NY, USA

© Springer Nature Switzerland AG 2019   201
A. B. Yanke, B. J. Cole (eds.), *Joint Preservation of the Knee*,
https://doi.org/10.1007/978-3-030-01491-9_13

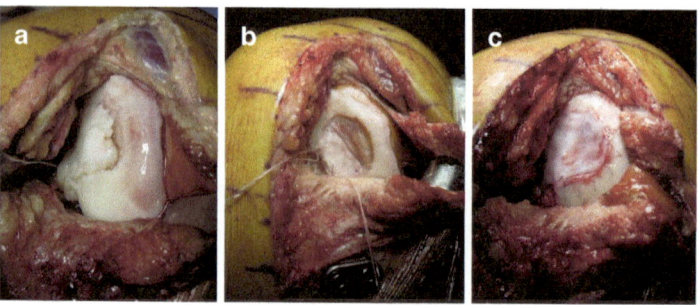

FIGURE 13.1 (a–c) Intraoperative photographs from initial ACI sandwich procedure demonstrating the MFC osteochondral defect (a), preliminary placement of the deep collagen membrane after bone grafting (b), and final graft construct after cell injection and fixation of the superficial collagen membrane with circumferential 6-0 resorbable sutures (c)

while ascending stairs and experienced a pop over the medial aspect of the right knee. Since that time, he also experienced recurrent knee swelling and intermittent catching.

Physical Assessment

The patient presented with a BMI of 25.8. Examination of the right knee revealed a subtle valgus mechanical alignment consistent with prior valgus-producing high tibial osteotomy. He had a nonantalgic gait. Knee range of motion was 0–135° with no effusion. He had a stable ligamentous examination to Lachman, posterior drawer, and varus and valgus stress at 0° and 30° of knee flexion. Patellofemoral examination revealed mild crepitation, normal patellar mobility, and no J-sign. There was tenderness to palpation along the medial joint line and over the MFC.

Diagnostic Studies

Anterior-posterior (AP) and lateral radiographs revealed evidence of a well-healed high tibial osteotomy with retained hardware (Arthrex Puddu locking plate, Naples, FL;

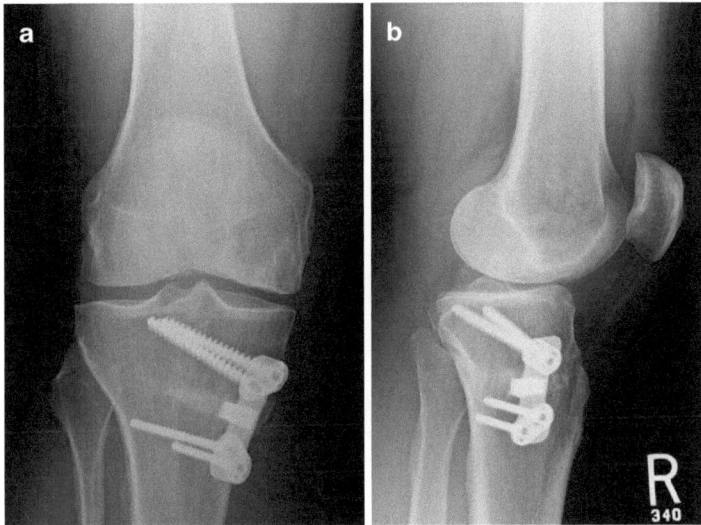

FIGURE 13.2 (**a, b**) Standing AP (**a**) and lateral (**b**) radiographs of the right knee obtained at representation in 2017 demonstrating subtle medial joint space narrowing and large subchondral cyst at the medial aspect of the MFC

Fig. 13.2a, b). Standing AP radiograph (Fig. 13.2a) revealed subtle medial compartment joint space narrowing without significant progression compared to 1 year after initial reconstruction (Fig. 13.3a, b). Compared to films obtained 1 year after his initial reconstruction, there was an evolution of new cortical irregularity along the MFC with a large subchondral cyst at the medial margin of the MFC. MRI redemonstrated the large subchondral cyst and showed an adjacent chondral defect measuring 2 cm × 2 cm (Fig. 13.4a, b).

Diagnosis

The patient was diagnosed with an osteochondral lesion involving the MFC as a result of ACI graft delamination.

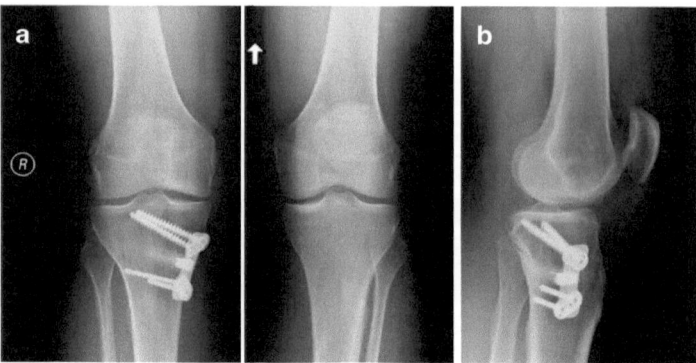

FIGURE 13.3 (**a, b**) Standing bilateral AP (**a**) and lateral (**b**) radiographs of the patient's operative right lower extremity obtained in 2011, 1 year following initial reconstruction

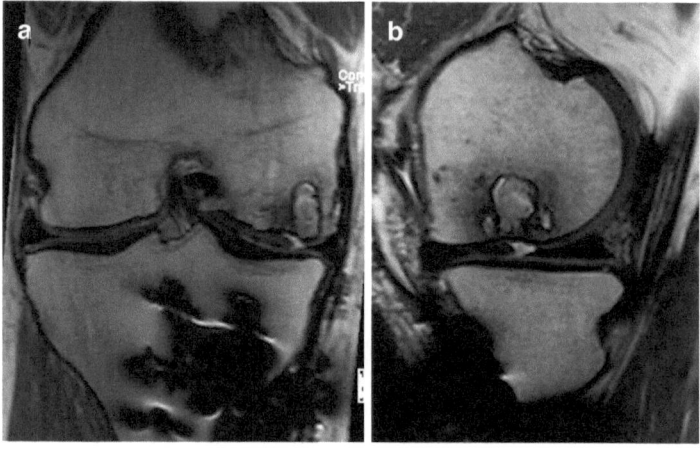

FIGURE 13.4 (**a, b**) Coronal (**a**) and sagittal (**b**) proton density MRI slices demonstrating a full-thickness chondral defect involving the MFC, large underlying subchondral cyst, and intact medial meniscus

Management Options

Cases of revision cartilage repair can be very challenging. Prior attempts at cartilage repair often result in compromised subchondral bone and increased lesion size. Notably, 30–50%

of patients who have undergone marrow stimulation techniques (MST, microfracture or subchondral drilling) present with altered subchondral bone [1]. Surgical options for larger lesions with damaged subchondral bone include the ACI "sandwich" technique with bone grafting, osteochondral autograft (OAT) mosaicplasty, osteochondral allograft (OCA) transplantation, unicompartmental knee arthroplasty (UKA), and, more recently, biphasic biomimetic osteochondral scaffolds such as Agili-C (Cartiheal Ltd., Israel) and MaioRegen (FinCeramica S.p.A., Italy). Considering the patient's young age, well-preserved tibiofemoral joint space, and lack of osteoarthritis, it was deemed appropriate to pursue another attempt at cartilage restoration (as opposed to arthroplasty). This case involved failure of prior ACI "sandwich" technique with significant subchondral changes, and, as such, it was felt prudent to utilize an osteochondral restorative procedure. Although promising, biomimetic osteochondral scaffolds like Agili-C and MaioRegen remain investigational and only available in Europe through clinical trials. Both mosaicplasty and osteochondral allograft transplantation are viable options for lesions with damaged subchondral bone; however, mosaicplasty demonstrates inferior results in lesions >3 cm^2, as well as increased concerns over donor site morbidity [2].

Surgical Technique

Due to the large lesion size and the extent of damage to the underlying bone, the decision was made to perform autologous bone grafting to address the large subchondral cyst and osteochondral allograft transplantation to address the osteochondral defect. Examination under anesthesia redemonstrated a stable ligamentous exam. Utilizing the prior anterior surgical incision, a medial parapatellar arthrotomy was performed, and a large osteochondral defect was identified on the MFC measuring 24 mm in its largest dimension (Fig. 13.5). A 2.4 mm guide pin was placed in the center of the defect, and this was over-reamed with a 24 mm diameter reamer to a depth of 8 mm. After reaming, a very large cyst over the medial aspect

206   A. J. Riff and A. H. Gomoll

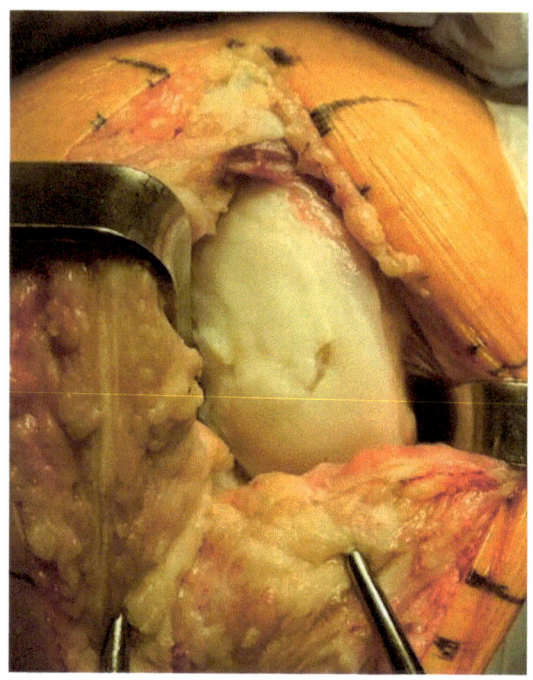

FIGURE 13.5 MFC following medial parapatellar arthrotomy demonstrating delaminated ACI graft

of the defect was identified (Fig. 13.6). The cyst was evacuated with a curette, and an OATS harvester was used to create a cylindrical cavity of 10 mm diameter. A corresponding 10 mm autograft plug was harvested from the medial epicondyle and placed into the cavity and impacted until it was flush (Fig. 13.7). A 24 mm x × 8 mm cylindrical osteochondral allograft was fashioned at the back table. Prior to placement, the bony portion of the graft was perforated multiple times with a 0.7 mm Kirshner wire to facilitate bony ingrowth and thoroughly washed with a pulsatile lavage to clear marrow elements to minimize immunogenicity. A Jamshidi needle was used to obtain bone marrow aspirate from the medial epicondyle, which was applied to the graft's subchondral bone to further optimize the healing environment. The graft was then placed

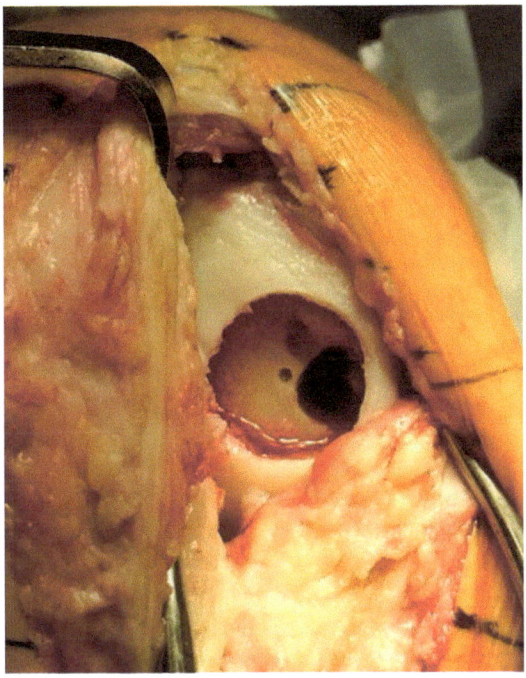

FIGURE 13.6 Initial lesion preparation included placement of a central guide pin which was over-reamed with a 24 mm reamer to a depth of 8 mm. Reaming revealed a medial subchondral cyst measuring 10 mm in diameter

into the recipient socket and reduced with manual pressure until it was seated flush with the surrounding MFC (Fig. 13.8). It was deemed to be mechanically stable and no further fixation was utilized.

Clinical Pearls/Pitfalls
When performing osteochondral allograft transplantation for large osteochondral defects, there are a number of important technical strategies to minimize graft immunogenicity, improve graft placement, and optimize

graft incorporation. Grafts should be treated with sustained pulsatile lavage with saline admixed with bacitracin prior to implantation to flush out marrow elements from the bony portion of the graft that contribute most to graft immunogenicity. When compared to a pulsatile saline lavage, a combined saline and high-pressure carbon dioxide lavage more effectively clears marrow elements in the deep zone of osteochondral allografts [3]. Overly aggressive recipient site reaming can result in thermal necrosis of the underlying bone and an excessively deep socket, which necessitates a graft with larger bony component (increasing graft immunogenicity). The use of bone marrow aspirate concentrate or platelet-rich plasma to the allograft subchondral bone may enhance biologic graft incorporation [4]. When inserting the graft, a freer elevator or dental pick can be helpful to "shoehorn" the graft into place. Strong impaction of the graft may compromise chondrocyte viability, and manual placement is preferred. If the graft is determined to be unstable after placement or if >40% of the graft is unshouldered (in the case of peripheral defects), adjunctive fixation with headless screws or a biocomposite implant is recommended. If the graft is incongruous with the surrounding articular surface after final impaction, the edges can be carefully contoured with a No. 15 blade for minor localized incongruity or removal of the plug with addition of bone graft to the socket or removal of bone from the plug, for more significant incongruity to optimize articular congruity. The latter is preferred as using a blade will remove the superficial zone of the cartilage which is important for several reasons.

Literature Review and Discussion

Patients with failed cartilage repair present a challenging problem. Prior to embarking on a revision procedure, it is essential to explore reasons for failure. Several host factors have been

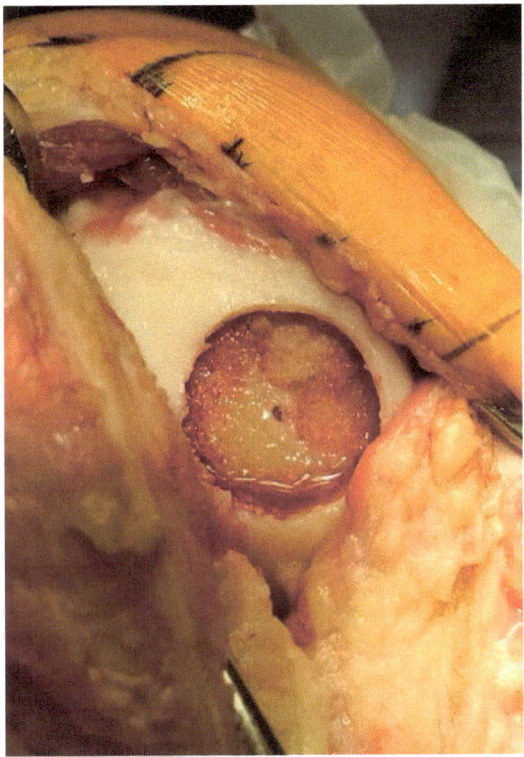

FIGURE 13.7 Further lesion preparation included placement of a 10 mm core of autologous bone from the medial epicondyle and application of bone marrow aspirate concentrate to further optimize the healing environment

identified that confer a poor prognosis with cartilage repair such as high demand level, worker compensation status, age >30 years, and BMI >30 kg/m² [5]. In these patients, it is important to have a discussion of goals of care, and the decision to proceed with revision cartilage repair procedure should be made with caution (particularly if the risk factors cannot be modified). Furthermore, a comorbid condition such as malalignment, instability, or meniscal deficiency can lead to premature degradation of primary cartilage repair tissue. Cartilage lesions with concomitant malalignment, instability

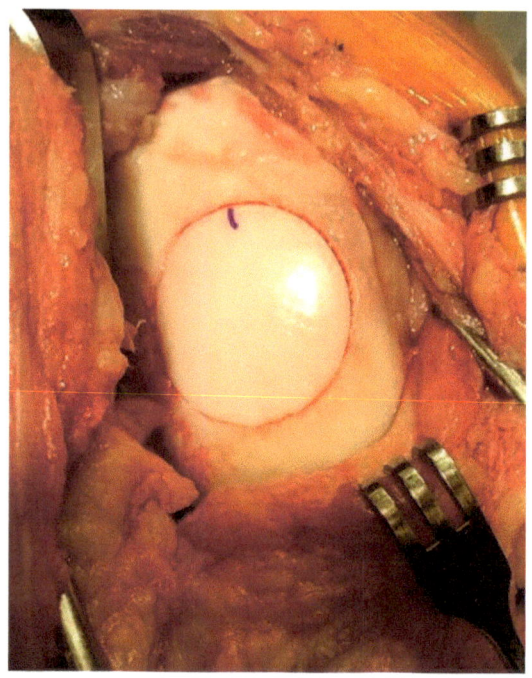

FIGURE 13.8 MFC after placement of the osteochondral allograft. The graft is flush with surrounding MFC. In light of excellent press-fit stability, no additional fixation was utilized

caused by ACL deficiency, or meniscal deficiency should be managed with concomitant procedures to optimize the intra-articular environment. To assess for these conditions, a careful physical exam should be performed to assess ligamentous status and static and dynamic alignment. Standing mechanical axis radiographs should be obtained to evaluate limb alignment. MRI can also be helpful to evaluate the integrity of the meniscus, size of the cartilage lesion, and quality of the opposing chondral surface. Of note, MRI should not be used in isolation to predict lesion size. Gomoll and colleagues demonstrated in a retrospective review that MRI may underestimate lesion size by 47–377% (depending on lesion location) when compared with intraoperative findings [6]. Staging arthroscopy or requesting old operative reports and arthroscopic images are both useful strategies to determine the post-debridement dimensions of the lesion in question.

When selecting a revision cartilage repair technique, surgeons should select a technique that it is effective in treating large lesions and damaged subchondral bone. Successful cartilage repair requires recapitulation of the tissue composition, zonal architecture, and material properties of the articular cartilage-subchondral bone unit [7]. Cartilage repair options for larger lesions with compromised subchondral bone include OAT/mosaicplasty, ACI "sandwich" technique with bone grafting, OCA transplantation, and, more recently, biphasic biomimetic osteochondral scaffolds (Agili-C, Cartiheal, Kfar Saba, Israel and MaioRegen Fin-Ceramica Faenza SpA, Italy).

OAT mosaicplasty is an attractive option for revision cartilage repair as it allows immediate restoration of the articular cartilage-subchondral bone unit with autologous tissue (which removes concerns regarding graft availability, graft expense, and disease transmission). Nevertheless, the results of mosaicplasty for large lesions (>3 cm^2) have been less favorable than ACI and OCA. Solheim and colleagues reported a poor long-term outcome (defined as a Lysholm score of 64 or less or having had a knee replacement) in 57% of mosaicplasty patients with lesions >3 cm^2 in size [2]. Bentley and colleagues performed a randomized trial comparing mosaicplasty and ACI for lesions with an average size of 4 cm^2 [8]. The authors reported a failure rate at 10 years of 55% in the mosaicplasty group compared to just 17% in the ACI group. Gudas and colleagues performed a randomized controlled trial comparing mosaicplasty and microfracture for small and medium lesions (<4 cm^2), noting significant improvement in ICRS scores for both techniques and reduced failure with mosaicplasty compared to microfracture at 10 years post-op (14% vs. 38%) [9]. As such, osteochondral autograft remains a viable revision cartilage repair technique for lesions <2–3 cm^2; however, ACI or OCA should be favored for larger lesions.

ACI has been broadly demonstrated to be an effective treatment for full-thickness chondral defects of the knee, with authors consistently reporting good to excellent outcomes in more than 80% of patients. However, due to technical-, patient-, and lesion-specific factors, it remains difficult to determine the optimal place for ACI in the algorithm for treating chondral defects of the knee joint. ACI has displayed favorable results for large lesions; however, the results of ACI following failed cartilage repair in the literature have been controversial. Pestka and colleagues reported a dramatically higher rate of clinical failure in patients with prior marrow stimulation (25% vs. 3.6%) in a matched pair series of 56 patients (28 undergoing primary ACI, 28 with history of marrow stimulation) [10]. Similarly, Zaslav and fellow contributors to the STAR (Study of the Treatment of Articular Repair) clinical trial reported a high rate of clinical failure in ACI patients with history of prior debridement (26%) and marrow stimulation (25%) [11]. Minas and colleagues performed a large-scale series of 321 patients comparing clinical failure rates among ACI patients who had undergone either primary ACI or ACI following failed MST (with failure defined as persistent symptoms in the setting of MRI evidence of graft delamination, surgical removal of 25% of graft area, repeat cartilage procedure, or prosthetic replacement) [12]. The authors reported a dramatically higher rate of clinical failure in the MST cohort compared with those treated with primary ACI (26% vs. 8%). The authors suggested that prior marrow stimulation may result in unfavorable thickening of the subchondral bone and may promote formation of an intralesional osteophyte, both of which compromise graft incorporation. Nevertheless, the authors also noted that in a small cohort, they performed careful lesion prep with a microbur to thin the thickened subchondral bone and that this technique seemed to result in a trend toward reduced failure rate. For the use of ACI in the setting of deep osteochondral lesions, Jones and Peterson proposed the ACI sandwich technique which involves initial placement of bone graft and "sandwiching" the autologous chondrocytes between two membranes on the surface to separate the cells from the underlying bone graft and marrow space. Although limited results are available on this technique, Minas and colleagues reported survival in 87% of ACI sandwich procedures and 90% good/excellent satisfaction at 5 years [13].

Gracitelli and colleagues evaluated the results of osteo-chondral allograft transplantation after failed cartilage repair (163 patients with history of MST, OAT, or ACI) [14]. The authors reported a reoperation rate of 42%; however, graft survivorship was 82% at 10 years, and 89% of patients reported being "extremely satisfied" or "satisfied." Another manuscript from Gracitelli and colleagues compared the results of primary OCA with OCA s/p MST and reported comparable clinical outcomes, clinical failure rates, and patient satisfaction among both groups [15]. Rosa and colleagues performed a recent systematic review of revision cartilage repair techniques and concluded that OCA transplantation is the most reliable treatment in the setting of failed cartilage repair [16].

Off-the-shelf osteochondral scaffolds are an exciting frontier in the treatment of large osteochondral defects as they promise improved accessibility compared to OCA without concern for immunogenicity. MaioRegen (Fin-Ceramica Faenza SpA, Italy) is a tri-layered biomimetic osteochondral scaffold first introduced for clinical use in 2011 in Europe. The superficial layer consists of type I equine collagen, the intermediate layer of 60% equine collagen and 40% magnesium-enriched HA (Mg-HA), and the deep layer of 30% equine collagen and 70% Mg-HA. The scaffold has been shown to induce subchondral trabecular bone regeneration in an equine model [17]. Agili-C (Cartiheal, Israel) is a porous bioabsorbable biphasic scaffold derived from coral, to which HA is added. It contains (1) a bone phase composed of calcium carbonate in an aragonite crystalline form and (2) a cartilage phase composed of modified aragonite and HA [18]. Aragonite possesses a nano-rough surface and porous architecture which permit cell adhesion and proliferation. Kon and colleagues reported complete histologic restoration of hyaline cartilage and subchondral bone in six of seven goats 12 months following treatment with Agili-C [19]. While these products offer promise for revision cartilage repair in the future, to date human patients have only been treated in phase IV clinical trials in Europe.

The revision cartilage repair situation is truly a salvage situation, and patients must be counseled that all available treatment options are fraught with moderate rates of failure and high rates of revision surgery. Multiple studies in the literature have suggested inferior outcomes of ACI following MST compared to primary ACI. The literature comparing primary OCA with OCA s/p MST is limited, but what exists seems to suggest results are unaffected by prior surgery. For patients who have failed a prior MST, we would recommend obtaining an MRI to evaluate for the presence of an intralesional osteophyte or subchondral cystic change. If those anatomic changes are encountered, it is likely wise to favor OCA; however, in their absence the surgeon may proceed with either OCA or ACI.

References

1. Mithoefer K, Williams RJ, Warren RF, Potter HG, Spock CR, Jones EC, Wickiewicz TL, Marx RG. The microfracture technique for the treatment of articular cartilage lesions in the knee. A prospective cohort study. J Bone Joint Surg Am. 2005;87:1911–20.
2. Solheim E, Hegna J, Øyen J, Harlem T, Strand T. Results at 10 to 14 years after osteochondral autografting (mosaicplasty) in articular cartilage defects in the knee. Knee. 2013;20:287–90.
3. Meyer MA, et al. Effectiveness of lavage techniques in removing immunogenic elements from osteochondral allografts. Cartilage. 2017;8(4):369–73.
4. Stoker AM, et al. Bone marrow aspirate concentrate versus platelet rich plasma to enhance osseous integration potential for osteochondral allografts. J Knee Surg. 2018;31(4):314–20.
5. Chahal J, Thiel GV, Hussey K, Cole BJ. Managing the patient with failed cartilage restoration. Sports Med Arthrosc Rev. 2013;21:62–8.

6. Gomoll AH, Yoshioka H, Watanabe A, Dunn JC, Minas T. Preoperative measurement of cartilage defects by MRI underestimates lesion size. Cartilage. 2011;2:389–93.

7. Cook JL, Gomoll AH, Farr J. Commentary on "third-generation autologous chondrocyte implantation versus mosaicplasty for knee cartilage injury: 2-year randomized trial". J Orthop Res. 2016;34:557–8.

8. Bentley G, Biant LC, Vijayan S, Macmull S, Skinner JA, Carrington RWJ. Minimum ten-year results of a prospective randomised study of autologous chondrocyte implantation versus mosaicplasty for symptomatic articular cartilage lesions of the knee. J Bone Joint Surg Br. 2012;94:504–9.

9. Gudas R, Gudaitė A, Pocius A, Gudienė A, Čekanauskas E, Monastyreckiene E, Basevičius A. Ten-year follow-up of a prospective, randomized clinical study of mosaic osteochondral autologous transplantation versus microfracture for the treatment of osteochondral defects in the knee joint of athletes. Am J Sports Med. 2012;40:2499–508.

10. Pestka JM, Bode G, Salzmann G, Sudkamp NP, Niemeyer P. Clinical outcome of autologous chondrocyte implantation for failed microfracture treatment of full-thickness cartilage defects of the knee joint. Am J Sports Med. 2012;40:325–31.

11. Zaslav K, Cole B, Brewster R, DeBerardino T, Farr J, Fowler P, Nissen C. A prospective study of autologous chondrocyte implantation in patients with failed prior treatment for articular cartilage defect of the knee: results of the Study of the Treatment of Articular Repair (STAR) clinical trial. Am J Sports Med. 2008;37:42–55.

12. Minas T, Gomoll AH, Rosenberger R, Royce RO, Bryant T. Increased failure rate of autologous chondrocyte implantation after previous treatment with marrow stimulation techniques. Am J Sports Med. 2009;37:902–8.

13. Minas T, Ogura T, Headrick J, Bryant T. Autologous chondrocyte implantation "Sandwich" technique compared with autologous bone grafting for deep osteochondral lesions in the knee. Am J Sports Med. 2017;16:036354651773800.

14. Gracitelli GC, Meric G, Pulido PA, McCauley JC, Bugbee WD. Osteochondral allograft transplantation for knee lesions after failure of cartilage repair surgery. Cartilage. 2014;6:98–105.

15. Gracitelli GC, Meric G, Briggs DT, Pulido PA, McCauley JC, Belloti JC, Bugbee WD. Fresh osteochondral allografts in the

knee: comparison of primary transplantation versus transplantation after failure of previous subchondral marrow stimulation. Am J Sports Med. 2015;43:885–91.

16. Rosa D, Di Donato S, Balato G, D'Addona A, Smeraglia F, Correra G, Di Vico G. How to manage a failed cartilage repair: a systematic literature review. Joints. 2017;05:093–106.

17. Kon E, Mutini A, Arcangeli E, Delcogliano M, Filardo G, Nicoli Aldini N, Pressato D, Quarto R, Zaffagnini S, Marcacci M. Novel nanostructured scaffold for osteochondral regeneration: pilot study in horses. J Tissue Eng Regen Med. 2010;4:300–8.

18. Kon E, Robinson D, Verdonk P, Drobnic M. A novel aragonite-based scaffold for osteochondral regeneration: early experience on human implants and technical developments. Injury. 2016;47:S27.

19. Kon E, Filardo G, Shani J, Altschuler N, Levy A, Zaslav K, Eisman JE, Robinson D. Osteochondral regeneration with a novel aragonite-hyaluronate biphasic scaffold: up to 12-month follow-up study in a goat model. J Orthop Surg Res. 2015;10:81.

Chapter 14
Medial Meniscus Allograft Transplantation in the Setting of Revision Anterior Cruciate Ligament Reconstruction

Trevor R. Gulbrandsen, Katie Freeman, and Seth L. Sherman

Case Presentation

This patient is a 24-year-old female with a complex history relating to recurrent right knee pain and instability. As a 15-year-old high school soccer athlete, she sustained a contact injury resulting in an anterior cruciate ligament (ACL) rup-

The original version of this chapter was revised. A correction to this chapter is available at https://doi.org/10.1007/978-3-030-01491-9_19

T. R. Gulbrandsen
Department of Orthopaedic Surgery, University of Iowa Hospitals and Clinics, Iowa City, IA, USA

K. Freeman
Department of Orthopedic Surgery and Rehabilitation, University of Nebraska Medical Center, Omaha, NE, USA

S. L. Sherman (✉)
Department of Orthopaedic Surgery, University of Missouri, Columbia, MO, USA

Missouri Orthopaedic Institute, Columbia, MO, USA
e-mail: shermanse@health.missouri.edu

ture and medial meniscus tear. This was treated with hamstring autograft ACL reconstruction and medial meniscal repair at an outside institution. She returned to sport but a year later sustained a noncontact injury with re-rupture of the ACL. This was treated with revision ACL reconstruction using allograft and partial medial meniscectomy. She again returned to sport but at the age of 18 sustained another noncontact injury with a third ACL rupture. This was again treated with re-revision ACL allograft and subtotal medial meniscectomy. The patient's knee never returned to normal following this surgery. She presented to our clinic with 1 year of insidious worsening right knee pain and instability even with daily life activity. Her right knee "gives way" and has diffuse but mostly medial-based pain and activity-related swelling. This problem is significantly affecting her overall quality of life.

On physical examination, the patient had a BMI of 24. She has near neutral alignment and walks with a non-antalgic gait. She has adequate dynamic strength and is able to squat with reasonable symmetry. Involved side demonstrates well-healed incisions, good quadriceps tone, and ROM that is 10-0-140 and equal to the opposite limb. Anterior drawer test is grossly positive. Lachman test is a grade 3B; pivot shift is a grade 3. Posterior sag and posterior drawer are negative. There is tenderness to palpation along the medial joint line with a negative McMurray test. Varus and valgus stress at 0° and 30° is stable. Prone dial test is symmetric at 30° and 90°. Distal compartments are soft and otherwise neurovascularly intact.

Weight-bearing AP, PA flexion, and lateral and Merchant view radiographs demonstrated a posteriorly placed nonanatomic ACL tibial tunnel with suggestion of tunnel widening. There was some early narrowing of the medial compartment. The mechanical axis view demonstrates neutral alignment. Lateral tibial x-ray demonstrates normal tibial slope. Magnetic resonance imaging showed evidence of medial meniscus deficiency (Fig. 14.1).

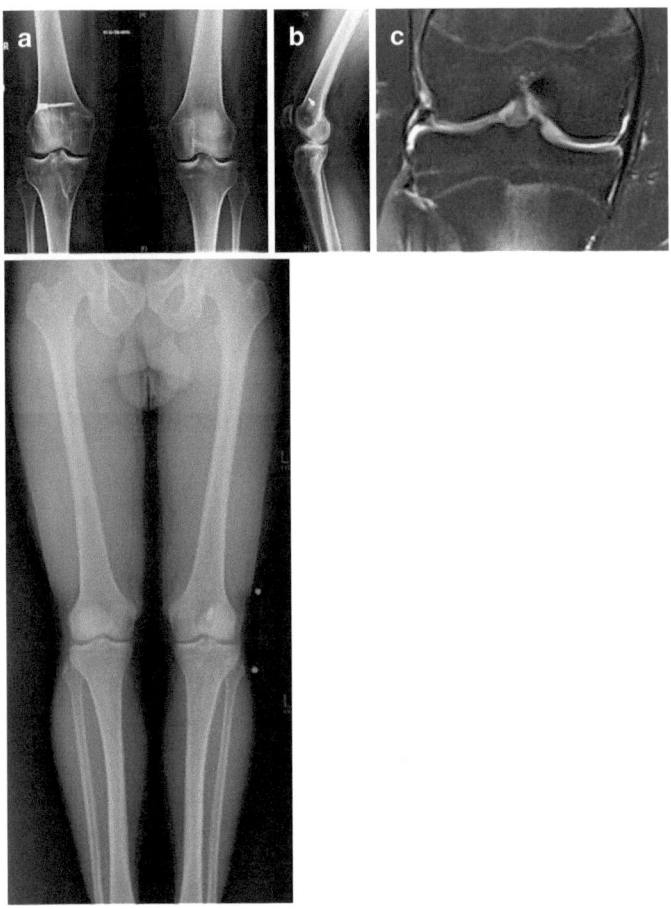

FIGURE 14.1 Preoperative Rosenberg (**a**) and lateral radiographs (**b**) showing previous ACL reconstruction button. Preoperative coronal MRI showing meniscus deficiency and healthy articular cartilage (**c**). Preoperative mechanical axis radiograph demonstrating normal alignment

Diagnosis/Assessment

The patient's clinical presentation is consistent with attritional failure of her third ACL reconstruction and symptomatic medial meniscal deficiency. Her alignment in both the coronal and sagittal planes is neutral without varus or increased tibial slope. She does not have any obvious large, focal full-thickness cartilage defects. Lateral and patellofemoral compartments are unremarkable.

The patient has several risk factors for failure of her prior ACL reconstructions including young age, high activity level, early return to play, prior graft choices, tunnel position, underlying hyperlaxity, and medial meniscus deficiency. Regarding graft choices, primary ACL reconstruction with hamstring is commonly performed, but there are concerns with this choice regarding graft laxity and increased failure rate, particularly in young female athletes with small hamstring grafts and underlying hyperlaxity. For revision and re-revision, there is also concern that allograft ACL reconstruction may have a higher failure rate than revision using autograft tissue. For both the primary and revision settings, ACL tunnel position is critical and likely nonanatomic in this case. Additionally, there is concern for tibial ACL tunnel widening that may require bone grafting prior to any definitive salvage intervention. Underlying hyperlaxity is a clinical problem that may influence outcome and should be addressed at the time of repeat revision surgery. Medial meniscal deficiency is a major cause of ACL reconstruction failure. The medial meniscus is an important secondary stabilizer to anterior translation whereby medial meniscal deficiency puts undue stress on the ACL graft and may lead to recurrent laxity and failure. This should also be addressed at the time of repeat revision.

Management

Given her complex problem list, staging arthroscopy is a reasonable option to consider for this patient. Staging will allow careful examination under anesthesia with a focus on confirming ACL functional instability and identifying missed laxity of her secondary stabilizers (i.e., posteromedial, posterolateral). ROM assessment will ensure symmetry with the opposite limb or allow for treatment of arthrofibrosis before definitive revision surgery. Regarding the ACL reconstruction, prior graft material and/or hardware in the path of future revision should be removed. Tunnels should be evaluated and debrided with bone grafting performed as indicated.

Arthroscopy will also confirm medial meniscus deficiency and allow for initial preparation of 2–3 mm rim of healthy meniscus for future meniscus allograft transplantation (MAT). Additionally, arthroscopy will rule out concomitant cartilage pathology that may require treatment at the definitive intervention. If there is malalignment present, realignment osteotomy (i.e., valgus-producing HTO, slope-decreasing HTO, biplanar HTO) should be performed at index procedure following arthroscopy. This is not indicated for the above patient.

EUA confirmed preserved ROM including symmetric hyperlaxity to 10°. Lachman and pivot remained grade 3 B and grade 3, respectively. Other secondary stabilizers were intact. On staging arthroscopy, there was notable tricompartment synovitis and scar adhesions that were lysed. The previous ACL allograft was lax and functionally incompetent. This was removed to better evaluate ACL tunnels. The femoral tunnel was vertical and not within the ACL footprint and could be left alone as it would not interfere with revision surgery. The tibial tunnel was posterior to the anatomic footprint and would also not require bone grafting because it would not significantly overlap with our revision tunnel. The medial meniscus had evidence of deficiency following prior meniscectomy, particularly in the mid-body (Fig. 14.2). A small meniscal root flap tear was debrided. The meniscus was prepared to a healthy rim of 2–3 mm of remnant tissue. Chondroplasty was performed for a small, less than 2 cm^2, grades 2–3 unstable cartilage lesion of the medial femoral condyle. The medial tibial plateau had diffuse grade 1 softening with an area posterior of grade 2 changes that was left alone. Lateral and patellofemoral compartments were unremarkable.

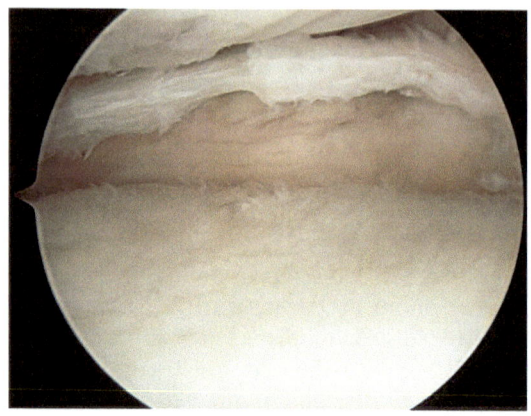

FIGURE 14.2 Medial compartment with severe meniscus deficiency

The patient recovered uneventfully from staging arthroscopy. She was able to WBAT with a compression sleeve, wean her crutches over 1–2 weeks, and regain full ROM. After obtaining insurance approval and finding an acceptable size-age-matched MAT graft, she underwent definitive salvage intervention 3 months after staging arthroscopy. Pre-surgical planning is documented below.

Problem List

Repeat revision ACL reconstruction: Tunnels are nonanatomic and avoidable with standard drilling techniques. Graft choice will be soft tissue-only quadriceps autograft fixed with suspensory fixation using an all-inside technique.

Medial meniscal deficiency: MAT using fresh frozen size- and age-matched allograft tissue. Bone plug MAT for the medial side can avoid the ACL footprint and preserve bone stock since the anterior and posterior insertions are farther apart and obliquely oriented on the medial side.

MFC chondral lesion: <2 cm2 and not full thickness. If progressed to full thickness, OAT autograft vs. consignment osteochondral allograft performed through mini-arthrotomy after MAT can be considered. It likely would not need to be addressed if no progression.

Hyperlaxity: In the revision setting, this can be managed with the addition of a lateral extra-articular tenodesis, performed using either a strip of iliotibial band or allograft tissue.

Surgical Technique

General anesthesia was performed along with a single-shot adductor canal nerve block.

Quadriceps harvest was performed with the use of a tourniquet. The tourniquet was deflated following harvest and not used for the remainder of the case. A 10 mm double blade was used to harvest a 70 mm soft tissue-only full-thickness quadriceps graft. The extensor mechanism was repaired with running 0 vicryl suture. The ACL graft was prepared on the back table (QuadLink construct using TightRope suspensory fixation). The femoral graft diameter was 9.5 mm and tibial diameter 10.5 mm. The graft was pretensioned on the back table.

Arthroscopy was then initiated, and a lysis of adhesions was done to improve access and visualization. There was no evidence of disease progression on the cartilage surfaces and no indication for cartilage restoration, which was not performed. Attention was turned to the medial compartment. The deep medial collateral ligament was trephinated with a spinal needle, which was performed in order to gain improved access to the compartment. A reverse notchplasty was performed with a power rasp. The meniscus remnant was debrided to a 2–3 mm rim of healthy stable meniscus. A flip cutter was brought in through the medial portal to the posterior root insertion, and a 9.5 mm × 10 mm socket was reamed. A shuttle suture was then passed.

The femoral revision ACL tunnel was then prepared. The flexible reamer was brought into the knee through the anteromedial portal. A 9.5 mm × 30 mm socket was reamed. It was recognized that the lateral femoral cortex was weakened by prior surgery. Decision was made to utilize an extended femoral TightRope button to ensure adequate suspensory fixation.

The femoral ACL guidewire was left in place, and attention was turned to the approach and preparation for the lateral extra-articular tenodesis. A 6 cm incision was made along the lateral aspect of the knee, and the iliotibial band was split. The lateral collateral ligament (LCL) was identified, and a guidewire was placed posterior and proximal to the origin of the LCL for the lateral extra-articular tenodesis.

AP and lateral plane radiographs were then obtained with fluoroscopy to confirm the position. The guidewire was over-reamed to accommodate the tenodesis graft. Shuttle sutures for the femoral ACL and lateral tenodesis were passed at this time.

Attention was then turned to the tibia. A flipcutter was used to create a 10.5 mm × 28 mm tibial ACL socket, and a shuttle suture was passed. With the knee in hyperflexion, a high anteromedial portal was established to prepare the anterior medial meniscal root insertion. A guidewire was placed in the anatomic origin of the anterior root of the medial meniscus and was over-reamed in an antegrade fashion to create a 9 mm × 10 mm socket. An ACL guide was used to shuttle a suture into this socket from the medial aspect of the tibia. Zone-specific cannulas were then used with an inside-out technique to shuttle two sutures through the junction of the mid-meniscus remnant with the anterior and posterior horns, respectively. These would be used during graft passage and fixation (Figs. 14.3 and 14.4).

The meniscus transplant had been previously prepared. The bone plugs were 9 mm × 3 mm and loaded with suspensory cortical suture ×2 for the anterior and posterior meniscal root. Two labral tapes were placed at the junction of the mid-meniscus with the anterior and posterior horn, respectively. A passport cannula was placed medially and MAT shuttle sutures were retrieved. The meniscus transplant was shuttled uneventfully into the joint, and posterior root suspensory cortical fixation was provisionally secured (Figs. 14.5 and 14.6).

The anterior suspensory cortical fixation was then provisionally secured for the anterior root. There was no appreciable graft mismatch. Hybrid meniscus fixation was performed with combination of all-inside for the posterior horn, inside-out for the mid-body, and outside-in for the anterior horn. FastFix was used posteriorly. The three inside-out

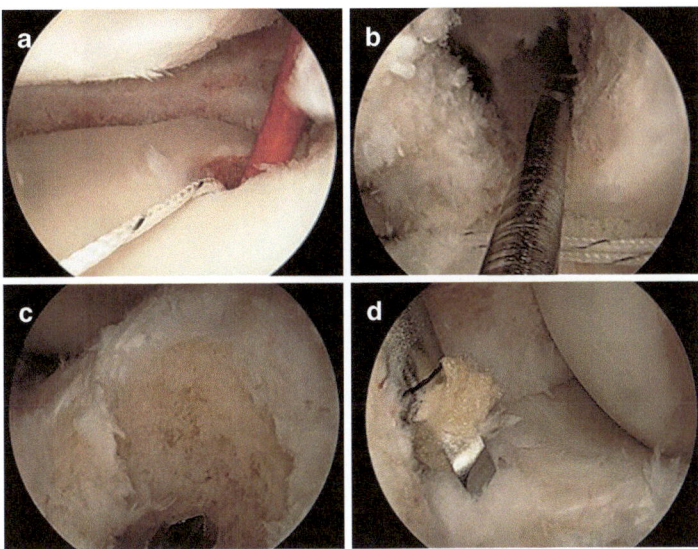

FIGURE 14.3 (**a**) Posterior meniscal tunnel using ACL guide to pass shuttle stitch. (**b**) Femoral ACL tunnel. (**c**) Tibial ACL tunnel. (**d**) Low-Profile Reamer through accessory high AM portal in deeper flexion

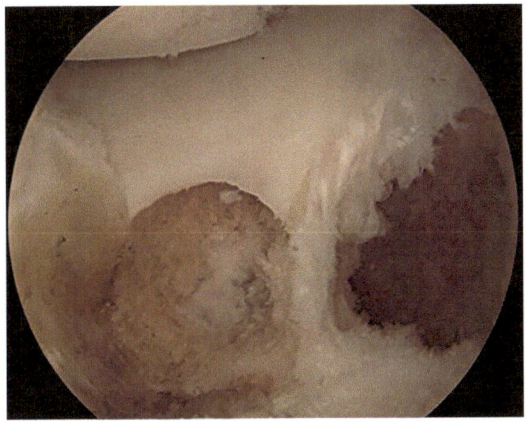

FIGURE 14.4 Anterior meniscal tunnel (left tunnel) in proximity to the femoral ACL tunnel (right tunnel)

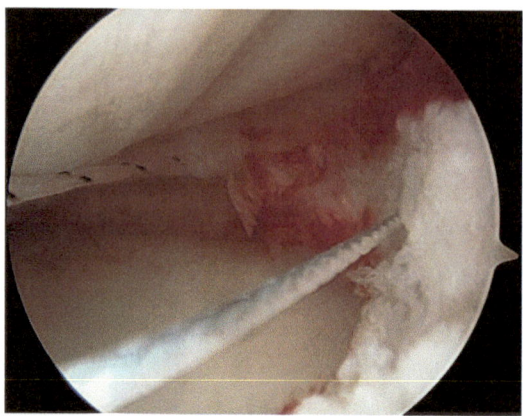

FIGURE 14.5 Shuttling sutures for the medial meniscus allograft

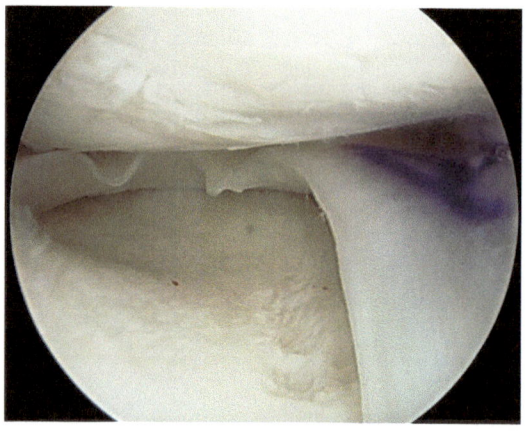

FIGURE 14.6 MAT in place in the medial compartment

FiberWire sutures and the labral tapes from the MAT were retrieved through a medial-based incision. The suture pairs were tied in extension, and the labral tapes were secured to the tibia to reproduce the meniscotibial ligaments. Outside-in technique was used to pass a no. 2 FiberWire in a horizontal mattress fashion through the anterior horn of the meniscus that was tied over the capsule. The MAT was probed and determined to be stable throughout a ROM arc with no need for further fixation.

Attention was turned to the ACL reconstruction. Shuttle sutures were passed through the passport cannula, which was subsequently removed. The femoral suspensory cortical sutures were shuttled through the anteromedial portal and out the lateral based incision. The femoral button was docked on the lateral cortex using direct and fluoroscopic visualization. The quadriceps autograft was then pulled into the femoral socket. The knee was cycled and brought into full extension where the tibial button was placed and secured. Lachman and pivot shift demonstrated good stability. Direct visualization demonstrated that the ACL graft had good physiologic tension without any graft impingement in extension. There was at least 20 mm of graft in both the femoral and tibial tunnels.

Finally, attention was turned to the lateral extra-articular tenodesis. The semitendinosus graft was prepared with a suspensory cortical fixation suture. The suspensory cortical suture was shuttled into the femoral tunnel and secured on the far medial cortex. The graft was provisionally brought into the femoral tunnel. The graft was then looped under the LCL and brought to a point midway between Gerdy's tubercle and the fibular head, approximately 1.5 cm distal to the joint line. The graft was secured in this location using a SwiveLock anchor with the knee at 30°. The graft was finally tensioned on the femoral side using the suspensory cortical fixation device. The graft demonstrated favorable anisometry, tight in extension and loose in flexion (Figs. 14.7 and 14.8).

Outcome

This patient has had an expected gradual recovery with mild stiffness in terminal flexion. At 7 months postoperative, she was making excellent subjective and objective gains. She had good quadriceps tone, no effusion, no tenderness, and near-full extension that was lacking 5–10° of terminal flexion. At 9 months she had continual recovery with her outcomes

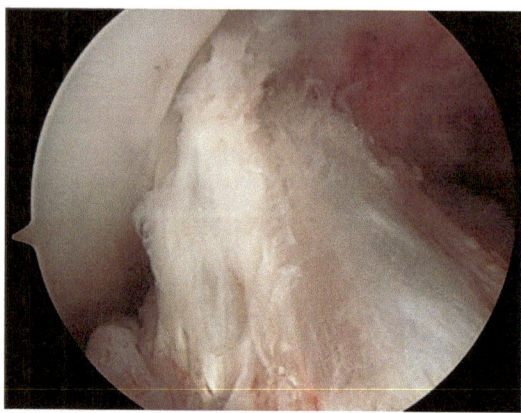

FIGURE 14.7 Quadriceps ACL autograft

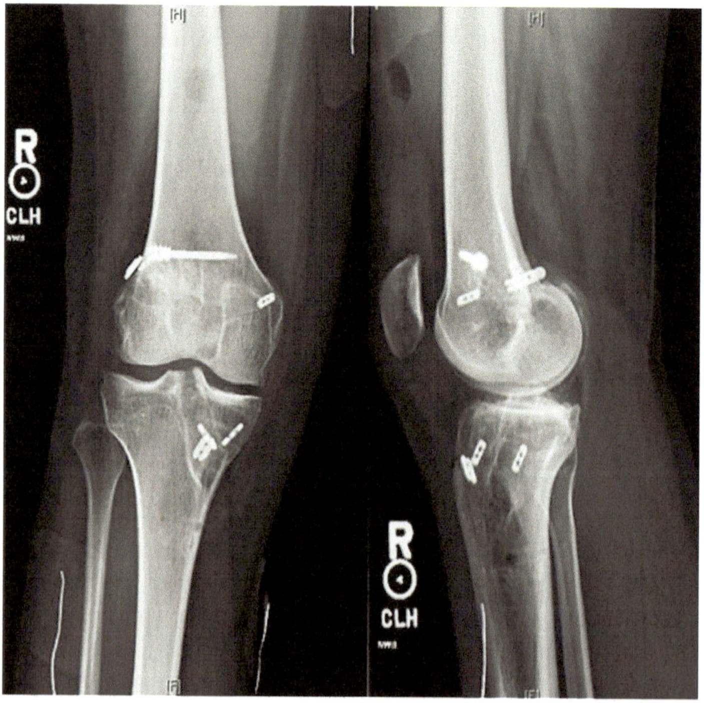

FIGURE 14.8 Postoperative AP and lateral radiographs showing quadriceps autograft suspensory cortical buttons and medial meniscal suspensory cortical fixation placement

scores that were a Single Assessment Numeric Evaluation (SANE) value of 25 and a Visual Analogue Scale (VAS) of 3.4.

Literature Review

The medial meniscus has a conferred mid-body attachment to the deep medial collateral ligament as well as adjacent anchoring of the posterior horn to the PCL in the intercondylar area. Due to these important attachments, the medial meniscus plays a unique role in stabilization in regard to anterior translation, especially in the ACL-deficient state [1, 2].

Untreated ligamentous instability (i.e., ACL, PCL, PLC, MCL) is a contraindication for meniscal allograft transplantation due to the increased risk factor of failure of the transplant. Furthermore, due to the previously described stabilizing role of the medial meniscus, meniscal deficiency could lead to increased stress forces on the ACL reconstruction [3]. In 1995, Van Arkel and de Boer were the first to suggest the benefits of combined ACL reconstruction and MAT, indicating that the ACL could provide knee stability and the MAT could decrease the risk of ACL graft failure [4]. Since then, ACL and medial MAT arthroscopic surgical techniques have dramatically improved, resulting in more successful outcomes.

Although there have been few long-term follow-up studies on combined ACL reconstruction and medial MAT, there have been several short-term follow-up reports that have confirmed the benefit of combined ACL reconstruction and MAT. Sekiya et al. looked at the clinical outcomes of 28 patients after combined ACLR and MAT with an average follow-up of 2.8 years. Twenty-one of those 28 had medial MAT/ACLR. On follow-up, these patients had improved clinical outcome scores including Activities of Daily Living Scale of the Knee Outcome Survey score of 89.9, Sports Activities Scale score of 80.0, and Lysholm score of 92.5. On radiographic studies there was no significant difference in joint space narrowing between the transplanted compartment and that of the contralateral knee [5].

Graf et al. reported an 8.5-year follow-up of clinical and radiographic outcomes in eight patients who underwent combined ACLR and medial MAT: six consisted of patellar tendon allograft ACLs, and two consisted of patellar tendon autograft. Using IKDC symptom evaluation, they reported improvement in subjective clinical outcome scores with two normal scores, five nearly normal scores, and one abnormal score. They additionally reported five normal scores, one nearly normal score, and two abnormal scores on the IKDC functional test assessment. Significantly, six of the eight patients reported that they were extremely pleased with the function of their knee and were able to participate in recreational sports [6].

Furthermore, Saltzman et al. reported the benefit of concomitant ACLR and MAT in enhancing objective knee stability. They reported a 5-year follow-up of 40 patients on clinical and radiographic outcomes after concomitant ACLR and MAT. Thirty-three (82.5%) of the 40 consisted of medial MAT. There were significant improvements in both patient-reported outcomes and clinical outcome scores. On the final follow-up, the mean medial joint space height decreased from 5.2 ± 1.1 mm preoperatively to 4.5 ± 0.8 mm ($p = 0.02$). There were no significant differences in ligament laxity on 30Ib and maximum manual strength. There were, however, eight (24%) reported graft failures (one patient requiring revision MAT, six patients progressing to total knee arthroplasty, and one patient requiring revision ACLR/MAT) [7].

When deciding on the best surgical technique for concomitant primary or revision ACL reconstruction with medial MAT, several factors must be considered including adequate anatomic footprint restoration, preserved bone stock, and fixation strategy. The medial meniscus has a wide separation of the anterior and posterior horns in the sagittal plane. Additionally in the axial plane, the horn attachments have an oblique trajectory. Due to these anatomical factors, modified surgical techniques using bone plugs have advantages in the medial compartment. The bone plug technique provides flexibility to adjust for small graft size mismatch and helps to restore the horns to anatomic location while sustaining bone stock preservation. Though technically demanding, the trough meniscus transplant technique can be performed in conjunction with ACL reconstruction as well, even in the lateral compartment.

As described in this case, medial MAT with concomitant ACL reconstruction can be a successful procedure providing radiographic and clinical improvements with proper patient selection and preoperative planning.

Clinical Pearls
- Recognition of risk factors for failure of the previous ACL reconstruction is a critical first step in the workup of these complex patients (i.e., graft choice, tunnel position, meniscal deficiency, malalignment, unrecognized secondary stabilizer injury, etc.).
- Workup must include thorough H&P including evaluation of prior surgical reports, weight-bearing x-rays including assessment of sagittal and coronal alignment, and advanced imaging study (i.e., MRI).
- Staging arthroscopy can be advantageous. This will allow for careful EUA, lysis of adhesions, removal of hardware, tunnel bone grafting, and precise evaluation of chondral or meniscal lesions. Realignment osteotomy may be performed at the time of staging arthroscopy, as indicated.
- Second-stage surgery includes all intra-articular work including revision ACL reconstruction and medial MAT. The medial MAT should be completed prior to placing and tensioning the ACL graft. Cartilage restoration may also be performed during this stage.
- In general, bone plug medial MAT is preferred for these combined cases as it is technically easier, bone stock preserving, and ACL tunnel sparing and can accommodate for graft size mismatch better than

trough techniques. The use of soft tissue ACL auto-graft and suspensory cortical fixation is also advantageous in these combined cases with closely drilled tunnels.

- Appropriate counseling and realistic patient expectations are *critical*. Combined ACL reconstruction and medial MAT is a salvage procedure. The goal is functional stability and pain relief for daily life and improvement of quality of life. Sporting goals are secondary and may not be achievable. Durability may be placed at significant risk with high-impact loading, which should likely be avoided. These procedures do not last forever and should be considered as bridges for future intervention including eventual arthroplasty.

References

1. Śmigielski R, Becker R, Zdanowicz U, et al. Medial meniscus anatomy—from basic science to treatment. Knee Surg Sports Traumatol Arthrosc. 2015;23:8.
2. Allen CR, Wong EK, Livesay GA, Sakane M, Fu FH, Woo SL. Importance of the medial meniscus in the anterior cruciate ligament-deficient knee. J Orthop Res. 2000;18(1):109–15.
3. Deledda D, Rosso F, Cottino U, Bonasia DE, Rossi R. Results of meniscectomy and meniscal repair in anterior cruciate ligament reconstruction. Joints. 2015;3(3):151–7.
4. van Arkel ER, de Boer HH. Human meniscal transplantation. Preliminary results at 2 to 5-year follow-up. J Bone Joint Surg Br. 1995;77:589–95.
5. Sekiya JK, Giffin JR, Irrgang JJ, Fu FH, Harner CD. Clinical outcomes after combined meniscal allograft transplantation and anterior cruciate ligament reconstruction. Am J Sports Med. 2003;31:896–906.

6. Graf KW Jr, Sekiya JK, Wojtys EM. Long-term results after combined medial meniscal allograft transplantation and anterior cruciate ligament reconstruction: minimum 8.5-year follow-up study. Arthroscopy. 2004;20:129–40.

7. Saltzman BM, Meyer MA, Weber AE, Poland SG, Yanke AB, Cole BJ. Prospective clinical and radiographic outcomes after concomitant anterior cruciate ligament reconstruction and meniscal allograft transplantation at a mean 5-year follow-up. Am J Sports Med. 2017;45:550–62.

Chapter 15
Tibiofemoral Cartilage Defect with Malalignment

Christian Lattermann and Burak Altintas

Chief Complaint

Medial knee pain

History of Present Illness

The patient is a 34-year-old otherwise healthy and athletic, non-smoking female who is a passionate water skier and teacher presents with 2 years of atraumatic pain in the medial side of the knee. She reports temporary swelling of the joint and pain after activity and sometimes during weight-bearing along the medial aspect. She denies any feeling of instability. She has occasional swelling and stiffness that resolve overnight. She reports having a partial medial meniscectomy 10 years ago. Nonoperative treatment with ice, elevation, and anti-inflammatory medications did not provide lasting relief.

C. Lattermann (✉)
Brigham and Women's Hospital, Harvard Medical School,
Boston, MA, USA
e-mail: clattermann@bwh.harvard.edu

B. Altintas
Steadman Philippon Clinic, Vail, CO, USA

© Springer Nature Switzerland AG 2019
A. B. Yanke, B. J. Cole (eds.), *Joint Preservation of the Knee*,
https://doi.org/10.1007/978-3-030-01491-9_15

Pearls
- History of partial meniscectomy: Partial meniscectomy is a risk factor for chondral degeneration. Particularly pain after activity is an indicator of possible degenerative changes rather than an acute injury.

Physical Examination

The patient has a normal BMI of 23.5. She walks with a normal gait and gross macroscopic alignment of the lower extremity shows varus deformity. The right knee has no effusion, soft tissue swelling, erythema, or warmth. The range of motion is from 0° to 135°. There is tenderness to palpation over the medial compartment diffusely more along the proximal tibia than the joint line. Meniscal tests (flexion, compression, rotation) are negative. There is good patellofemoral tracking without crepitus. The ligamentous examination shows no abnormalities. The neurovascular examination is within normal limits.

Pearls
- Medial-sided symptoms: Medial-sided symptoms may have their origin in the joint but can also come from other medial structures such as pes anserine bursitis, a meniscal cyst, or medial collateral ligament injury. A comprehensive exam is important to delineate if this is specific to the joint line or proximal or distal to the joint. Questions related to the pain before, during, and after activity are an important discriminator regarding acute and chronic as well as stable and unstable meniscal injuries. Finally, medial

overload can also cause generalized medial-sided pain. Inspection of the gait and alignment should be done in all cases.
- Effusion: Any effusion is suspicious for chondral damage. Effusions that are not self-limited may be more synovial irritation and can happen with OA, RA, or severe overloading. Effusions that resolve overnight and reoccur with specific events may be structurally related to a chondral or meniscus injury.

Imaging

Imaging with standard x-rays of the knee (AP and lateral) is obtained to evaluate for avascular necrosis, osseous lesions, or joint space narrowing. In this case, the plain radiographs show low-grade medial joint space narrowing (2 mm). The long-leg alignment (MTP-2) view shows varus malalignment of 6°. Due to the normal joint space on radiographs, an MRI was ordered to assess the articular cartilage and meniscus status and showed a 2 cm^2 chondral defect in the medial femoral condyle with an intact subchondral bone plate. There were also findings consistent with a prior partial medial meniscectomy. There is no evidence of damage to the lateral meniscus or the ligaments.

Pearls
- Varus malalignment: Alignment plays an important role in decision-making, as malalignment can predispose to overloading on either side of the joint. A clinical diagnosis of axial deformity should be verified with a single leg weight-bearing (MTP-2) long-leg alignment x-ray.

Approach to Treatment

The following aspects should be considered in this young active patient with persistent symptoms related to a symptomatic cartilage lesion of the medial femoral condyle with varus malalignment and prior meniscal deficiency:

1. Evaluating alignment is crucial for the treatment planning. This patient has a varus deformity with a concomitant chondral lesion on the medial side. The choice to include osteotomy typically requires the weight-bearing line to be in the affected joint compartment.
2. The patient is status post partial medial meniscectomy, which puts her at increased risk of early medial osteoarthritis. If the diagnostic arthroscopy shows a re-rupture of the medial meniscus, this should be debrided judiciously. If a subtotal or total meniscectomy is needed, meniscus transplantation should be considered due to the young age of this patient. The patient should be counseled regarding having a higher risk of advanced medial osteoarthritis in the future with a need of joint replacement surgery. It should be clearly conveyed that this procedure is performed to alleviate her symptoms and prevent an early replacement surgery.
3. Though the evidence can be inconsistent, treating the cartilage lesion in conjunction with the malalignment is typically recommended. The type of cartilage modality that is chosen is likely secondary to the fact that it should be addressed in some way.
4. Patient's ability and willingness for compliance should not be noted. Especially, the limited weight-bearing following the osteotomy should be discussed carefully.

In case of a combination of malalignment with cartilage abnormalities, the primary objective should be the correction of the alignment. A thorough analysis of the long-leg standing radiographs must be done to determine how to correct the deformity. The genu varum arises typically from the tibia; however the distal femoral angle should be measured as well.

If the origin is from the proximal tibia, either a medial open-wedge or lateral closing-wedge high tibial osteotomy (HTO) can be performed. The movement of the tibia into valgus reduces the forces acting onto the medial compartment, at the expense of increased lateral cartilage stress. Therefore it should be kept in mind that overcorrection can lead to rapid degeneration in the lateral compartment [1]. A recent study by Tsukada et al. showed no significant differences in terms of the ratio of cartilage repair tissue in the medial compartment between 17 overcorrected knees with mean deformity of $15° \pm 1°$ and 54 moderately corrected knees with mean deformity of $10° \pm 2°$ after open-wedge HTO [2].

With appropriate patient selection, accurate preoperative planning, modern surgical fixation techniques, and rapid rehabilitation, it is an effective biological treatment for degenerative disease, deformity, and knee instability and also as an adjunct to other complex joint surfaces and meniscal cartilage surgeries [3]. Bonasia et al. analyzed prognostic factors and showed that advanced age, possibly obesity and failure to regain adequate postoperative motion, may predispose to early failure. On the other hand, younger patients with good knee function and only mild degenerative joint disease appear to be ideal candidates for this procedure [4]. In critical or borderline indications, the temporary use of an unloading valgus producing knee brace may well predict future outcome of HTO surgery in terms of expectable postoperative pain relief [5]. A lateral closing-wedge HTO is usually performed for osteoarthritis patients with no morphotype alterations and with light or moderate deformity. However, it is more difficult to change the tibial slope. Additional factors that influence the choice of osteotomy include age, bone quality, patellar height, and functional demand. Patients at risk for nonunion, such as patients with a high BMI or smokers, should be strongly considered for closing-wedge osteotomy, if as surgical candidates at all [6]. Relative and absolute contraindications for osteotomy include significant osteoarthritis and cartilage/meniscus lesion in the contralateral compartment, bone loss of more than 3 mm in the affected compartment with high risk of subsequent joint instability, reduced range of motion with more than 10° extension loss, less than 90° of knee flexion, more than 20° of need for correction, advanced knee instability, morbid obesity, smoking and rheumatoid arthritis, or other systemic joint disease [7]. The relationship of smoking and outcomes from articular cartilage surgery in the knee suggests an overall negative influence [8]. Regarding cartilage regeneration, a recent study demonstrated cartilage regeneration after opening-wedge valgus HTO, which was affected by BMI, preoperative cartilage degeneration grade, and postoperative limb alignment. The authors underlined that patient selection based on BMI rather than age should be considered [9].

The preservation of the tibiofibular joint and the posterolateral structures along with easier adjustment of the tibial slope are the main advantages of the medial open-wedge HTO. The disadvantages lie in the risk of correction loss and nonunion together with longer rehabilitation due to limited weight-bearing. On the other hand, lateral closing-wedge HTO allows earlier weight-bearing and has less risk of nonunion and loss of correction. However, closing-wedge osteotomy alters the tibial shape, which can complicate subsequent arthroplasty [6]. Complications include neurovascular injuries (peroneal nerve), as the most serious ones, along with non-/malunion, infection, deep vein thrombosis, and intraoperative fracture of the tibial plateau [10].

Retrospective analysis of 533 patients revealed favorable midterm results after valgus HTO in varus osteoarthritis even in older patients with a high degree of cartilage damage [11]. Jung et al. demonstrated that the degenerated cartilage of the medial femoral condyle and medial tibial plateau could be partially or entirely covered by newly regenerated cartilage at 2 years after adequate correction of varus deformity by medial opening-wedge HTO without cartilage regeneration strategies [12]. However, these results should be interpreted with caution due to short-term follow-up and sole macroscopic evaluation without histology. Other studies with short-term follow-up reported promising results [13, 14]. Bode et al.

analyzed the outcome in 51 patients and reported a survival rate of over 96% at 5 years, concluding HTO as a reliable treatment option with satisfying and stable clinical outcome following 60 months [15]. Hantes et al. demonstrated that medial open-wedge HTO with a locking plate is an effective joint preservation method to treat medial compartment osteoarthritis in active patients younger than 45 years with satisfactory clinical and radiological results along with a 95% survival rate 12 years postoperatively [16]. A study on sporting activity following HTO for the treatment of medial compartment knee osteoarthritis in the active patient demonstrated favorable clinical results and allowed patients to return to sports and recreational activities similar to the preoperative level [17].

Despite the abundance of literature favoring the utilization of open-wedge HTO for varus knee deformity, Kanamaya et al. showed improved JOA scores after short-term follow-up following closing-wedge osteotomy [18]. Furthermore, a recent study comparing both techniques demonstrated favorable clinical outcomes for patients who underwent a closed-wedge osteotomy after a mean follow-up of 7.9 years [19].

The chondral damage of the medial compartment in patients with repairable chondral defects and no established OA should be addressed at the time of osteotomy [20]. In the United States, HTO was performed at a significantly higher rate in conjunction with autologous chondrocyte implantation and open osteochondral allograft [21]. However, in this chapter, we will focus on marrow stimulating therapy. Parker et al. showed in an MRI follow-up study on patients following medial opening-wedge HTO that after a non-weight-bearing period, the rate of change in the medial compartment changed from negative to positive, indicating the potential for articular cartilage recovery secondary to an improved mechanical environment [22]. Early results following HTO with an external fixator and microfracture for the varus knee with medial chondral wear in 33 patients led to significant improvements in WOMAC and Lysholm scores [23]. The combination of HTO and chondral resurfacing on 91 knees with a minimum follow-up of 5 years was deemed effective in the treatment of severe medial osteoarthritis and varus malalignment as a high survival rate of 95.2% was found indicating that arthroplasty can be initially postponed in most of these patients [24]. On the contrary, another study showed that subchondral drilling had no effect on the outcome at 2 years after medial open-wedge HTO [25]. Akizuki et al. showed that 64% of the regenerated tissue following abrasion arthroplasty for medial compartment osteoarthritis with eburnation in patients undergoing HTO consisted of fibrocartilage at around 12 months after surgery. However, there was no difference in the clinical outcome at 2–9 years postoperatively between the patients with and without concomitant cartilage therapy [26].

A survivorship analysis showed 91% survivorship at 7 years with patients who proceeded to knee arthroplasty after combined HTO/microfracture had a mean delay of 81.3 months. The authors noted that patients with medial meniscus injury at surgery were 9.2 times more likely to undergo arthroplasty than patients without [27]. This underlines the importance of providing the patient in our case scenario with sufficient information as her history of partial meniscectomy puts her at increased risk for failure. Harris et al. could show in 18 patients undergoing varus or valgus osteotomy combined with meniscal transplantation and articular cartilage surgery a statistically significant and clinically meaningful improvement in clinical outcome scores at long-term follow-up. Although there was a low rate of cartilage or meniscal revision (or both) and total knee arthroplasty, there was a high rate of reoperation [28]. This underlines the importance of meniscal preservation in this patient population.

Kim et al. showed microfracture with collagen augmentation was superior to that after microfracture in terms of the cartilage repair quality in patients undergoing HTO despite the clinical results not reflecting this difference in tissue repair after 1 year [29]. The histological evaluation of the articular cartilage from the medial compartment after arthroscopic subchondral drilling followed by postoperative intra-articular injections of autologous peripheral blood stem cells and hyaluronic acid with concomitant medial open-wedge HTO in patients with varus deformity of the knee joint demonstrated regenerate that closely resembled the native articular cartilage [30]. Another study showed that intra-articular injection of cultured mesenchymal stem cells is effective in improving both short-term clinical and MOCART outcomes in patients undergoing HTO and microfracture for varus knees with cartilage defects [31]. However, studies with longer follow-up are needed to add more substantial evidence to these newer treatment methods.

The advantages and disadvantages of the techniques can be depicted in Table 15.1.

TABLE 15.1 Different therapeutic approaches

Technique	Advantages	Disadvantages
Marrow stimulation procedure without osteotomy	Easy to perform Uncomplicated postoperative rehabilitation	Short-term benefit Only temporary relief
Cartilage procedure with osteotomy	Long-lasting functional outcome Treatment of the underlying cause Possible conversion to other treatment options later on, if needed	Strict postoperative rehabilitation with limited weight-bearing Enhanced risk of complications including nonunion
Unicondylar knee replacement	Early symptom relief	Burns the bridges for any reconstruction in the future High likelihood that the patient will need a revision replacement surgery at some point in the future

Technique Description

Due to the abovementioned arguments, the preferred treatment for this patient is an arthroscopy followed by a high tibial valgus osteotomy. The patient is positioned supine on the operating table. During diagnostic arthroscopy, a full-thickness 10 mm by 20 mm chondral lesion of the medial femoral condyle within the weight-bearing zone in extension is identified (Fig. 15.1). After confirming the absence of any ligamentous lesion, a microfracture procedure is performed (Fig. 15.2). The stability testing of the medial meniscus with the probe does not show any re-rupture, which would require further treatment (Fig. 15.3).

Following the arthroscopy, a 7–8 cm incision is made between the tibial tuberosity and the posteromedial border of the tibial joint line (Fig. 15.4). The sartorius fascia is incised longitudinally above the semitendinosus attachment in the pes anserinus. After releasing the hamstrings from the tibia and partially detaching the superficial medial collateral ligament, a Hohmann retractor is inserted along the posterior tibia. Agneskirchner et al. could show in a biomechanical study that a complete release of the distal fibers of the MCL is necessary after valgus opening-wedge HTO for effective decompression of the medial joint space [32]. The utilization of the Hohmann retractor serves for the protection of the neurovascular structures in the posterior compartment. Under fluoroscopic control, a 2 mm Kirschner wire is introduced at the metaphyseal-diaphyseal transition zone of the medial tibia toward the tip of the fibular head (Fig. 15.5). It is important to stop drilling as soon as the lateral cortex is reached in order not to injure the peroneal nerve. Another Kirschner wire is placed parallel to the first one along the planned osteotomy level. Next, a calibrated saw is used for the horizontal cut with an end approximately 1 cm medial to the lateral cortex. It is important to complete the osteotomy of the posterior cortex. Then, an anterior ascending cut is made posterior to the tibial tuberosity (TT). Care must be taken not to injure the patellar tendon or induce a detachment of the TT. The TT fragment should have

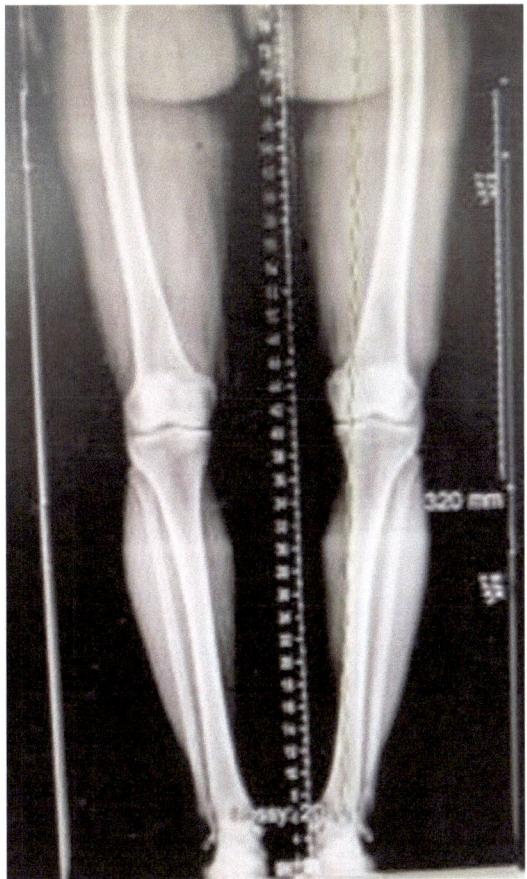

FIGURE 15.1 Long-leg alignment film indicating varus malformation of the left knee

a minimum thickness of about 10 mm to minimize the risk of fracture (Fig. 15.6). Despite the usefulness of the calibrated saw, an image intensifier should be utilized as needed to make the correct cuts. With growing experience, the surgeon will be able to limit the dose of radiation to the patient. After the completion of the osteotomy, an osteotomy chisel is inserted into the transverse osteotomy above the Kirschner wires up to

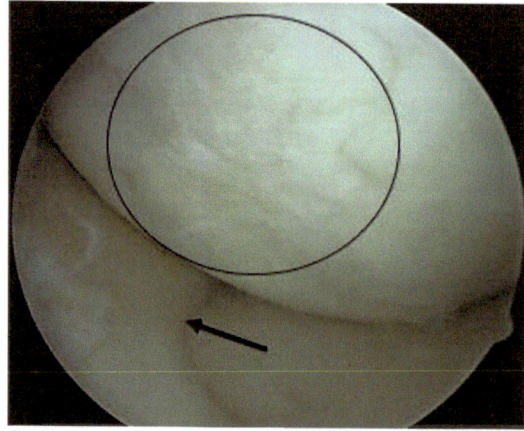

FIGURE 15.2 Grade 3a chondral lesion on medial femoral condyle of the left knee (circle indicating 2 × 2 cm area). Arrow indicating normal anterior and middle contour of the medial meniscus

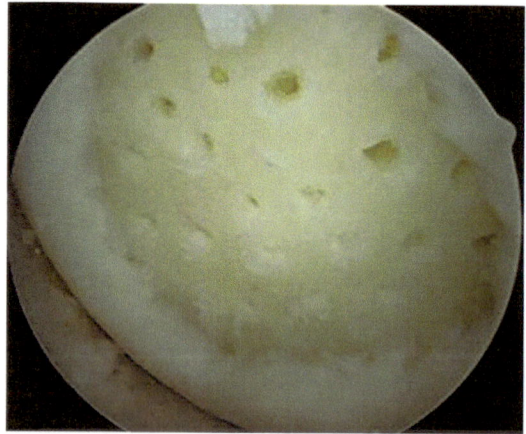

FIGURE 15.3 Microfracture treatment of the chondral defect after debridement of the defect to the subchondral bone and stabilization of the edges

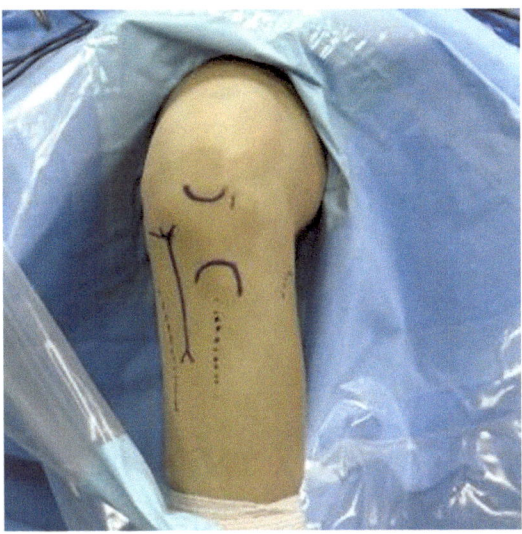

FIGURE 15.4 Medial-sided incision approximately from the joint line to about 2–3 cm distal of the tibial tubercle

the lateral bony hinge with careful hammering. Then a second osteotomy chisel is inserted between the first chisel and the guidewires. Additional chisels are inserted between the first two for gradual spreading of the osteotomy. The desired correction is achieved using a spreader introduced into the most posterior part of the osteotomy site. This enables the creation of a trapezoidal gap to minimize the risk of tibial slope increment. As shown in a 3D finite element model, joint line obliquity of more than 5° induces excessive shear stress in the tibial articular cartilage. Thus, attention should be paid to joint line congruity [33]. After adequate correction, the chisels are removed, and the alignment can be checked with the help of a rod connecting the center of the femoral head with the ankle joint center under image intensifier. Next, a 4.5 mm locking plate is inserted subcutaneously on the medial proximal tibia.

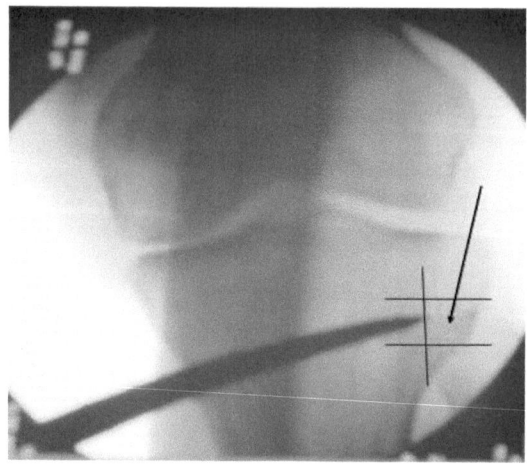

FIGURE 15.5 Under fluoroscopy the guidewire is inserted to be positioned in the lateral target zone. It should be located within 1 cm of the lateral cortex between the tip of the fibula and the base of the fibula. This will protect against lateral breakout. The osteotome (visible here) will follow the guidewire

The shaft portion must be in line with the tibial diaphysis to avoid overhang in the anteroposterior direction. The plate must bridge the osteotomy, and the proximal part must be positioned parallel to the slope approximately 1 cm subchondral to the joint line. After the correct positioning, the plate is secured by insertion of a Kirschner wire into the central drill sleeve in the proximal portion. After fixation of the proximal part of the plate with locking screws, the distal part is fixed with the knee in full extension (Fig. 15.7). If needed, the lateral hinge can be compressed with the help of a cortical screw before the fixation of the distal part. Once the fixation was finished, the spreader is removed. The osteotomy gap can be filled with allograft bone or autograft. A systematic review of opening-wedge osteotomies showed good short-term to midterm outcomes with acceptable complication rates. The lowest rates of delayed union/nonunion were in autograft bone-filled

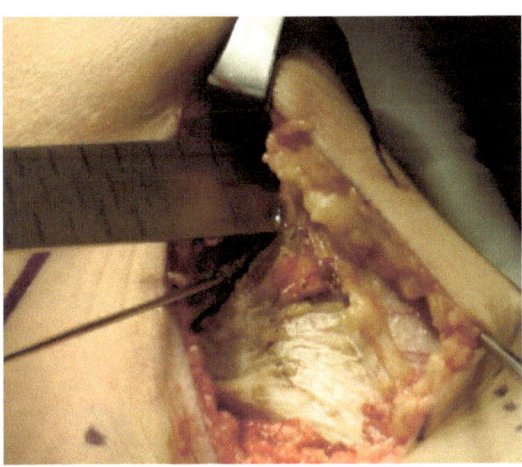

FIGURE 15.6 With the guidewire positioned, the biplanar osteotomy is begun using an Army-Navy retractor to elevate the patellar tendon and carefully scoring the tubercle toward the osteotomy plane in a slightly a-/p-angled position. The osteotomy should be positioned such that the tubercle is not thinner than 1 cm to prevent fracture of the tubercle

osteotomies [34]. After the procedure, the medial collateral ligament and the hamstring tendons will be covered by the plate.

Postoperative Rehabilitation Protocol

Following surgery, the patient is mobilized with partial weight-bearing (10–15% of current weight) on crutches for 6 weeks followed by gradual increase of weight-bearing in the following weeks. Quadriceps strengthening exercises are started immediately. She is placed on continuous passive motion without limitation for 6 weeks at 4 hours per day. Concomitant physiotherapy is initiated with focus on reducing the inflammation.

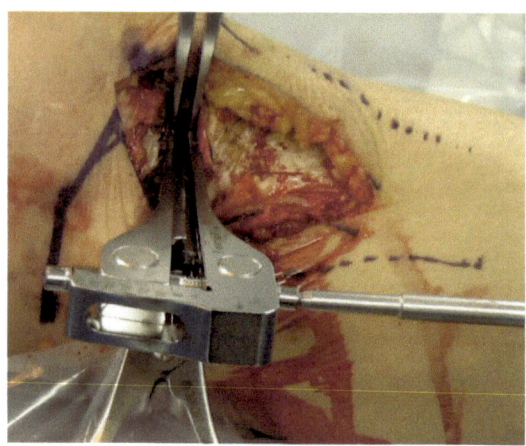

FIGURE 15.7 The osteotomy plane is carefully cut up to within 1 cm of the lateral cortex and a wedge (in this case a variable pitch wedge) is inserted to open up the osteotomy to the predetermined angle or mm distance. Then the fixation of choice can be utilized to secure the osteotomy in place. It is important that the osteotomy cleft is equal all along or wider posteriorly than an anteriorly in order not to decrease the posterior tibial slope

References

1. Amis AA. Biomechanics of high tibial osteotomy. Knee Surg Sports Traumatol Arthrosc. 2013;21(1):197–205. https://doi.org/10.1007/s00167-012-2122-3.
2. Tsukada S, Wakui M. Is overcorrection preferable for repair of degenerated articular cartilage after open-wedge high tibial osteotomy? Knee Surg Sports Traumatol Arthrosc. 2017;25(3):785–92. https://doi.org/10.1007/s00167-015-3655-z.
3. Smith JO, Wilson AJ, Thomas NP. Osteotomy around the knee: Evolution, principles and results. Knee Surg Sports Traumatol Arthrosc. 2013;21(1):3–22. https://doi.org/10.1007/s00167-012-2206-0.
4. Bonasia DE, Dettoni F, Sito G, et al. Medial opening wedge high tibial osteotomy for medial compartment overload/arthritis in the varus knee. Am J Sports Med. 2014;42(3):690–8. https://doi.org/10.1177/0363546513516577.

5. Minzlaff P, Saier T, Brucker PU, Haller B, Imhoff AB, Hinterwimmer S. Valgus bracing in symptomatic varus malalignment for testing the expectable "unloading effect" following valgus high tibial osteotomy. Knee Surg Sports Traumatol Arthrosc. 2015;23(7):1964–70. https://doi.org/10.1007/s00167-013-2832-1.

6. Gomoll AH, Filardo G, Almqvist FK, et al. Surgical treatment for early osteoarthritis. Part II: Allografts and concurrent procedures. Knee Surg Sports Traumatol Arthrosc. 2012;20(3):468–86. https://doi.org/10.1007/s00167-011-1714-7.

7. Gomoll AH, Angele P, Condello V, et al. Load distribution in early osteoarthritis. Knee Surg Sports Traumatol Arthrosc. 2016;24(6):1815–25. https://doi.org/10.1007/s00167-016-4123-0.

8. Kanneganti P, Harris JD, Brophy RH, Carey JL, Lattermann C, Flanigan DC. The effect of smoking on ligament and cartilage surgery in the knee. Am J Sports Med. 2012;40(12):2872–8. https://doi.org/10.1177/0363546512458223.

9. Kumagai K, Akamatsu Y, Kobayashi H, Kusayama Y, Koshino T, Saito T. Factors affecting cartilage repair after medial opening-wedge high tibial osteotomy. Knee Surg Sports Traumatol Arthrosc. 2017;25(3):779–84. https://doi.org/10.1007/s00167-016-4096-z.

10. Gardiner A, Gutiérrez Sevilla GR, Steiner ME, Richmond JC. Osteotomies about the knee for tibiofemoral malalignment in the athletic patient. Am J Sports Med. 2010;38(5):1038–47. https://doi.org/10.1177/0363546509335193.

11. Floerkemeier S, Staubli AE, Schroeter S, Goldhahn S, Lobenhoffer P. Outcome after high tibial open-wedge osteotomy: A retrospective evaluation of 533 patients. Knee Surg Sports Traumatol Arthrosc. 2013;21(1):170–80. https://doi.org/10.1007/s00167-012-2087-2.

12. Jung W-H, Takeuchi R, Chun C-W, et al. Second-look arthroscopic assessment of cartilage regeneration after medial opening-wedge high tibial osteotomy. Knee Surg Sports Traumatol Arthrosc. 2014;30(1):72–9. https://doi.org/10.1016/j.arthro.2013.10.008.

13. Niemeyer P, Koestler W, Kaehny C, et al. Two-year results of open-wedge high tibial osteotomy with fixation by medial plate fixator for medial compartment arthritis with varus malalignment of the knee. Arthroscopy. 2008;24(7):796–804. https://doi.org/10.1016/j.arthro.2008.02.016.

14. Niemeyer P, Schmal H, Hauschild O, Von Heyden J, Sdkamp NP, Kstler W. Open-wedge osteotomy using an internal plate fixator in patients with medial-compartment gonar-

thritis and varus malalignment: 3-year results with regard to preoperative arthroscopic and radiographic findings. Arthroscopy. 2010;26(12):1607–16. https://doi.org/10.1016/j.arthro.2010.05.006.

15. Bode G, von Heyden J, Pestka J, et al. Prospective 5-year survival rate data following open-wedge valgus high tibial osteotomy. Knee Surg Sports Traumatol Arthrosc. 2015;23(7):1949–55. https://doi.org/10.1007/s00167-013-2762-y.

16. Hantes ME, Natsaridis P, Koutalos AA, Ono Y, Doxariotis N, Malizos KN. Satisfactory functional and radiological outcomes can be expected in young patients under 45 years old after open wedge high tibial osteotomy in a long-term follow-up. Knee Surg Sports Traumatol Arthrosc. 2017. https://doi.org/10.1007/s00167-017-4816-z.

17. Salzmann GM, Ahrens P, Naal FD, et al. Sporting activity after high tibial osteotomy for the treatment of medial compartment knee osteoarthritis. Am J Sports Med. 2009;37(2):312–8. https://doi.org/10.1177/0363546508325666.

18. Kanamiya T, Naito M, Hara M, Yoshimura I. The influences of biomechanical factors on cartilage regeneration after high tibial osteotomy for knees with medial compartment osteoarthritis: Clinical and arthroscopic observations. Arthroscopy. 2002;18(7):725–9. https://doi.org/10.1053/jars.2002.35258.

19. van Egmond N, van Grinsven S, van Loon CJM, Gaasbeek RD, van Kampen A. Better clinical results after closed- compared to open-wedge high tibial osteotomy in patients with medial knee osteoarthritis and varus leg alignment. Knee Surg Sports Traumatol Arthrosc. 2016;24(1):34–41. https://doi.org/10.1007/s00167-014-3303-z.

20. Schultz W, Göbel D. Articular cartilage regeneration of the knee joint after proximal tibial valgus osteotomy: a prospective study of different intra- and extra-articular operative techniques. Knee Surg Sports Traumatol Arthrosc. 1999;7(1):29–36. https://doi.org/10.1007/s001670050117.

21. Montgomery SR, Foster BD, Ngo SS, et al. Trends in the surgical treatment of articular cartilage defects of the knee in the United States. Knee Surg Sports Traumatol Arthroscz. 2014;22(9):2070–5. https://doi.org/10.1007/s00167-013-2614-9.

22. Parker DA, Beatty KT, Giuffre B, Scholes CJ, Coolican MRJ. Articular cartilage changes in patients with osteoarthritis after osteotomy. Am J Sports Med. 2011;39(5):1039–45. https://doi.org/10.1177/0363546510392702.

23. Sterett WI, Steadman JR. Chondral resurfacing and high tibial osteotomy in the varus knee. Am J Sports Med. 2004;32(5):1243–9. https://doi.org/10.1177/0363546503259301.
24. Schuster P, Schulz M, Mayer P, Schlumberger M, Immendoerfer M, Richter J. Open-wedge high tibial osteotomy and combined abrasion/microfracture in severe medial osteoarthritis and varus malalignment: 5-year results and arthroscopic findings after 2 years. Arthrosc J Arthrosc Relat Surg. 2015;31(7):1279–88. https://doi.org/10.1016/j.arthro.2015.02.010.
25. Jung W-H, Takeuchi R, Chun C-W, Lee J-S, Jeong J-H. Comparison of results of medial opening-wedge high tibial osteotomy with and without subchondral drilling. Arthrosc J Arthrosc Relat Surg. 2015;31(4):673–9. https://doi.org/10.1016/j.arthro.2014.11.035.
26. Akizuki S, Yasukawa Y, Takizawa T. Does arthroscopic abrasion arthroplasty promote cartilage regeneration in osteoarthritic knees with eburnation? A prospective study of high tibial osteotomy with abrasion arthroplasty versus high tibial osteotomy alone. Arthrosc J Arthrosc Relat Surg. 1997;13(1):9–17. https://doi.org/10.1016/S0749-8063(97)90204-8.
27. Sterett WI, Steadman JR, Huang MJ, Matheny LM, Briggs KK. Chondral resurfacing and high tibial osteotomy in the varus knee. Am J Sports Med. 2010;38(7):1420–4. https://doi.org/10.1177/0363546509360403.
28. Harris JD, Hussey K, Wilson H, et al. Biological knee reconstruction for combined malalignment, meniscal deficiency, and articular cartilage disease. Arthrosc J Arthrosc Relat Surg. 2015;31(2):275–82. https://doi.org/10.1016/j.arthro.2014.08.012.
29. Kim MS, Koh IJ, Choi YJ, Pak KH, In Y. Collagen augmentation improves the quality of cartilage repair after microfracture in patients undergoing high tibial osteotomy: a randomized controlled trial. Am J Sports Med. 2017;45(8):1845–55. https://doi.org/10.1177/0363546517691942.
30. Saw K-Y, Anz A, Jee CS-Y, Ng RC-S, Mohtarrudin N, Ragavanaidu K. High tibial osteotomy in combination with chondrogenesis after stem cell therapy: a histologic report of 8 cases. Arthrosc J Arthrosc Relat Surg. 2015;31(10):1909–20. https://doi.org/10.1016/j.arthro.2015.03.038.
31. Wong KL, Lee KBL, Tai BC, Law P, Lee EH, Hui JHP. Injectable cultured bone marrow-derived mesenchymal stem cells in varus knees with cartilage defects undergoing high tibial osteotomy: A prospective, randomized controlled clinical trial with

2 years' follow-up. Arthroscopy. 2013;29(12):2020–8. https://doi.org/10.1016/j.arthro.2013.09.074.

32. Agneskirchner JD, Hurschler C, Wrann CD, Lobenhoffer P. The effects of valgus medial opening wedge high tibial osteotomy on articular cartilage pressure of the knee: a biomechanical study. Arthroscopy. 2007;23(8):852–61. https://doi.org/10.1016/j.arthro.2007.05.018.

33. Nakayama H, Schröter S, Yamamoto C, et al. Large correction in opening wedge high tibial osteotomy with resultant joint-line obliquity induces excessive shear stress on the articular cartilage. Knee Surg Sports Traumatol Arthroscz. 2017:1–6. https://doi.org/10.1007/s00167-017-4680-x.

34. Lash NJ, Feller JA, Batty LM, Wasiak J, Richmond AK. Bone grafts and bone substitutes for opening-wedge osteotomies of the knee: a systematic review. Arthroscopy. 2015;31(4):720–30. https://doi.org/10.1016/j.arthro.2014.09.011.

Chapter 16
Tibial Cartilage Defects

Kevin C. Wang, Rachel M. Frank, and Brian J. Cole

Case Presentation

History

A 56-year-old gentleman presented to the office with a chief complaint of several months of left, lateral knee pain. He states that the knee pain has been gradual in onset with no specific inciting event. Since its onset, the pain has been slowly worsening. The pain is generally localized to the lateral side of the knee with occasional episodes of medial-sided pain. He reports occasional swelling in the knee, often related to activity. He rates his average pain as 3/10 but states that the pain is worse with any sort of weight-bearing activities, especially with pivoting,

K. C. Wang
Department of Orthopedics, Icahn School of Medicine
at Mount Sinai, New York, NY, USA

R. M. Frank
Department of Orthopaedic Surgery, University of Colorado
School of Medicine, Aurora, CO, USA

B. J. Cole (✉)
Department of Orthopedic Surgery, Rush University Medical
Center, Chicago, IL, USA
e-mail: brian.cole@rushortho.com

© Springer Nature Switzerland AG 2019
A. B. Yanke, B. J. Cole (eds.), *Joint Preservation of the Knee*,
https://doi.org/10.1007/978-3-030-01491-9_16

twisting, and going up and down stairs. The pain is usually worse toward the end of the day after ambulating on it. He will occasionally feel catching or have locking symptoms while ambulating. The patient denies any pain behind the kneecap. Therefore his presentation could be summarized as unicompartmental, weight-bearing pain that is associated with swelling.

The patient was initially treated with anti-inflammatories as needed and underwent a series of hyaluronic acid injections as well. These resulted in some relief, but did not provide a satisfactory reduction in symptoms. He has not had any steroid injections or previous surgical procedures on his knee, and he has not engaged in any regimented physical therapy sessions.

Physical Examination

On physical examination, the patient was 5 feet, 9 inches tall, weighed 184 pounds (body mass index of 27.2), was in no apparent distress, and could ambulate without apparent difficulty. He had a mild effusion in the left knee with mild tenderness to palpation along the lateral joint line. He had active range of motion from 0° to 125° with no catching or clicking. The patient's motor strength was 5/5 in the quadriceps and had no visible atrophy. There was no tenderness to palpation along the lateral femoral condyle and only mild pain with lateral joint line palpation.

Diagnostic Imaging

X-rays were obtained and reviewed in the office and revealed well-preserved joint spaces with no evidence of medial or lateral joint space narrowing (Fig. 16.1). There was no evidence of patellofemoral arthrosis. MRI revealed a localized chondral defect in the lateral tibial plateau with evidence of subchondral edema (Fig. 16.2). The remaining structures including the lateral meniscus and femoral cartilage appeared intact.

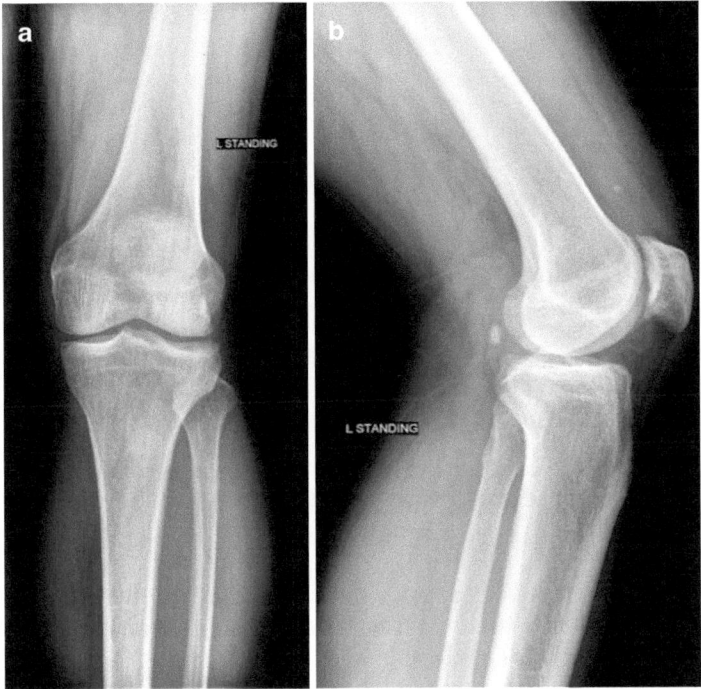

FIGURE 16.1 Preoperative plan standing AP (**a**) and lateral (**b**) radiography

Management and Treatment Options

The patient's findings were consistent with a localized chondral defect of the lateral tibial plateau. The location of this defect on imaging was consistent with the patient's clinical presentation and physical exam findings, and the possible treatment options, including continued conservative treatment, were discussed with the patient. The treatment plan was a diagnostic arthroscopy for index evaluation and, if the findings were consistent with an isolated tibial plateau defect, marrow stimulation of the defect with BioCartilage (Arthrex) and platelet-rich plasma (PRP) augmentation.

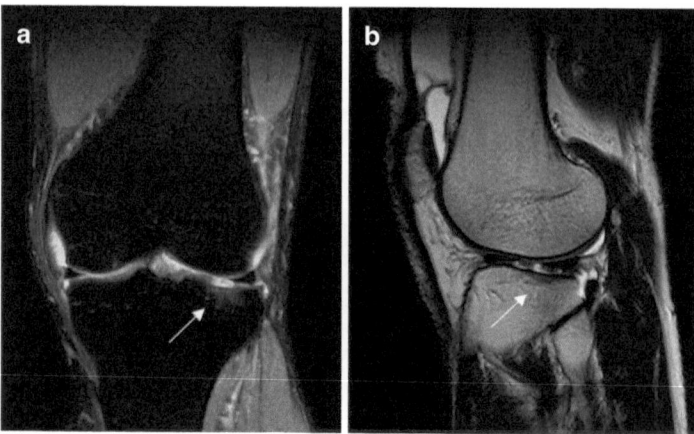

FIGURE 16.2 Preoperative coronal (**a**) and sagittal (**b**) magnetic resonance imaging demonstrating an isolated tibial plateau articular cartilage injury (white arrow) and associated bone edematous changes

Other treatment options for tibial plateau defects include microfracture alone, matrix-associated autologous chondrocyte implantation (MACI) with fibrin glue, and osteochondral allograft or autograft. MACI techniques should only be considered if the practitioner is comfortable using this treatment methodology for other indications, as it can be a technically challenging procedure that requires specialized equipment. In the tibial plateau, geometry, exposure, and access present challenging hurdles for osteochondral allograft or autograft applications, and practitioners should proceed with caution if considering these techniques. These also would typically require an open approach including takedown of the distal MCL.

In patients with articular cartilage defects of any kind, it is important to consider and address concomitant pathology when indicated. While the majority of published research for these indications addresses lesions of the femoral condyle, it is likely that similar principles apply in the treatment of tibial plateau lesions, and the following pathologies are concomitantly addressed in the senior author's practice. In tibial lesions with a bipolar component, a corresponding femoral condyle cartilage defect, the bipolar pathology should be addressed. Additionally, patients with ligamentous instability and meniscal pathology should undergo concomitant ligament reconstruction or meniscal allograft transplantation (MAT) to improve the chance of a successful outcome.

Surgical Technique

Diagnostic Arthroscopy

The diagnostic arthroscopy was performed through standard inferomedial and inferolateral portals. The knee was examined for meniscal, ligamentous, and articular cartilage pathology. Specifically, the femoral condyle, meniscus, and tibial plateau were evaluated on the lateral side. A degenerative medial meniscal tear of about 10% was identified and debrided, and a degenerative lateral meniscal tear of between 10% and 20% was identified and debrided. A trochlear defect that was approximately 20 mm × 20 mm was identified. This was debrided to a stable rim but otherwise left untreated given its inconsistency with the patient's clinical presentation. An area of delamination was identified on the lateral tibial plateau and measured to be approximately 15 mm long and 6 mm wide (Fig. 16.3). This was debrided down to a stable rim utilizing a 4.5 mm rotary shaver and a curette.

FIGURE 16.3 An intraoperative arthroscopic image of an isolated tibial plateau chondral defect prior to preparation of the defect

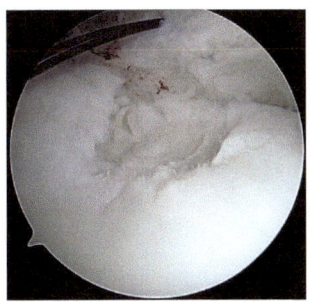

Marrow Stimulation

Prior to marrow stimulation, the calcified layer was debrided with an angled curette. The rim was debrided with a shaver to establish stable, vertical walls at the border of the defect. An arthroscopic K-wire was utilized to create atraumatic perforations in the subchondral plate to allow access to bone marrow mesenchymal stem cells. These holes were spaced 2–3 mm apart avoiding confluence to minimize the likelihood of ectopic bone formation (Fig. 16.4).

Application of BioCartilage and PRP

The microfracture site was dried with neurosurgical patties to optimize the adherence of the BioCartilage and PRP mixture (Fig. 16.5a). Blood pressure and tourniquet control were utilized to minimize bleeding into the area (Fig. 16.5b). The BioCartilage/PRP mixture was prepared outside of the knee and introduced within the defect taking care not to overfill the defect. A Freer elevator was utilized to flatten the surface of the BioCartilage/PRP mixture to lie slightly below the level of the surrounding articular cartilage. After appropriately applying the BioCartilage/PRP mixture, fibrin glue was applied over the top of the mixture taking care not to

FIGURE 16.4 An arthroscopic image of a tibial plateau lesion after preparation via curettage and subchondral bone perforation via drilling

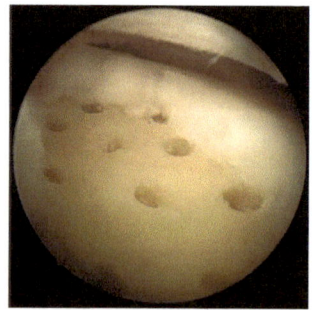

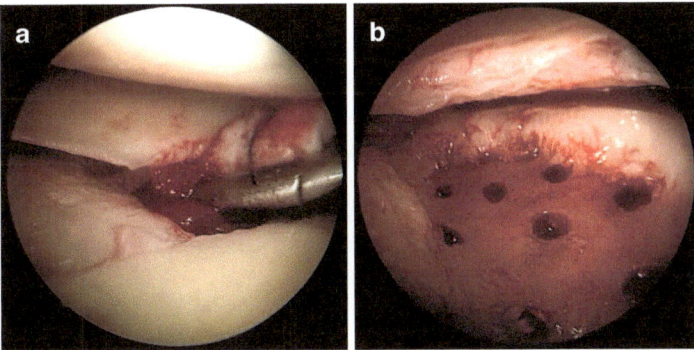

FIGURE 16.5 (**a**) An arthroscopic image of a tibial plateau chondral defect after preparation being adequately dried for optimal BioCartilage adhesion. (**b**) An arthroscopic image of a fully prepared tibial chondral lesion prior to BioCartilage application

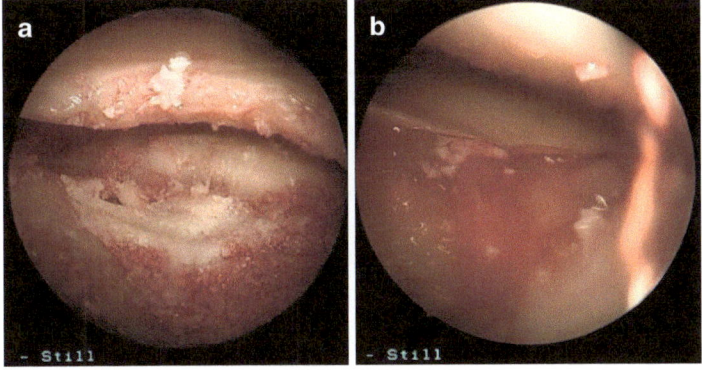

FIGURE 16.6 An arthroscopic image of an isolated tibial plateau lesion after being filled with the BioCartilage/PRP mixture (**a**) and after sealing the defect with fibrin glue (**b**)

over-apply the glue to reduce the risk of adherence to opposing surfaces. The fibrin glue was allowed to cure for 7 min prior to range of motion testing to minimize the risk of dislodgement (Fig. 16.6).

Postoperative Care

The patient was made nonweight-bearing immediately post-operatively with a 1-week delay in continuous passive motion (CPM) because of the application of BioCartilage. After 1 week, CPM was initiated for 6 hours a day with passive and active range-of-motion (ROM) exercises that were allowed as tolerated. At 6 weeks postoperatively, weight-bearing was slowly initiated with a steady increase of 25% weekly. Advanced strengthening exercises were initiated at 8 weeks postoperatively with further progression of weight-bearing activities as tolerated. Functional activity was started at 6 months postoperatively, and return to full activity was allowed at 8 months with physician clearance.

Literature Review

While there have been publications on the treatment methods and outcomes for treating cartilage lesions of the knee, these primarily focus on lesions of the femoral condyles and patellofemoral joint with few investigations specifically detailing treatment of the tibial plateau [1]. This paucity of available literature leaves surgeons with little clinical guidance on the treatment of these kinds of defects. While microfracture surgery is generally the first line of treatment for articular cartilage defects given its relative technical simplicity and low complication rates, the long-term outcomes have been questioned [2–4]. Additionally, osteochondral grafts (both autograft and allograft) have demonstrated success in cartilage defects of the knee, specifically for defect of the femoral head and patellofemoral joint involving the subchondral bone [5, 6], but the geometry and anatomical restrictions imposed by tibial plateau defects present unique challenges when pursuing these kinds of treatment [7–9]. While osteochondral grafts have shown positive outcomes for more severe tibial plateau cartilage defects, the technical challenges and potential for injury to surrounding structures when using these approaches necessitate caution.

In addition to direct treatment of the cartilage lesions, mechanical realignment may be an effective management strategy for tibial plateau defects, with high tibial osteotomy (HTO) used to reduce mechanical loading of diseased compartments [9]. A recent investigation has shown improved International Cartilage Repair Society (ICRS) cartilage grading in 34.6% of medial tibial plateau cartilage lesions in patients treated with HTO alone. Patient-reported outcome scores were also significantly improved in these patients at final follow-up; however, these did not correlate with the ICRS grading [10]. This literature suggests that HTO, both in isolation and as a concomitant procedure, can be an effective treatment for tibial plateau lesions, specifically those of the medial compartment, when varus malalignment is identified. While the patient in the current case example did not suffer from malalignment, in cases with varus malalignment, HTO should be strongly considered.

Given concerns regarding the long-term durability of microfracture – often attributed to the development of mechanically inferior fibrocartilage – new adjunct treatments have been developed with the hope of improving hyaline cartilage regeneration and improving the long-term durability of microfracture [2, 11]. In an animal model, BioCartilage (Arthrex, Naples, FL), a minced allogeneic cartilage product, combined with platelet-rich plasma, a promising biologic, has been shown to facilitate the generation of hyaline cartilage compared to microfracture alone. Similar results have also been shown with bone marrow aspirate concentrate (BMAC) [12]. Clinical outcomes remain to be determined, but the use of BioCartilage/PRP or BMAC to augment microfracture has been shown to improve hyaline cartilage regeneration in translational studies. These treatment strategies may potentially improve the long-term durability of microfracture treatment by affecting the type of cartilage fill.

Though clinical evidence for appropriate treatment of tibial plateau lesions is limited, the same principles for cartilage defect treatment apply here. As outlined above, care should be taken to utilize a technique that is logistically reasonable without adding increased risk. Therefore, treatments in this arena should focus on microfracture augmentation and cell-based treatments.

Tips and Tricks

- Avoid excessive application of BioCartilage/PRP mixture, as this can be easily dislodged by shear stresses if it stands proud over the surrounding cartilage margins.
- High tibial osteotomy should be strongly considered in cases with medial compartment involvement in the setting of varus malalignment.
- Order of operations:
  - Standard anterolateral arthroscopic approach.
  - Diagnostic arthroscopy.
  - Debridement of symptomatic articular cartilage lesions.
  - Microfracture of bare subchondral plate.
  - Evacuate saline from the knee and dry the microfracture site.
  - Prepare BioCartilage/PRP mixture.
  - Apply BioCartilage/PRP mixture and spread evenly, taking care not to exceed the height of the surrounding articular cartilage rim.
  - Apply fibrin glue to fix the BioCartilage/PRP mixture.
  - Close in standard fashion.

References

1. Wajsfisz A, Makridis KG, Djian P. Arthroscopic retrograde osteochondral autograft transplantation for cartilage lesions of the tibial plateau: a prospective study. Am J Sports Med. 2013;41(2):411–5.
2. Frank RM, Cotter EJ, Nassar I, Cole B. Failure of bone marrow stimulation techniques. Sports Med Arthrosc Rev. 2017;25(1):2–9.
3. Cole BJ, Pascual-Garrido C, Grumet RC. Surgical management of articular cartilage defects in the knee. J Bone Joint Surg Am. 2009;91(7):1778–90.
4. Miller BS, Briggs KK, Downie B, Steadman JR. Clinical outcomes following the microfracture procedure for chondral defects of the knee: a longitudinal data analysis. Cole BJ, Kercher JS, editors. Cartilage. 2010;1(2):108–12.

5. Frank RM, Lee S, Levy D, Poland S, Smith M, Scalise N, et al. Osteochondral allograft transplantation of the knee: analysis of failures at 5 years. Am J Sports Med. 2017:036354651667607.

6. Oliver-Welsh L, Griffin JW, Meyer MA, Gitelis ME, Cole BJ. Deciding how best to treat cartilage defects. Orthopedics. 2016;39(6):343–50.

7. Gross AE, Shasha N, Aubin P. Long-term followup of the use of fresh osteochondral allografts for posttraumatic knee defects. Clin Orthop. 2005;NA(435):79–87.

8. Ronga M, Grassi FA, Bulgheroni P. Arthroscopic autologous chondrocyte implantation for the treatment of a chondral defect in the tibial plateau of the knee. Arthrosc J Arthrosc Relat Surg. 2004;20(1):79–84.

9. Ueblacker P, Burkart A, Imhoff AB. Retrograde cartilage transplantation on the proximal and distal tibia. Arthrosc J Arthrosc Relat Surg. 2004;20(1):73–8.

10. Kim K-I, Seo M-C, Song S-J, Bae D-K, Kim D-H, Lee SH. Change of chondral lesions and predictive factors after medial open-wedge high tibial osteotomy with a locked plate system. Am J Sports Med. 2017:036354651769486.

11. Fortier LA, Chapman HS, Pownder SL, Roller BL, Cross JA, Cook JL, et al. BioCartilage improves cartilage repair compared with microfracture alone in an equine model of full-thickness cartilage loss. Am J Sports Med. 2016;44(9):2366–74.

12. Fortier LA, Potter HG, Rickey EJ, Schnabel LV, Foo LF, Chong LR, et al. Concentrated bone marrow aspirate improves full-thickness cartilage repair compared with microfracture in the equine model. J Bone Jt Surg Am. 2010;92(10):1927–37.

Part IV
Review and Evidence

Chapter 17
Evidence-Based Treatment of Articular Cartilage Lesions in the Knee

Kyle R. Duchman and Jonathan C. Riboh

Introduction

Articular cartilage lesions of the knee are a common finding at the time of knee arthroscopy [1, 2], and they tend to be particularly prevalent in young, athletic patient populations [3]. While the natural history of isolated articular cartilage lesions in the knee remains an area of ongoing debate [4, 5], the utilization of surgical management in the United States to treat these lesions has increased significantly in recent years [6, 7]. Despite the increased surgical utilization and impressive amount of literature dedicated to articular cartilage lesions in the knee, there remain more questions than answers when it comes to treatment of these lesions due in large part

K. R. Duchman
Department of Orthopaedic Surgery, University of Iowa Hospitals and Clinics, Iowa City, IA, USA

J. C. Riboh (✉)
Department of Orthopaedic Surgery, Duke University Medical Center, Durham, NC, USA
e-mail: jonathan.riboh@duke.edu

© Springer Nature Switzerland AG 2019   269
A. B. Yanke, B. J. Cole (eds.), *Joint Preservation of the Knee*,
https://doi.org/10.1007/978-3-030-01491-9_17

to the limited amount of high-level evidence on the topic [8]. The following will review the best available evidence for treatment of articular cartilage lesions in the knee while providing an update on current reparative and restorative treatment options, recommended treatment algorithms, special considerations in the competitive athlete, and future directions for research and clinical improvement.

Quality of the Current Literature: What Is the Best Available Evidence?

Despite a relatively high volume of primary clinical literature, the quality of clinical studies dedicated to articular cartilage lesions of the knee remains low. Limitations in study quality were recognized over a decade ago [9]. Today, the same methodological flaws, including a lack of consistency with outcome reporting and failure to track outcomes across domains, continue to plague the primary literature [10]. Of the available literature on articular cartilage lesions in the knee, approximately 76% can be classified as Level IV evidence, with only 8% and 7% of studies classified as Level I or II evidence, respectively [8]. Furthermore, the quality of evidence on the topic has failed to improve with time, despite previous recognition of the shortcomings in the literature. Because of these limitations, results of clinical studies are rightfully interpreted with caution, and consensus statements for or against specific treatments are lacking.

Currently Available Techniques for Cartilage Restoration in the Knee

Bone Marrow Stimulation

Bone marrow stimulation techniques include transarticular or retrograde drilling and microfracture, with microfracture most frequently used to address articular cartilage lesions in the knee. Microfracture, originally described in the 1990s by

Dr. Richard Steadman, results in the production of Type I fibrocartilage by accessing marrow mesenchymal stem cells through penetration of the subchondral bone [11]. Due in part to its long track record, widespread availability of instrumentation, relative technical ease compared to other cartilage restoration procedures, and the fact that it is a single-stage procedure, microfracture remains one of the most commonly employed reparative cartilage techniques for the knee [6]. Still, there remains concern that the improvement in short-term outcomes following microfracture deteriorates over time [12], potentially due to the fact that the procedure fails to histologically replicate hyaline cartilage [13].

While the technical aspects of microfracture have remained largely unmodified since its original description, there has been a growing interest in the use of adjuncts with microfracture. Enhanced microfracture techniques, or the so-called microfracture plus, which typically consists of the addition of acellular matrix products with or without stem cell or peripheral blood additives, have been explored in hopes of improving histological and clinical outcomes (Fig. 17.1). Despite promising early results [14–16], these modifications remain relatively new, and the longevity of outcomes compared to microfracture alone or other cartilage restoration techniques needs further exploration.

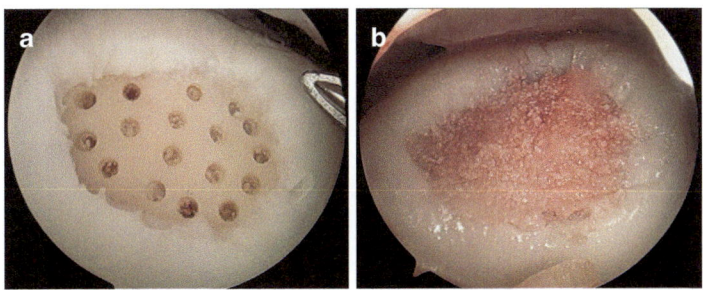

Figure 17.1 (a) Large trochlear cartilage defect arthroscopically prepared to a circumferential stable rim and penetration of subchondral bone with microfracture awls. (b) Using dry arthroscopic techniques, acellular cartilage matrix is applied to the prepared defect prior to sealing with fibrin glue

Cell-Based Therapies

Available cell-based therapies for articular cartilage lesions of the knee include autologous chondrocyte implantation (ACI) or particulated juvenile cartilage allograft. ACI has been available for several decades and, over time, has went through several derivations. ACI is a two-stage procedure, requiring an initial arthroscopic biopsy to harvest chondrocytes for isolation and expansion by proprietary means, followed by implantation of the cells during a second surgical procedure [17]. Containing expanded cells was initially a challenge, and several generations of ACI techniques required a periosteal patch or collagen membrane to contain cells [18]. Recently, matrix-induced ACI became available for use in the United States, supplanting many of the technical challenges associated with earlier ACI techniques (Fig. 17.2) [19]. ACI

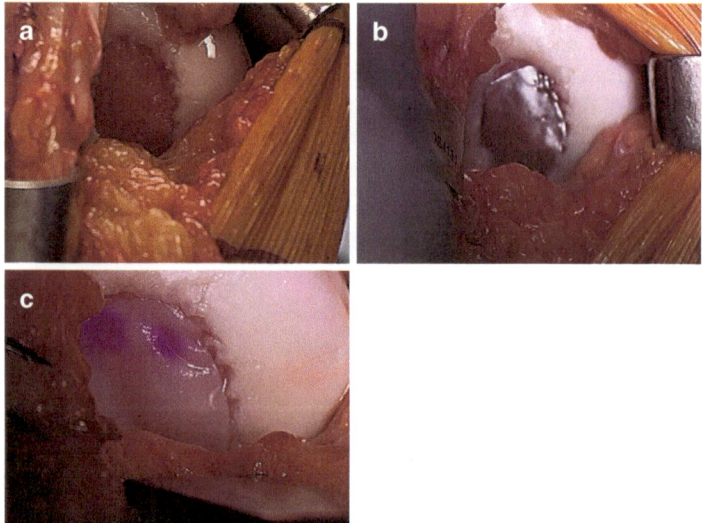

Figure 17.2 (a) Large medial femoral condyle defect after removal of calcified cartilage layer through a medial parapatellar arthrotomy. (b) The defect is sized using a foil impression, which will aid with sizing the matrix containing chondrocytes on the back table. (c) The matrix is implanted in the prepared defect prior to sealing with fibrin glue

has shown the ability to produce "hyaline-like" cartilage [13] and is useful for large lesions with low risk of donor site morbidity. Multiple generations of the procedure have shown promising clinical outcomes [20], although the two-stage requirement of the procedure remains the major downside.

Particulated allograft cartilage is an off-the-shelf product that can be used to address articular cartilage lesions in the knee during a single stage without donor site morbidity [21, 22]. As a new procedure, there remain insufficient randomized or comparative studies to guide specific indications [23]. Basic science studies have suggested that particulated juvenile cartilage allograft may provide an improved ability to restore articular cartilage surfaces as compared to adult allograft cartilage [24]. As new products become available, it will be important to consider the effect of donor age on outcomes in clinical studies. While the limited morbidity and technical ease associated with the procedure are promising, further clinical studies are needed to better determine the clinical applications for particulated allograft cartilage procedures to address articular cartilage lesions in the knee.

Osteochondral Autograft Transfer

Osteochondral autograft transfer (OAT) provides the ability to replace the entire osteochondral unit with local autogenous tissue from non-weight-bearing portions of the knee [25]. OAT can be particularly useful for articular cartilage lesions with an underlying cystic component or necrotic regions of the bone. Additionally, OAT allows for transfer of hyaline cartilage to the articular cartilage lesion, providing the most predictable histologic outcome for all cartilage restoration procedures [13]. However, the procedure can be technically demanding, as achieving a flush graft that is neither proud nor depressed is imperative to restore native contact pressures that do not put the graft or adjacent cartilage at risk [26]. The application of OAT is limited primarily by lesion size, as locations for local autologous tissue are limited primarily to the lateral border of the lateral femoral condyle proximal to the sulcus terminalis or intercondylar notch.

Even with careful graft harvest, donor site morbidity remains a concern [27, 28]. Despite providing the most consistent histologic outcomes, OAT is clearly limited by the size of the articular cartilage lesion as well as the technically demanding nature of the procedure. Given the fact that OAT has not shown clear superiority to other cartilage restoration procedures in studies using pooled data [29, 30], the benefits of transfer of healthy articular cartilage to a damaged region must be weighed with the potential for donor site morbidity.

Osteochondral Allograft Transplantation

Fresh osteochondral allograft transplantation has recently gained popularity as a surgical option for treatment of large articular cartilage lesions in the knee mainly due to improved allograft processing techniques and more widespread availability of grafts in the United States. The procedure is not limited by lesion size, nor does it result in donor site morbidity while potentially restoring the hyaline surface in the knee (Fig. 17.3) [31, 32]. However, as a fresh allograft tissue, concerns over graft immunogenicity and transmission of infectious disease have been raised [33]. Additionally, additional imaging procedures may be needed to obtain appropriately sized allografts [34, 35]. Recent studies have highlighted the importance of graft and chondrocyte viability at the time of implantation as a potentially important factor influencing both clinical and histologic outcomes [36]. In order to optimize chondrocyte viability, graft implantation should not be excessively delayed, and surgeons should understand the processing and storage techniques of their respective tissue bank [37–39]. Because of this, both patients and surgeons need to have flexibility to accommodate scheduling when appropriate size-matched tissue becomes available. Despite promising results in non-comparative studies [40], it will be important to carefully track outcomes and the potential factors that may predict outcomes, including chondrocyte viability, carefully in order to better define its role in the treatment of articular cartilage lesions in knee.

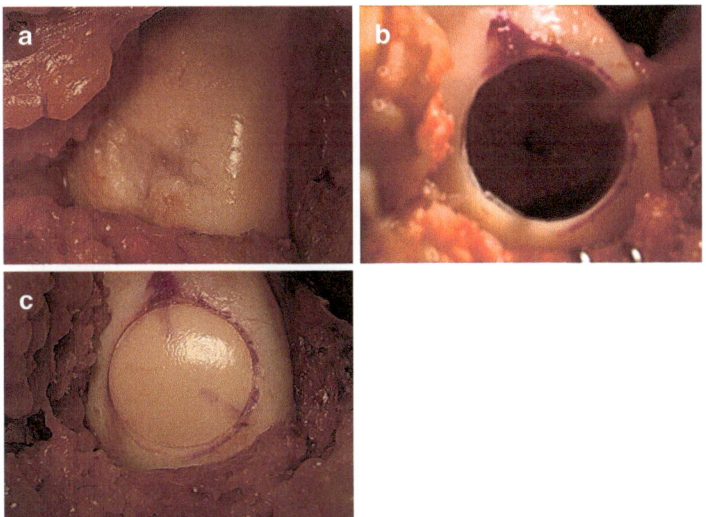

FIGURE 17.3 (**a**) Medial femoral condyle with large area of grade III and IV chondromalacia viewed through a medial parapatellar arthrotomy. (**b**) The lesion is prepared with a cylindrical reamer placed over a guide pin in the center of the lesion. (**c**) After preparation on the back table, the matching cylindrical allograft is implanted with interference fit

Randomized Control Trials: Comparison of Cartilage Restoration Techniques

The number of randomized, prospective, comparative, clinical trials focused on treatment of articular cartilage lesions in the knee is limited, with Level III and IV studies making up the majority of the available literature [8]. Even when considering the higher-level randomized studies, many of them are limited by small sample size, unpredictable patient crossover, and poor patient follow-up, which in some cases does not allow the studies to be considered Level I based on follow-up <80% [41]. Additionally, many of these studies are the result of evaluation of the same cohort or subgroup of the same cohort at multiple timepoints, which artificially increases the volume of available high-quality studies. Still, these studies provide the best available evidence to guide treatment decisions for articular cartilage lesions in the knee. The majority of available comparative studies compare variable generations of ACI with microfracture (Table 17.1) [42–50]. There are fewer studies comparing microfracture to OAT [51–54], variable generations of ACI to OAT [55–58], various generations of ACI to each other [59–61], and more recently, microfracture to enhanced microfracture ("microfracture plus") [15, 16, 62, 63]. Within these comparative categories, there is no consensus outcome, particularly when independently comparing studies from different cohort. This general finding is corroborated by two recently performed systematic reviews made up of comparative studies investigating reoperation and clinical outcomes and short- and midterm follow-up. Both systematic reviews found no difference in reoperation or clinical outcomes when comparing microfracture, OAT, and various ACI techniques [29, 30]. However, there was a trend toward improved histologic cartilage repair and lower reoperation rates with more long-term follow-up for advanced cartilage repair techniques, including OAT and collagen membrane ACI [30].

Notably missing from the comparative studies is osteochondral allograft transplantation, which, to date, has not been compared to any other reparative or restorative cartilage procedure in the knee. Additionally, there are no multi-armed randomized studies that compare more than two treatment techniques. Pediatric patients are also underrepresented, as only one study is dedicated to patients ≤18 years of age [53]. Because of this, it should come as no surprise that definitive indications, treatment algorithms, and outcomes are lacking for the diverse group of patients with articular cartilage lesions of the knee. Future studies should aim to incorporate osteochondral allograft transplantation as a treatment option while also stratifying by patient age and activity level in order to better define the indications and outcomes for these procedures.

TABLE 17.1 Randomized, prospective, comparative clinical studies on restorative procedures for articular cartilage lesions in the knee

Author	Year	Treatments	Patients (n)	Mean follow-up (months)	Mean patient age (years)	Summary of outcomes
Basad et al. [42]	2010	MACI vs. MFx	60	24	35.3	MACI clinically superior to MFx
Crawford et al. [43]	2012	MACI vs. MFx	30	26	40	MACI clinically superior to MFx
Knutsen et al. [44][a]	2004	pACI vs. MFx	80	24	32.2	Equivalent clinical and histologic outcomes
Knutsen et al. [45][a]	2007	pACI vs. MFx	80	60	32.2	Equivalent clinical and radiographic outcomes
Knutsen et al. [46][a]	2016	pACI vs. MFx	80	180	32.2	Equivalent clinical outcomes
Saris et al. [47][b]	2008	pACI vs. MFx	118	18	33.9	pACI superior histologic outcomes to MFx
Saris et al. [48][b]	2009	pACI vs. MFx	118	36	33.9	pACI superior clinical outcomes to MFx
Van Assche et al. [49][b]	2010	pACI vs. MFx	67	24	31	Equivalent functional outcomes

(continued)

TABLE 17.1 (continued)

Author	Year	Treatments	Patients (n)	Mean follow-up (months)	Mean patient age (years)	Summary of outcomes
Vanlauwe et al. [50]	2011	pACI vs. MFx	118	60	33.9	pACI clinically superior to MFx, dependent on acuity
Gudas et al. [51][c]	2005	MFx vs. OAT	57	37.1	24.5	OAT clinically superior to MFx
Gudas et al. [52][c]	2012	MFx vs. OAT	29	120	24.5	OAT clinically superior to MFx
Gudas et al. [53][c]	2009	MFx vs. OAT	47	50.4	14.4	OAT clinically superior to MFx
Ulstein et al. [54]	2014	MFx vs. OAT	25	1176	32.2	Equivalent clinical and radiographic outcomes
Bentley et al. [55][d]	2003	mACI vs. OAT	100	19	31.3	mACI arthroscopically superior to OAT
Bentley et al. [56][d]	2012	mACI vs. OAT	100	120	31.3	mACI clinically superior to OAT
Dozin et al. [57]	2005	pACI vs. OAT	47	6	28.7	Equivalent clinical outcomes

Study	Year	Comparison	N	Follow-up (months)	Age	Outcome
Horas et al. [58]	2003	pACI vs. OAT	40	24	33.4	OAT clinically superior to pACI
Bartlett et al. [59]	2005	mACI vs. MACI	91	12	33.6	Equivalent clinical, arthroscopic, and histologic outcomes
Gooding et al. [60]	2006	pACI vs. mACI	68	24	30.5	Equivalent clinical outcomes
Zeifang et al. [61]	2010	pACI vs. MACI	21	24	29.3	Equivalent clinical outcomes
Anders et al. [62]	2013	MFx vs. MFx+	38	24	38	Equivalent clinical outcomes
Koh et al. [26]	2016	MFx vs. MFx+	80	24	39	MFx + improved radiographic outcomes
Stanish et al. [15]	2013	MFx vs. MFx+	80	12	36.2	Equivalent clinical outcomes
Volz et al. [16]	2017	MFx vs. MFx+	47	60	37	MFx + clinically superior to MFx+

MACI matrix-induced autologous chondrocyte implantation (ACI), *mACI* membrane patch ACI, *MFx* microfracture, *MFx +* enhanced microfracture, *OAT* osteochondral autograft transfer, *pACI* periosteal patch ACI
[a,b,c,d]Same cohort or subgroup of same cohort

Treatment-Based Algorithms for Articular Cartilage Lesions in the Knee

In light of the limited high-level evidence to guide treatment decisions for articular cartilage lesions of the knee, many of the available recommendations are expert opinion from high-volume surgeons in the field, although few evidence-based studies do tend to shape commonly referenced treatment algorithms [64, 65]. When approaching the patient with an articular cartilage lesion in the knee, the ultimate goal of the procedure should be to provide a solution tailored to the individual patient. That is, is the cartilage procedure to be considered palliative, reparative, or restorative? [66] While treatment options for these definitions often overlap rather than neatly fall into a single category, it is important to consider the differences when starting to make treatment decisions. Microfracture, for example, is considered a reparative procedure, whereas the hyaline and hyaline-like surface produced by OAT, osteochondral allograft transplantation, or ACI move toward the restorative realm. A variety of patient factors, including age, sex, activity level, body mass index (BMI), and history of previous surgery, are frequently considered, as are lesion factors, including location, size, depth, and containment [64, 67]. While the effect of age on the outcome of cartilage procedures has been called into question [64, 65], separating age from activity level remains a challenge, and age has typically remained an important part of treatment algorithms. While not truly related to the articular cartilage lesion, other factors including limb alignment, status of the meniscus, and ligamentous stability, must all be considered and concomitantly addressed, if needed [66].

Understanding patient goals and limitations of the available reparative and restorative techniques is paramount to achieve successful outcomes. In general, restorative procedures are favored for the young, active patient. Lesions with significant bone loss or cystic change are best treated with replacement of the entire osteochondral unit using OAT or osteochondral allograft transplantation. OAT is typically limited to lesions $\leq$2–3 cm^2 due to limited amounts of autologous tissue available and to limited donor site morbidity, whereas osteochondral allograft transplantation is ideal for larger-sized lesions [67–70]. ACI and other cell-based therapies, such as particulated juvenile cartilage allograft, are better suited for surface lesions without significant bone loss, although techniques for bone grafting with overlying ACI have been described [71, 72]. ACI is best used for lesions $\geq$2–3 cm^2, in the young, active patient population, with similar indications for particulated juvenile cartilage allograft albeit with a much shorter track record compared with various ACI generations [23]. Microfracture is typically used for lesions <2 cm^2 in young, active individuals or for larger lesions in older individuals with lower activity levels given the relative technical ease and low morbidity of the procedure. From a technical standpoint, microfracture requires a stable rim of adjacent cartilage in order to maintain a clot for formation of fibrocartilage. Because of this, in areas where it is not possible to obtain a stable rim of adjacent cartilage or the contour of the surface is unfavorable, which is often the case in the patellofemoral joint, other procedures, including ACI, OAT, or osteochondral allograft transplantation, may be considered.

These guidelines should serve to provide a framework for approaching the variety of patients that present with articular cartilage lesions in the knee. While high-level clinical evidence for these guidelines is limited, the technical aspects of the procedure and specific characteristics of the lesion often guide treatment. It is important, however, to individualize treatment strategies for patients in order to meet their individual goals and optimize outcomes.

The Effect of Concomitant Procedures

Creating a stable and biomechanically favorable environment for cartilage repair is critical to the success of reparative and restorative cartilage procedures in the knee [67, 73].

Ligamentous laxity, meniscal insufficiency, and malalignment create a biologically and biomechanically unfavorable environment for cartilage repair. The negative effects of malalignment and meniscal deficiency on cartilage contact pressures in the knee have been previously elucidated in the laboratory [74, 75], while ligamentous insufficiency can create excessive shear forces that place healing cartilage at risk [76]. A single non-randomized comparative study has suggested improved clinical outcomes for ACI performed in conjunction with valgus-producing high tibial osteotomy (HTO) for medial compartment cartilage lesions in the setting of minimal malalignment (<5° varus) compared to ACI alone [77]. Other studies have shown durable results and good to excellent clinical results for medial compartment cartilage lesions treated with microfracture and valgus-producing HTO [78, 79]. While the negative effects of malalignment on cartilage repair and restoration are commonly acknowledged, the degree of acceptable malalignment remains a topic of debate, although most agree that the magnitude of correction, when performed, should yield a neutral or slightly overcorrected mechanical axis [67].

Similarly, meniscal transplantation for meniscal deficiency combined with cartilage restoration procedures has provided optimistic results [80]. Most importantly, several studies have investigated a combination of procedures performed concomitantly with articular cartilage procedures, including osteotomy and/or meniscal transplantation, confirming the safety and efficacy of the concomitant surgical approach [81, 82]. However, when performing concomitant procedures, it is important to understand the rehabilitation goals and postoperative restrictions for each procedure performed in order to create a rehabilitation protocol that does not compromise outcomes. While the clinical data on the effect of osteotomy and meniscal transplantation performed in conjunction with articular cartilage procedures in the knee are limited, the reported safety of these procedures should encourage further clinical research on their efficacy.

Articular Cartilage Repair and Restoration in Children and Adolescents

The amount of high-quality literature dedicated to articular cartilage lesions of the knee in children, not including excision, drilling, or fixation of osteochondritis dissecans lesions, is very limited. A single randomized control trial compared OAT with microfracture in patients ≤18 years of age and noted clinical superiority of OAT, although both provided encouraging clinical results from 4-year follow-up [53]. Even in this cohort, distinguishing between a traumatic articular cartilage injury and osteochondritis dissecans lesion is difficult, and this remains a challenge when critically evaluating literature on the topic throughout the pediatric literature. Other cartilage procedures, including microfracture, ACI, and osteochondral allograft transplantation, have shown short-term efficacy when used in the pediatric patient [83–86]. A unique finding in pediatric patients undergoing cartilage restoration procedures in the knee is the positive influence of early clinical presentation on outcomes [87], thus emphasizing the importance of access to care in this dependent patient population. Overall, while the goal of treatment of articular cartilage lesions in the young, active patient is aimed at restoration of the cartilage surface, the data to support long-term cartilage restoration is lacking to make definitive conclusions.

Return to Sport in the Competitive Athlete

Injuries to the articular cartilage of the knee are relatively common in competitive athlete and may occur with a greater frequency compared to the general population [3]. Due to the high biomechanical and physiologic demands of the competitive athlete and the negligible ability of articular cartilage to heal on its own [70, 88], reparative and restorative procedures are often performed in order to allow athletes to return to their preinjury level of function. Part of the difficulty in evaluating the impact of articular cartilage procedures on return to sport is the fact that they are often performed concomitantly with other procedures [89]. Thus, determining the independent effect of articular cartilage procedures, whether positive or negative, remains elusive. Several recent systematic reviews with meta-analysis have investigated the ability of athletes undergoing a variety of cartilage restoration procedures to return to sport. In these studies, return to sport rates range between 60% and 90% [89–91]. While all these studies relied on predominantly Level III and IV studies, the aggregate data does show a trend toward improved return to sport for athletes undergoing OAT, followed by ACI, and, finally, microfracture [90, 91]. Although not consistently represented in systematic reviews, osteochondral allograft transplantation has provided return to sport rates of 75–90% in individual series, providing optimism for this option in the future [92–94].

Aggregate data provides the best data on return to sport for athletes following surgery for articular cartilage lesions of the knee with relatively promising short-term results. As has been mentioned previously, the durability of these outcomes remains largely unknown. Additionally, while outcomes following articular cartilage procedures in the knee are limited by heterogeneity and a lack of consistent long-term follow-up, several reasons for not returning to sport, including graduation or psychologic reasons, may not accurately reflect function or dysfunction, thus further limiting conclusions when using return to sport as a primary outcome.

Conclusion

A variety of surgical options exist to address articular cartilage injuries in the knee with favorable short-term outcomes. However, the best available literature fails to provide evidence on the long-term outcomes of these procedures, nor can it provide definitive treatment recommendations due to the lack of superiority of one technique over others. In general, restorative procedures are favored for young, active individuals, as this, in theory, provides the best option for long-term health of the joint. While recent developments have improved the technical challenges associated with articular cartilage repair in the knee, the quality of literature has not similarly improved. Moving forward, well-designed, multi-armed randomized control trials will certainly add to our knowledge on this complex topic, as will consistent outcome reporting with granular reporting of specific data elements of interest, such as the presence or absence of concomitantly performed procedures.

References

1. Aroen A, Loken S, Heir S, et al. Articular cartilage lesions in 993 consecutive knee arthroscopies. Am J Sports Med. 2004;32(1):211–5.
2. Widuchowski W, Widuchowski J, Trzaska T. Articular cartilage defects: study of 25,124 knee arthroscopies. Knee. 2007;14(3):177–82.
3. Flanigan DC, Harris JD, Trinh TQ, Siston RA, Brophy RH. Prevalence of chondral defects in athletes' knees: a systematic review. Med Sci Sports Exerc. 2010;42(10):1795–801.
4. Shelbourne KD, Jari S, Gray T. Outcome of untreated traumatic articular cartilage defects of the knee: a natural history study. J Bone Joint Surg Am. 2003;85-A(Suppl 2):8–16.
5. Widuchowski W, Widuchowski J, Faltus R, et al. Long-term clinical and radiological assessment of untreated severe cartilage damage in the knee: a natural history study. Scand J Med Sci Sports. 2011;21(1):106–10.
6. McCormick F, Harris JD, Abrams GD, et al. Trends in the surgical treatment of articular cartilage lesions in the United States: an analysis of a large private-payer database over a period of 8 years. Arthroscopy. 2014;30(2):222–6.
7. Montgomery SR, Foster BD, Ngo SS, et al. Trends in the surgical treatment of articular cartilage defects of the knee in the United States. Knee Surg Sports Traumatol Arthrosc. 2014;22(9):2070–5.

8. Harris JD, Erickson BJ, Abrams GD, et al. Methodologic quality of knee articular cartilage studies. Arthroscopy. 2013;29(7):1243–1252.e1245.

9. Jakobsen RB, Engebretsen L, Slauterbeck JR. An analysis of the quality of cartilage repair studies. J Bone Joint Surg Am. 2005;87(10):2232–9.

10. Makhni EC, Meyer MA, Saltzman BM, Cole BJ. Comprehensiveness of outcome reporting in studies of articular cartilage defects of the knee. Arthroscopy. 2016;32(10):2133–9.

11. Steadman JR, Rodkey WG, Briggs KK. Microfracture: its history and experience of the developing surgeon. Cartilage. 2010;1(2):78–86.

12. Mithoefer K, McAdams T, Williams RJ, Kreuz PC, Mandelbaum BR. Clinical efficacy of the microfracture technique for articular cartilage repair in the knee: an evidence-based systematic analysis. Am J Sports Med. 2009;37(10):2053–63.

13. DiBartola AC, Everhart JS, Magnussen RA, et al. Correlation between histological outcome and surgical cartilage repair technique in the knee: a meta-analysis. Knee. 2016;23(3):344–9.

14. Fortier LA, Chapman HS, Pownder SL, et al. BioCartilage improves cartilage repair compared with microfracture alone in an equine model of full-thickness cartilage loss. Am J Sports Med. 2016;44(9):2366–74.

15. Stanish WD, McCormack R, Forriol F, et al. Novel scaffold-based BST-CarGel treatment results in superior cartilage repair compared with microfracture in a randomized controlled trial. J Bone Joint Surg Am. 2013;95(18):1640–50.

16. Volz M, Schaumburger J, Frick H, Grifka J, Anders S. A randomized controlled trial demonstrating sustained benefit of Autologous Matrix-Induced Chondrogenesis over microfracture at five years. Int Orthop. 2017;41(4):797–804.

17. Brittberg M, Lindahl A, Nilsson A, Ohlsson C, Isaksson O, Peterson L. Treatment of deep cartilage defects in the knee with autologous chondrocyte transplantation. N Engl J Med. 1994;331(14):889–95.

18. Batty L, Dance S, Bajaj S, Cole BJ. Autologous chondrocyte implantation: an overview of technique and outcomes. ANZ J Surg. 2011;81(1–2):18–25.

19. Jacobi M, Villa V, Magnussen RA, Neyret P. MACI – a new era? Sports Med Arthrosc Rehabil Ther Technol. 2011;3(1):10.

20. Goyal D, Goyal A, Keyhani S, Lee EH, Hui JH. Evidence-based status of second- and third-generation autologous chondrocyte

implantation over first generation: a systematic review of level I and II studies. Arthroscopy. 2013;29(11):1872–8.

21. Farr J, Cole BJ, Sherman S, Karas V. Particulated articular cartilage: CAIS and DeNovo NT. J Knee Surg. 2012;25(1):23–9.

22. Farr J, Yao JQ. Chondral defect repair with particulated juvenile cartilage allograft. Cartilage. 2011;2(4):346–53.

23. Riboh JC, Cole BJ, Farr J. Particulated articular cartilage for symptomatic chondral defects of the knee. Curr Rev Musculoskelet Med. 2015;8(4):429–35.

24. HD A, Martin JA, Amendola RL, et al. The potential of human allogeneic juvenile chondrocytes for restoration of articular cartilage. Am J Sports Med. 2010;38(7):1324–33.

25. Hangody L, Rathonyi GK, Duska Z, Vasarhelyi G, Fules P, Modis L. Autologous osteochondral mosaicplasty. Surgical technique. J Bone Joint Surg Am. 2004;86-A(Suppl 1):65–72.

26. Koh JL, Wirsing K, Lautenschlager E, Zhang LO. The effect of graft height mismatch on contact pressure following osteochondral grafting: a biomechanical study. Am J Sports Med. 2004;32(2):317–20.

27. Ahmad CS, Guiney WB, Drinkwater CJ. Evaluation of donor site intrinsic healing response in autologous osteochondral grafting of the knee. Arthroscopy. 2002;18(1):95–8.

28. LaPrade RF, Botker JC. Donor-site morbidity after osteochondral autograft transfer procedures. Arthroscopy. 2004;20(7):e69–73.

29. Mundi R, Bedi A, Chow L, et al. Cartilage restoration of the knee: a systematic review and meta-analysis of level 1 studies. Am J Sports Med. 2016;44(7):1888–95.

30. Riboh JC, Cvetanovich GL, Cole BJ, Yanke AB. Comparative efficacy of cartilage repair procedures in the knee: a network meta-analysis. Knee Surg Sports Traumatol Arthrosc. 2017;25:3786–99.

31. Gross AE, Kim W, Las Heras F, Backstein D, Safir O, Pritzker KP. Fresh osteochondral allografts for posttraumatic knee defects: long-term followup. Clin Orthop Relat Res. 2008;466(8):1863–70.

32. LaPrade RF, Botker J, Herzog M, Agel J. Refrigerated osteoarticular allografts to treat articular cartilage defects of the femoral condyles. A prospective outcomes study. J Bone Joint Surg Am. 2009;91(4):805–11.

33. Friedlaender GE, Horowitz MC. Immune responses to osteochondral allografts: nature and significance. Orthopedics. 1992;15(10):1171–5.

34. Bernstein DT, O'Neill CA, Kim RS, et al. Osteochondral allograft donor-host matching by the femoral condyle radius of curvature. Am J Sports Med. 2017;45(2):403–9.

35. Highgenboten CL, Jackson A, Aschliman M, Meske NB. The estimation of femoral condyle size. An important component in osteochondral allografts. Clin Orthop Relat Res. 1989;246: 225–33.
36. Cook JL, Stannard JP, Stoker AM, et al. Importance of donor chondrocyte viability for osteochondral allografts. Am J Sports Med. 2016;44(5):1260–8.
37. Cook JL, Stoker AM, Stannard JP, et al. A novel system improves preservation of osteochondral allografts. Clin Orthop Relat Res. 2014;472(11):3404–14.
38. Qi J, Hu Z, Song H, et al. Cartilage storage at 4 degrees C with regular culture medium replacement benefits chondrocyte viability of osteochondral grafts in vitro. Cell Tissue Bank. 2016;17(3):473–9.
39. Williams SK, Amiel D, Ball ST, et al. Prolonged storage effects on the articular cartilage of fresh human osteochondral allografts. J Bone Joint Surg Am. 2003;85-a(11):2111–20.
40. Familiari F, Cinque ME, Chahla J, et al. Clinical outcomes and failure rates of osteochondral allograft transplantation in the knee: a systematic review. Am J Sports Med. 2017:363546517732531.
41. Wright JG, Swiontkowski MF, Heckman JD. Introducing levels of evidence to the journal. J Bone Joint Surg Am. 2003;85-a(1):1–3.
42. Basad E, Ishaque B, Bachmann G, Sturz H, Steinmeyer J. Matrix-induced autologous chondrocyte implantation versus micro-fracture in the treatment of cartilage defects of the knee: a 2-year randomised study. Knee Surg Sports Traumatol Arthrosc. 2010;18(4):519–27.
43. Crawford DC, DeBerardino TM, Williams RJ 3rd. NeoCart, an autologous cartilage tissue implant, compared with microfracture for treatment of distal femoral cartilage lesions: an FDA phase-II prospective, randomized clinical trial after two years. J Bone Joint Surg Am. 2012;94(11):979–89.
44. Knutsen G, Engebretsen L, Ludvigsen TC, et al. Autologous chondrocyte implantation compared with microfracture in the knee. A randomized trial. J Bone Joint Surg Am. 2004;86-a(3):455–64.
45. Knutsen G, Drogset JO, Engebretsen L, et al. A randomized trial comparing autologous chondrocyte implantation with microfracture. Findings at five years. J Bone Joint Surg Am. 2007;89(10):2105–12.
46. Knutsen G, Drogset JO, Engebretsen L, et al. A randomized multicenter trial comparing autologous chondrocyte implantation with microfracture: long-term follow-up at 14 to 15 years. J Bone Joint Surg Am. 2016;98(16):1332–9.

47. Saris DB, Vanlauwe J, Victor J, et al. Characterized chondrocyte implantation results in better structural repair when treating symptomatic cartilage defects of the knee in a randomized controlled trial versus microfracture. Am J Sports Med. 2008;36(2):235–46.
48. Saris DB, Vanlauwe J, Victor J, et al. Treatment of symptomatic cartilage defects of the knee: characterized chondrocyte implantation results in better clinical outcome at 36 months in a randomized trial compared to microfracture. Am J Sports Med. 2009;37(Suppl 1):10s–9s.
49. Van Assche D, Staes F, Van Caspel D, et al. Autologous chondrocyte implantation versus microfracture for knee cartilage injury: a prospective randomized trial, with 2-year follow-up. Knee Surg Sports Traumatol Arthrosc. 2010;18(4):486–95.
50. Vanlauwe J, Saris DB, Victor J, Almqvist KF, Bellemans J, Luyten FP. Five-year outcome of characterized chondrocyte implantation versus microfracture for symptomatic cartilage defects of the knee: early treatment matters. Am J Sports Med. 2011;39(12):2566–74.
51. Gudas R, Kalesinskas RJ, Kimtys V, et al. A prospective randomized clinical study of mosaic osteochondral autologous transplantation versus microfracture for the treatment of osteochondral defects in the knee joint in young athletes. Arthroscopy. 2005;21(9):1066–75.
52. Gudas R, Gudaite A, Pocius A, et al. Ten-year follow-up of a prospective, randomized clinical study of mosaic osteochondral autologous transplantation versus microfracture for the treatment of osteochondral defects in the knee joint of athletes. Am J Sports Med. 2012;40(11):2499–508.
53. Gudas R, Simonaityte R, Cekanauskas E, Tamosiunas R. A prospective, randomized clinical study of osteochondral autologous transplantation versus microfracture for the treatment of osteochondritis dissecans in the knee joint in children. J Pediatr Orthop. 2009;29(7):741–8.
54. Ulstein S, Aroen A, Rotterud JH, Loken S, Engebretsen L, Heir S. Microfracture technique versus osteochondral autologous transplantation mosaicplasty in patients with articular chondral lesions of the knee: a prospective randomized trial with long-term follow-up. Knee Surg Sports Traumatol Arthrosc. 2014;22(6):1207–15.
55. Bentley G, Biant LC, Carrington RW, et al. A prospective, randomised comparison of autologous chondrocyte implantation

versus mosaicplasty for osteochondral defects in the knee. J Bone Joint Surg Br. 2003;85(2):223–30.

56. Bentley G, Biant LC, Vijayan S, Macmull S, Skinner JA, Carrington RW. Minimum ten-year results of a prospective randomised study of autologous chondrocyte implantation versus mosaicplasty for symptomatic articular cartilage lesions of the knee. J Bone Joint Surg Br. 2012;94(4):504–9.

57. Dozin B, Malpeli M, Cancedda R, et al. Comparative evaluation of autologous chondrocyte implantation and mosaicplasty: a multicentered randomized clinical trial. Clin J Sport Med. 2005;15(4):220–6.

58. Horas U, Pelinkovic D, Herr G, Aigner T, Schnettler R. Autologous chondrocyte implantation and osteochondral cylinder transplantation in cartilage repair of the knee joint. A prospective, comparative trial. J Bone Joint Surg Am. 2003;85-a(2):185–92.

59. Bartlett W, Skinner JA, Gooding CR, et al. Autologous chondrocyte implantation versus matrix-induced autologous chondrocyte implantation for osteochondral defects of the knee: a prospective, randomised study. J Bone Joint Surg Br. 2005;87(5):640–5.

60. Gooding CR, Bartlett W, Bentley G, Skinner JA, Carrington R, Flanagan A. A prospective, randomised study comparing two techniques of autologous chondrocyte implantation for osteochondral defects in the knee: Periosteum covered versus type I/III collagen covered. Knee. 2006;13(3):203–10.

61. Zeifang F, Oberle D, Nierhoff C, Richter W, Moradi B, Schmitt H. Autologous chondrocyte implantation using the original periosteum-cover technique versus matrix-associated autologous chondrocyte implantation: a randomized clinical trial. Am J Sports Med. 2010;38(5):924–33.

62. Anders S, Volz M, Frick H, Gellissen J. A randomized, controlled trial comparing autologous matrix-induced chondrogenesis (AMIC(R)) to microfracture: analysis of 1- and 2-year follow-up data of 2 centers. Open Orthop J. 2013;7:133–43.

63. Koh YG, Kwon OR, Kim YS, Choi YJ, Tak DH. Adipose-derived mesenchymal stem cells with microfracture versus microfracture alone: 2-year follow-up of a prospective randomized trial. Arthroscopy. 2016;32(1):97–109.

64. Behery O, Siston RA, Harris JD, Flanigan DC. Treatment of cartilage defects of the knee: expanding on the existing algorithm. Clin J Sport Med. 2014;24(1):21–30.

65. Bekkers JE, Inklaar M, Saris DB. Treatment selection in articular cartilage lesions of the knee: a systematic review. Am J Sports Med. 2009;37(Suppl 1):148s–55s.

66. Alford JW, Cole BJ. Cartilage restoration, part 1: basic science, historical perspective, patient evaluation, and treatment options. Am J Sports Med. 2005;33(2):295–306.

67. Alford JW, Cole BJ. Cartilage restoration, part 2: techniques, outcomes, and future directions. Am J Sports Med. 2005;33(3):443–60.

68. Camp CL, Stuart MJ, Krych AJ. Current concepts of articular cartilage restoration techniques in the knee. Sports Health. 2014;6(3):265–73.

69. Cole BJ, Pascual-Garrido C, Grumet RC. Surgical management of articular cartilage defects in the knee. Instr Course Lect. 2010;59:181–204.

70. Murray IR, Benke MT, Mandelbaum BR. Management of knee articular cartilage injuries in athletes: chondroprotection, chondrofacilitation, and resurfacing. Knee Surg Sports Traumatol Arthrosc. 2016;24(5):1617–26.

71. Bhattacharjee A, McCarthy HS, Tins B, et al. Autologous bone plug supplemented with autologous chondrocyte implantation in osteochondral defects of the knee. Am J Sports Med. 2016;44(5):1249–59.

72. Vijayan S, Bartlett W, Bentley G, et al. Autologous chondrocyte implantation for osteochondral lesions in the knee using a bilayer collagen membrane and bone graft: a two- to eight-year follow-up study. J Bone Joint Surg Br. 2012;94(4):488–92.

73. Weber AE, Gitelis ME, McCarthy MA, Yanke AB, Cole BJ. Malalignment: a requirement for cartilage and organ restoration. Sports Med Arthrosc. 2016;24(2):e14–22.

74. Agneskirchner JD, Hurschler C, Wrann CD, Lobenhoffer P. The effects of valgus medial opening wedge high tibial osteotomy on articular cartilage pressure of the knee: a biomechanical study. Arthroscopy. 2007;23(8):852–61.

75. Lee SJ, Aadalen KJ, Malaviya P, et al. Tibiofemoral contact mechanics after serial medial meniscectomies in the human cadaveric knee. Am J Sports Med. 2006;34(8):1334–44.

76. Brittberg M, Peterson L, Sjogren-Jansson E, Tallheden T, Lindahl A. Articular cartilage engineering with autologous chondrocyte transplantation. A review of recent developments. J Bone Joint Surg Am. 2003;85-A(Suppl 3):109–15.

77. Bode G, Schmal H, Pestka JM, Ogon P, Sudkamp NP, Niemeyer P. A non-randomized controlled clinical trial on autologous chondrocyte implantation (ACI) in cartilage defects of the medial femoral condyle with or without high tibial osteotomy in patients with varus deformity of less than 5 degrees. Arch Orthop Trauma Surg. 2013;133(1):43–9.

292   K. R. Duchman and J. C. Riboh

78. Sterett WI, Steadman JR. Chondral resurfacing and high tibial osteotomy in the varus knee. Am J Sports Med. 2004;32(5):1243–9.
79. Sterett WI, Steadman JR, Huang MJ, Matheny LM, Briggs KK. Chondral resurfacing and high tibial osteotomy in the varus knee: survivorship analysis. Am J Sports Med. 2010;38(7):1420–4.
80. Rue JP, Yanke AB, Busam ML, McNickle AG, Cole BJ. Prospective evaluation of concurrent meniscus transplantation and articular cartilage repair: minimum 2-year follow-up. Am J Sports Med. 2008;36(9):1770–8.
81. Harris JD, Hussey K, Saltzman BM, et al. Cartilage repair with or without meniscal transplantation and osteotomy for lateral compartment chondral defects of the knee: case series with minimum 2-year follow-up. Orthop J Sports Med. 2014;2(10):2325967114551528.
82. Harris JD, Hussey K, Wilson H, et al. Biological knee reconstruction for combined malalignment, meniscal deficiency, and articular cartilage disease. Arthroscopy. 2015;31(2):275–82.
83. Cvetanovich GL, Riboh JC, Tilton AK, Cole BJ. Autologous chondrocyte implantation improves knee-specific functional outcomes and health-related quality of life in adolescent patients. Am J Sports Med. 2017;45(1):70–6.
84. Micheli LJ, Moseley JB, Anderson AF, et al. Articular cartilage defects of the distal femur in children and adolescents: treatment with autologous chondrocyte implantation. J Pediatr Orthop. 2006;26(4):455–60.
85. Murphy RT, Pennock AT, Bugbee WD. Osteochondral allograft transplantation of the knee in the pediatric and adolescent population. Am J Sports Med. 2014;42(3):635–40.
86. Steadman JR, Briggs KK, Matheny LM, Guillet A, Hanson CM, Willimon SC. Outcomes following microfracture of full-thickness articular cartilage lesions of the knee in adolescent patients. J Knee Surg. 2015;28(2):145–50.
87. DiBartola AC, Wright BM, Magnussen RA, Flanigan DC. Clinical outcomes after autologous chondrocyte implantation in adolescents' knees: a systematic review. Arthroscopy. 2016;32(9):1905–16.
88. Buckwalter JA. Articular cartilage: injuries and potential for healing. J Orthop Sports Phys Ther. 1998;28(4):192–202.
89. Harris JD, Brophy RH, Siston RA, Flanigan DC. Treatment of chondral defects in the athlete's knee. Arthroscopy. 2010;26(6):841–52.

90. Krych AJ, Pareek A, King AH, Johnson NR, Stuart MJ, Williams RJ 3rd. Return to sport after the surgical management of articular cartilage lesions in the knee: a meta-analysis. Knee Surg Sports Traumatol Arthrosc. 2017;25:3186–96.
91. Mithoefer K, Hambly K, Della Villa S, Silvers H, Mandelbaum BR. Return to sports participation after articular cartilage repair in the knee: scientific evidence. Am J Sports Med. 2009;37(Suppl 1):167s–76s.
92. Krych AJ, Robertson CM, Williams RJ 3rd. Return to athletic activity after osteochondral allograft transplantation in the knee. Am J Sports Med. 2012;40(5):1053–9.
93. McCarthy MA, Meyer MA, Weber AE, et al. Can competitive athletes return to high-level play after osteochondral allograft transplantation of the knee? Arthroscopy. 2017;33(9):1712–7.
94. Nielsen ES, McCauley JC, Pulido PA, Bugbee WD. Return to sport and recreational activity after osteochondral allograft transplantation in the knee. Am J Sports Med. 2017;45(7):1608–14.

Chapter 18
Emerging Technologies in Cartilage Restoration

Andrew J. Riff, Annabelle Davey, and Brian J. Cole

Injuries to articular cartilage are common and increasing in prevalence due to the rise in obesity and involvement in organized sports. However, due to limited vascularity and cellularity, articular cartilage possesses little capacity for spontaneous healing. If left untreated, articular cartilage injuries are one of the most common causes of permanent disability in athletes and may lead to widespread osteoarthritis. This increasing disease burden has prompted investigation into finding durable solutions to this challenging problem.

Over the last 25 years, surgical intervention for cartilage injury has increased dramatically, with the most broadly utilized techniques including marrow stimulation techniques (MST, including microfracture and subchondral drilling), autologous chondrocyte implantation (ACI), and osteochondral grafting (including osteochondral autograft transfer [OAT]

A. J. Riff (✉)
IU Health Physicians Orthopedics & Sports Medicine,
Indianapolis, IN, USA
e-mail: ariff@iuhealth.org

A. Davey
University of Vermont, College of Medicine, Burlington, VT, USA

B. J. Cole
Department of Orthopedic Surgery, Rush University Medical
Center, Chicago, IL, USA

© Springer Nature Switzerland AG 2019   295
A. B. Yanke, B. J. Cole (eds.), *Joint Preservation of the Knee*,
https://doi.org/10.1007/978-3-030-01491-9_18

and osteochondral allograft transplantation [OCA]). While each of these techniques has had a significant impact on the field of cartilage restoration, each has inherent drawbacks. Marrow stimulation is simple and inexpensive; however, it is limited by fibrocartilage repair tissue, poor durability, and poor results for larger lesions. ACI renders greater longevity and greater utility for larger lesions than microfracture; however, it is limited by its expense, two-stage nature, and the fact that it generates hyaline-like cartilage but not true hyaline cartilage. Osteochondral allografts offer immediate hyaline cartilage and the ability to restore subchondral bone; however, allografts are available in limited supply and have associated concerns regarding disease transmission and chondrocyte viability.

Due to the shortcomings of existing cartilage repair techniques, several new technologies have recently entered the global cartilage repair market. Many of these novel products are first introduced in Europe or Asia due to less strict regulatory standards than those required by the US Food and Drug Administration (FDA). A limited number of products are able to come to market quickly in the United States if they qualify as "minimally manipulated" or intended for "homologous use," as such products do not require the FDA market approval pathway. Recently developed techniques that have garnered enthusiasm include augmented microfracture, matrix-assisted autologous chondrocyte implantation (MACI), minced cartilage products, off-the-shelf osteochondral implants, matrix plus stem cell products, and injectable agents. In this chapter, we will discuss new techniques being investigated abroad or recently introduced in the United States and the rationale behind each of these innovations and summarize available evidence for these new technologies.

Augmented Marrow Stimulation Techniques

Marrow stimulation techniques (MST), including microfracture and subchondral drilling, have long been the primary treatment for articular cartilage lesions due to the relative ease and low cost. However, due to fibrocartilage repair tissue, MST has demonstrated inferior durability to more costly treatments [1]. In augmented MST, a matrix or scaffold is added to the defect following marrow stimulation to stabilize the mesenchymal clot and to improve mesenchymal stem cell (MSC) differentiation into more hyaline-like articular cartilage [2]. Augmented MST techniques include autologous matrix-induced chondrogenesis (AMIC), BST-CarGel, GelrinC, BioCartilage, and chondrotissue.

First described by Behrens and colleagues in 2010, AMIC was the first described augmented marrow stimulation technique. AMIC combines microfracture with the application of a porcine collagen I/III matrix (ChondroGide, Geistlich, Pharma AG) fixated with either autologous or allogeneic fibrin glue [3]. This technique can be employed either arthroscopically or following a mini-arthrotomy [4]. A retrospective case series of 21 patients with large chondral defects (>2 cm^2) treated with AMIC reported MRI evidence of high-quality repair tissue in 67% of patients and 76% patient satisfaction [5]. These results are noteworthy because large lesions have demonstrated poor results with conventional MST [1]. A multicenter RCT compared AMIC with conventional microfracture in 47 patients with a mean defect size of 3.6 +/− 1.6 cm^2. Patients were randomized to receive either microfracture alone, glued AMIC, or sutured AMIC. All three groups showed significant improvements in Cincinnati and ICRS scores from preoperative to 2-year follow-up; however, patient-reported outcomes remained favorable between 2- and 5-year follow-up in both AMIC-treated groups, while the results of isolated microfracture declined between the 2- and 5-year time points. Moreover, MRI results indicated more complete defect fill in both AMIC groups than the isolated microfracture group [4].

BST-CarGel (Piramal Life Sciences, Laval, Quebec, Canada) is a bioscaffold containing liquid chitosan and autologous whole blood. Chitosan is an abundant glucosamine polysaccharide derived from the exoskeleton of crustaceans and is favored as a scaffold due to its biocompatibility, biodegradability, and adhesive properties. BST-CarGel is typically applied to the microfracture site through a mini-arthrotomy after creating a "dry-field" by swabbing the lesion with gauze. In a multicenter randomized controlled trial, BST-CarGel was shown to have superior outcomes to micro-fracture at 1-year and at 5-year follow-up [6]. Eighty patients with symptomatic grade III or IV articular cartilage lesions were randomized to receive either conventional microfrac-ture or microfracture augmented with BST-CarGel. Second-look arthroscopy was performed at a year postoperatively, and tissue biopsies were obtained. The BST-CarGel cohort demonstrated superior ICRS scores by surgeon visualization, superior histological parameters, and harbored repair tissue with improved collagen organization based on polarized light microscopy. At 5-year follow-up, the BST-CarGel group dem-onstrated superior fill by 3D quantitative MRI findings and reduced T2 relaxation times (suggesting more organized collagen).

GelrinC (Regentis Biomaterials, Or Akiva, Israel) is an investigational hydrogel composed of polyethylene glycol di-acrylate (PEG-DA) and denatured fibrinogen. These two liquid materials are added to the defect following microfrac-ture and are cross-linked in situ with UV light, forming a semisolid biodegradable scaffold for MSCs. In one study conducted in Austria reporting on the MRI outcomes of 21 patients undergoing microfracture augmented with GelrinC, the quality of the cartilage in the defect was found to be the same as healthy cartilage after 24 months in 81% of the patients as determined by global T2 index [7]. Additionally, average MOCART score increased at each follow-up time point from 6 months to 24 months, indicating that cartilage quality improved over the course of the postoperative time points [7]. While early results are promising, longer-term comparative literature is still necessary. A multicenter, open-label, phase I/II clinical trial is ongoing at institutions in Belgium, Germany, Israel, the Netherlands, and Poland (NCT00989794).

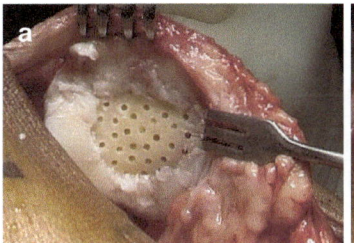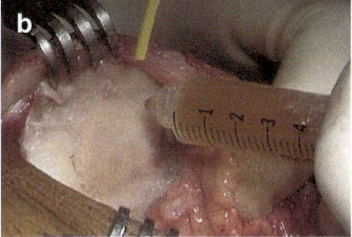

FIGURE 18.1 Central patellar chondral lesion measuring roughly 25 mm × 25 mm following lesion curettage and marrow stimulation (**a**) and application of BioCartilage and PRP (**b**)

BioCartilage (Arthrex, Inc., Naples, Florida) is a product made from dehydrated, micronized allogeneic cartilage that is designed to be implanted with platelet-rich plasma (PRP) (Fig. 18.1a, b). It contains components of hyaline cartilage extracellular matrix including type II collagen and proteoglycans that are thought to direct MSCs to produce higher-quality cartilage to fill the defect [2]. In a controlled laboratory study in an equine model, Fortier and colleagues demonstrated that microfracture augmented with BioCartilage and PRP was significantly better than microfracture alone in terms of ICRS histologic score and quantitative MRI T2 relaxation times at 13 months postoperatively [8]. There are currently no published clinical outcome studies in human subjects; however, Stannard and colleagues are currently conducting a single-center prospective cohort study comparing BioCartilage-augmented microfracture with microfracture in isolation (NCT02203071). BioCartilage is available for use in the United States.

Chondrotissue (BioTissue AG, Zurich, Switzerland) is a scaffold composed of polyglycolic acid (PGA) and hyaluronic acid (HA) immersed in PRP designed for application after marrow stimulation. In an ovine model, chondrotissue plus microfracture has been shown to improve the quality of repair tissue compared to isolated microfracture. Siclari and colleagues published a series of 52 patients with focal chondral lesions in the knee treated with chondrotissue-enhanced subchondral drilling, noting significant improvements in KOOS scores and histology (from 4 s-look biopsies) consistent with hyaline-like to hyaline repair tissue with increased proteoglycan content and type II collagen [9]. Released in 2007, chondrotissue is CE marked for use in Europe, but not commercially available in the United States.

Matrix-Assisted Autologous Chondrocyte Implantation

Introduced in 1987 and first published in 1994, autologous chondrocyte implantation (ACI) represented the first cell-based surgical technique for cartilage restoration. First-generation ACI was limited by the need for periosteal flaps, graft hypertrophy, and formation of hyaline-like cartilage. Second- and third-generation ACI techniques make use of three-dimensional matrices that eliminate the need for periosteal flaps and offer the promise of generating more natural hyaline cartilage. Although just recently approved by the FDA for use in the United States in December 2016, matrix-assisted autologous chondrocyte implantation (MACI) has been performed extensively in Europe and Australia since 1999 [10, 11]. MACI products are made by application of cultured autologous chondrocytes to a substrate composed of a collagen hydrogel or membrane, a copolymer of polyglycolic or polylactic acid and polydioxanone, or HA. A multitude of MACI products have been investigated including Hyalograft C, cartilage regeneration system (CaReS), Novocart 3D, NeoCart, and Biocart, among others.

In use since 1999, Hyalograft C (Fidia Advanced Polymers, Abano Terme, Italy) was the first autologous tissue-engineered cartilage product to hit the market [11]. Hyalograft C is a MACI product utilizing a HYAFF-11 scaffold, a nonwoven, esterified derivative of hyaluronic acid designed to support in vitro growth of chondrocytes. Following cell harvest performed in the same manner as conventional ACI, the biopsy specimen is sent to Fidia Advanced Biopolymers for in vitro cell culture. After 4 weeks of cell culture, the cell-seeded matrix can be implanted via a mini-arthrotomy and fixated around the periphery with fibrin glue. Initial studies revealed that Hyalograft C was safe, biocompatible, and avoided adverse events associated with the periosteal flap. Brix and colleagues published a case series of 53 subjects treated with Hyalograft C at an average 9-year follow-up [11]. The authors noted excellent patient-reported outcomes and surviv-ability for simple cases (isolated defects <4cm^2-failure rate of 4%) but poor results of salvage cases (early osteoarthritic changes or bipolar lesions—failure rate of 88%). Although Hyalograft C represented one of the most broadly used matri-ces on the market, it was removed from the European market in 2013 by the European Medical Association (EMA) due to concerns about manufacturing practices and low-quality com-parative studies [12].

CaReS (Arthro Kinetics, Krems, Austria) is a MACI prod-uct based on type I collagen scaffold derived from rat tail tendons. Preparation of CaReS involves (1) isolation of chon-drocytes from the biopsy specimen using collagenase, (2) suspension of isolated chondrocytes in type I collagen from rat tail tendons, (3) polymerization of the chondrocyte-collagen mixture in 37 °C in a humidified atmosphere, and (4) culture in autologous serum for 10–13 days. To meet quality control standards, all specimens are required to display cell viability >80% and expression of type II collagen based on real-time PCR. CaReS implants can be manufactured to a custom height and area. Schneider and colleagues published a multicenter case series of 116 German patients treated with CaReS between 2003 and 2008 [13]. The authors noted sig-nificant improvement in all patient-reported outcomes and 80% patient satisfaction.

Novocart 3D (TeTeC, Reutlingen, Germany) is a bilay-ered type I collagen sponge containing chondroitin sulfate. After processing, harvested cells are seeded onto the scaf-fold and cultivated in homologous serum for 2 days, and the graft is returned to the treating hospital. An Austrian study of Novocart 3D in 28 patients demonstrated that all patients had significant improvement in patient-reported outcomes and most cases revealed complete defect fill by MRI [14]. Somewhat concerning, Niethammer and colleagues noted MRI evidence of graft hypertrophy 25% of patients (11/44) treated with Novocart 3D, with particular abundance in those with history of acute trauma or OCD. It has been used commercially in Europe since 2003 and as part of a phase III trial in the United States since 2014 (NCT01957722).

NeoCart (Histogenics, Waltham, MA) combines a biodegradable bovine type I collagen patch with autogenous chondrocytes and bioreactor technology (Fig. 18.2a–d). Bioreactor treatment aims to optimize oxygen concentration, pressure, and perfusion and has been shown to improve integration of chondrocytes with a collagen matrix compared to untreated constructs in an in vivo porcine model [15, 16]. A phase II randomized clinical trial comparing NeoCart and microfracture in 30 patients with grade III lesions of the femoral condyle demonstrated that NeoCart was superior to microfracture with regard to percentage of patients improved and improvement in KOOS pain [17]. A phase III trial comparing NeoCart with microfracture is currently enrolling (NCT01066702).

BioCart II (Histogenics, Waltham, MA) is MACI product generated by culturing harvested chondrocytes with autologous serum and fibroblast growth factor 2v1 before they are seeded into a fibrin-hyaluronan matrix. Cells cultured in a medium containing an FGF variant have demonstrated a tenfold increase in cell proliferation compared to those cultured without the growth factor [18]. MRI evaluation of six knees between 15 and 27 months following treatment with BioCart II revealed that BioCart II rendered repair tissue similar to hyaline cartilage based on T2 relaxation times and dGEMRIC analysis [19]. A multicenter phase II trial comparing BioCart II to microfracture has been ongoing since 2008 but remains unpublished (NCT00729716).

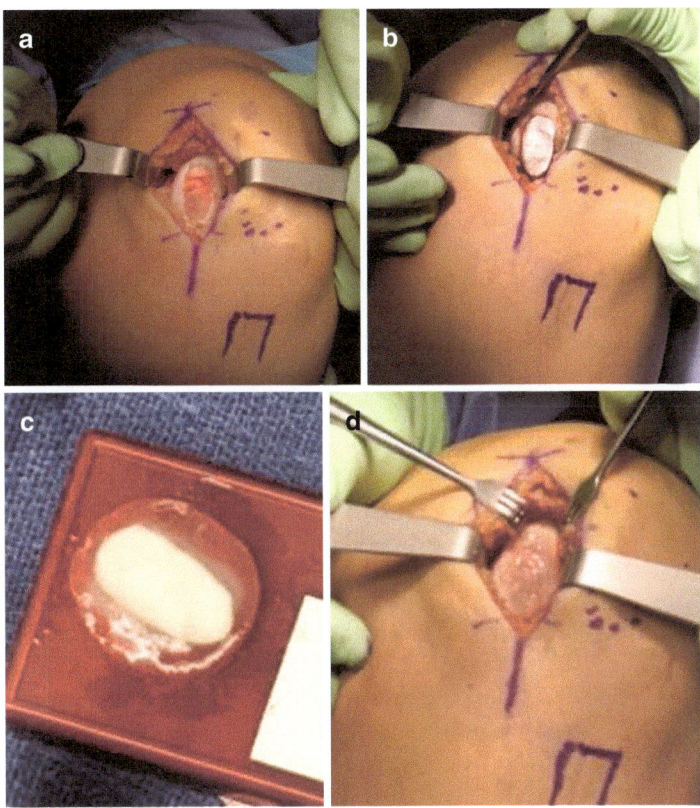

FIGURE 18.2 Large chondral lesion involving the medial femoral condyle measuring roughly 15 mm × 30 mm following lesion curettage (**a**). Lesion templating with aluminum foil (**b**). NeoCart graft preparation on the back table (**c**). NeoCart graft placement (**d**)

A recent systematic review of MACI techniques revealed that MACI results in hyaline-like histology in 38–75% of cases and better histology and patient-reported outcomes than microfracture [12]. This review highlighted the poor quality of the available literature and the need for future studies comparing different matrices to help surgeons in selecting the optimal graft choice for their patients.

Matrix plus Mesenchymal Stem Cells

In pursuit of a single-stage alternative to ACI, multiple products have emerged that combine mesenchymal stem cells (MSCs) with three-dimensional scaffolds. Proponents of these techniques theorize that coupling MSCs with the appropriate matrix and growth factors may offer a reliable method of generating durable hyaline-like cartilage. MSCs augment the quality of repair tissue by increasing the aggrecan concentration and enhancing cartilage firmness [20]. Products are available in this category utilizing both autologous (Hyalofast) and allogeneic (Cartistem) MSCs.

Hyalofast (Anika Therapeutics, Bedford, Massachusetts, USA) is a product that combines the HYAFF11 scaffold (the same scaffold used in Hyalograft C) with MSCs derived from bone marrow aspirate concentrate (BMAC). BMAC contains adult MSCs, platelets, cytokines, and growth factors (including platelet-derived growth factor [PDGF], transforming growth factor beta [TGFβ], and bone morphogenetic protein [BMP-2 and BMP-7]), which improve the healing milieu through their anabolic and anti-inflammatory properties [21–24]. MSCs constitute just 0.001% of nucleated cells in bone marrow aspirate; therefore, bone marrow aspirate is subjected to centrifugation to increase the MSC concentration. The Hyalofast technique involves templating the hyaluronan scaffold to the defect, soaking the scaffold with BMAC, and fixating it to surrounding cartilage with 6-0 PDS suture and/or fibrin glue. Gobbi and colleagues recently published a prospective matched cohort study comparing 25 patients treated with microfracture, and 27 patients were treated with Hyalofast [25]. At 2-year follow-up, a significantly greater proportion of the microfracture group had returned to pre-injury activity level, as determined by Tegner score. However, at 5-year follow-up, a significantly greater portion of the HA-BMAC group had returned to the pre-injury activity level [25]. The same group published a Level 2 cohort study comparing results of Hyalofast in patients >45 years of age with those <45 years of age [26]. At 4-year follow-up, both groups improved significantly in IKDC, KOOS, VAS, and Tenger scores, with no significant difference between the groups. As one would expect, patient-reported outcomes were superior in patients with lesion area <8 cm^2 and in patients with a single lesion as opposed to multiple lesions [26]. Hyalofast is commercially available in most European countries and some Asian and South American countries but is not available in the United States.

Multiple other strategies combining autologous stem cells and matrices are in early phases of clinical testing. There is interest in the use of a collagen matrix seeded with bioactive factors and adipose-derived stem cells (ADSCs). While there are not yet any clinical results, Calabrese and colleagues have demonstrated that ADSCs are able to completely differentiate into mature chondrocytes when combined with a type I collagen scaffold and chondrogenic inducing factors in vitro [27]. Dragoo and colleagues are currently enrolling patients in a multicenter RCT comparing ADSCs plus collagen scaffold with microfracture for isolated chondral lesions of the knee (NCT02090140).

The use of allogeneic stem cells in conjunction with a three-dimensional scaffold is another option that is being explored to avoid donor site morbidity. Cartistem (Medipost Co., Ltd., Korea) is a product that utilizes a sodium hyaluronate scaffold seeded with culture-expanded human umbilical cord blood-derived mesenchymal stem cells (hUBC-MSCs). The only available literature on Cartistem is a phase I/II single-center clinical trial of seven patients treated with either low-dose or high-dose hUBC-MSCs conducted in Korea [28]. Six of the seven patients consented to undergo second-look arthroscopy at 12-week follow-up, at which point the treating physician observed maturing cartilage in all six knees. VAS and IKDC scores improved in all subjects from preoperative level to 3-month follow-up and remained relatively stable from 3 months to 7 years [28]. This study suggests that Cartistem is safe and effective, but it is limited by its small sample size. Cole and Gomoll are currently conducting a phase I/II clinical trial investigating the safety and efficacy of Cartistem in 12 patients with full-thickness grade 3–4 articular cartilage defects of the knee which is expected to finish data collection in July of 2017 (NCT01733186).

Minced Cartilage Products

Minced cartilage repair is another treatment strategy that harnesses the theory of ACI in a single-stage alternative. This technique involves filling a chondral defect with a small amount of particulate hyaline cartilage secured with fibrin glue and often combined with a scaffold delivery system. Mincing cartilage into 1–2-mm^3 fragments allows the chondrocytes to escape from the extracellular matrix and to produce hyaline-like cartilage that will integrate with the surrounding native tissue [29]. Minced cartilage products utilizing both autologous (Cartilage Autograft Implantation System [CAIS]) and allogeneic (DeNovo Natural Tissue) cartilage have been investigated.

Cartilage Autograft Implantation System (CAIS) (DePuy Mitek, Raynham, Massachusetts, USA) is a proprietary technique which involves harvesting autologous cells from the intercondylar notch or trochlear border, mincing cartilage into 1–2-mm^3 fragments, securing minced fragments to a proprietary scaffold composed of polycaprolactone (35%) and PGA (65%) reinforced with PDO mesh, and fixating the implant to the defect using biodegradable anchors [30]. An initial randomized pilot study compared CAIS and microfracture in 29 patients with lesions involving the trochlea or femoral condyle [31]. At 24-month follow-up, both groups had a significant improvement in IKDC and KOOS scores from baseline, and the CAIS group had significantly higher scores than the microfracture group. Despite these promising results, the phase III multicenter randomized controlled trial (NCT00881023) was discontinued due to lack of enrollment and prohibitive expense [32].

DeNovo Natural Tissue (NT) (Zimmer Biomet, Warsaw, Indiana, USA) utilizes 1-mm^3 pieces of allogeneic cartilage from donors younger than 13 of age and secured with fibrin glue (Fig. 18.3a–d) [33]. The primary advantages of this technique relate to the fact that juvenile chondrocytes have a 100-fold increased ability to produce proteoglycans and that these cells do not stimulate an immunogenic response. The primary drawback of this technique is that DeNovo NT has a ~40-day shelf life and, as such, many surgeons will only perform this technique after performing a diagnostic arthroscopy making it a two-stage technique. While there are not yet any long-term outcome studies or Level I evidence, early clinical results are

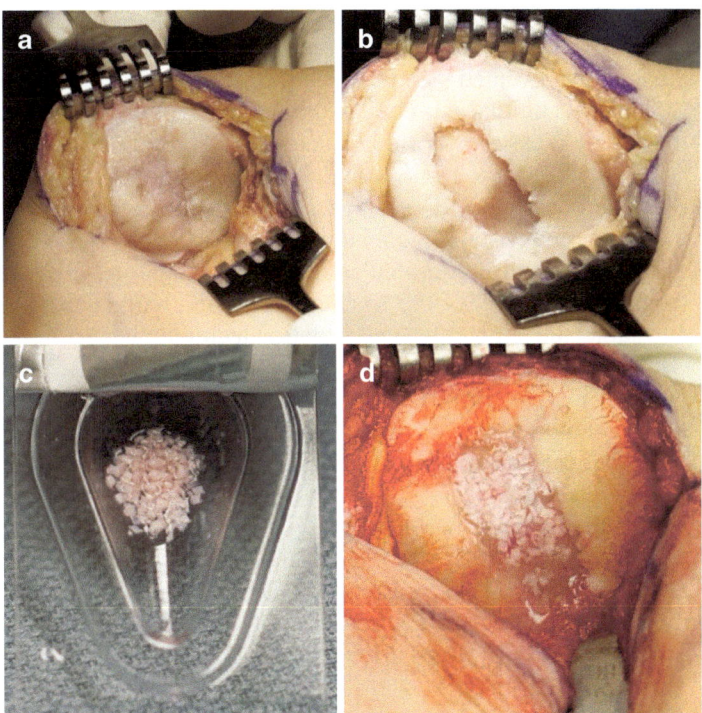

FIGURE 18.3 Central patellar lesion measuring 15 mm × 30 mm (**a**). Lesion following curettage to establish vertical walls (**b**). DeNovo NT graft in delivery packaging (**c**). Lesion following application of DeNovo NT with fibrin glue mixture (**d**)

extremely promising. In a case series of 25 patients with a mean femoral lesion size of 2.7 ± 0.8 cm^2, IKDC and KOOS clinical outcome scores showed significant improvements compared to baseline at 24 months after surgery [34]. Additionally, quantitative MRI results with T2 mapping demonstrated that the repair cartilage was of a similar composition to native cartilage after 2 years. Histologic results from biopsies taken from eight patients indicated that there was excellent integration of the transplant tissue with the native cartilage, although the biopsies contained both hyaline and fibrocartilage [34]. Additionally, in a retrospective Level IV case series, 17 patients with patellar chondral lesions who were treated with DeNovo NT were reviewed. Follow-up at a mean 8.2 months revealed significant improvement in KOOS score [35]. This technique is rapidly gaining popularity, with approximately 8700 cases performed since 2007 [29].

CartiONE (Orteq Ltd., London, UK) is a novel technique that combines minced cartilage, BMAC, and a commercially available scaffold in a single-step cartilage repair technique. In a 1 h time span, non-articular hyaline cartilage is harvested from the periphery of the trochlea or the intercondylar notch and subjected to patented cell-isolation technology, co-cultured with BMAC, and added to a commercially available scaffold prior to implantation. The rationale behind this technique is based on literature suggesting that trophic factors from MSCs help to increase chondrocyte proliferation and matrix formation [36]. The INSTRUCT clinical trial evaluated PROs, histologic outcomes, and radiologic outcomes of 40 patients treated with CartiONE for symptomatic cartilage defects in the knee (NCT01041885). This trial reported significant improvements in KOOS, IKDC, and VAS; consistent defect filling by MRI; and evidence of hyaline cartilage in most patients.

Off-the-Shelf Osteochondral Implants

Fresh osteochondral allograft (OCA) transplantation has emerged as a valuable and successful treatment for chondral and osteochondral defects with graft survivorship approaching

90% at 10 years [37, 38]. Despite the success of this technique, OCA remains limited by graft availability and concerns regarding disease transmission. Additionally, due to graft expense, many surgeons perform diagnostic arthroscopy prior to OCA transplantation making this a two-stage technique. Due to these limitations, stand-alone proprietary osteochondral implants have been developed that are readily available with prolonged shelf lives. Three off-the-shelf osteochondral implants are presently available on the market including Chondrofix, Cartiform, and ProChondrix. Although they contain no osteocytes on chondrocytes, two novel scaffolds (Maioregen and Agili-C) are also discussed in this section as they are used in isolation for the treatment of osteochondral defects.

Made available in 2012, Chondrofix (Zimmer Inc., Warsaw, IN) represented the first off-the-shelf osteochondral allograft. Chondrofix is a decellularized osteochondral allograft which is available in four precut sizes and offers a 2-year shelf life. Unfortunately, a prospective series of 32 patients treated with Chondrofix demonstrated a 72% failure rate within 2 years of implantation [39]. Although the authors did not speculate in their abstract on the cause of the high failure rate, it is probable that the lack of viable chondrocytes played a role.

Cartiform (Arthrex Inc., Naples, FL) and ProChondrix (AlloSource, Centennial, CO) represent two recently released, commercially available osteochondral allograft disc implants that contain viable chondrocytes. Since these implants are considered "minimally manipulated," they are available for use in the United States. Cartiform is a cryopreserved, viable osteochondral allograft (CVOCA) available in four sizes including 10 mm diameter, 20 mm diameter, 12x19mm, and 20x25mm. Cartiform contains full-thickness pores throughout its area that improve graft flexibility and allow the cryopreservation solution to penetrate the tissue to preserve cell viability throughout rather than just the surface of the graft. As a result, Cartiform possesses a 2-year shelf life when stored at −80 °C. Additionally, Cartiform has a minimal bone component which further improves graft flexibility to match the topography of the underlying bone. Released in 2016,

ProChondrix is a fresh chondral allograft composed of viable chondrocytes, matrix, and growth factors. ProChondrix is stored at 4 °C with 87.5% viability at the expiration of its 35-day shelf life. The grafts are available in 11-mm, 13-mm, 15-mm, 17-mm, and 20-mm diameter discs. Cartiform and ProChondrix have both been used as isolated grafts and in conjunction with marrow stimulation, which affords both a reparative response and restorative approach from the allograft. There is not currently a consensus about the need for concomitant marrow stimulation. In vitro histological evaluation of Cartiform in a goat model revealed that the graft retains viable chondrocytes, chondrogenic growth factors, and ECM proteins within intact hyaline cartilage and that when used in conjunction with microfracture results in improved cartilage regrowth compared to microfracture alone [40]. Clinical results in humans are presently unavailable.

Maioregen (Finceramica Faenza SpA, Faenza, Italy) is a tri-layered biomimetic osteochondral scaffold first introduced for clinical use in 2011 in Europe. The acellular scaffold was designed for the treatment of osteochondral defects. The superficial layer consists of type I equine collagen, the intermediate layer of 60% equine collagen and 40% magnesium-enriched HA (Mg-HA), and the deep layer of 30% equine collagen and 70% Mg-HA. The scaffold has been shown to induce subchondral trabecular bone regeneration in an equine model [41]. Berruto and colleagues recently published on the use of Maioregen in 11 patients for the treatment of spontaneous osteonecrosis of the knee (SPONK) [42]. While 2 of 11 ultimately underwent total knee arthroplasty, the remaining 9 patients had favorable results with significant improvements in Lysholm, IKDC, and VAS scores. Maioregen is not currently available in the United States; however, a phase IV clinical trial is recently completed in Europe (NCT01282034).

Agili-C (CartiHeal, Israel) is a porous bioabsorbable biphasic scaffold derived from coral, to which HA is added. It contains (1) a bone phase composed of calcium carbonate in an aragnite crystalline form and (2) a cartilage phase composed of modified aragonite and HA [43]. Aragonite possesses a nano-rough surface and porous architecture which permit cell adhesion and proliferation. Kon and colleagues reported complete histologic restoration of hyaline cartilage and subchondral bone in 6/7 goats 12 months following treatment with Agili-C for lesions measuring 6 mm in diameter and 10 mm in depth [44]. A multicenter European trial of 97 patients treated with tapered (n = 21) and cylindrical (76) implants revealed MRI findings 84% of patients with >75% defect fill and 90% with complete restoration of the cartilage interface [43]. Agili-C is not currently commercially available and is available only via a phase IV clinical trial in Europe (NCT02423629).

Injectable Agents

Traditional joint injections for osteoarthritis including corticosteroids or HA aim to decrease inflammation and improve symptoms without modifying the disease. Newer injectable agents including PRP, stem cells, and growth factors have recently become the focus of intensive study both to augment cartilage repair techniques and to delay progression of cartilage breakdown in osteoarthritis. The rationale behind these injections is to optimize the healing milieu within the joint by both increasing the concentration of favorable cytokines which increase glycosaminoglycan synthesis (IGF-1, FGF, and TGF-beta superfamily) and decreasing catabolic cytokines that contribute to osteoarthritis (IL-1, TNF, and IL-6, IL-7, and IL-8). Agents that have recently garnered attention include Orthokine/Regenokine, PRP, autologous and allogeneic MSCs, sprifermin (FGFR-18), and OP-1 (BMP7).

Much of the interest in injectable growth factors was sparked by reports of professional athletes traveling internationally for injections of Orthokine (Orthogen, Dusseldorf, Germany). Orthokine, now available in the United States as Regenokine, is autologous conditioned serum (ACS) which is procured from autologous blood that is incubated with boro-silicate glass spheres leading to increased levels of IL-1 receptor antagonist (IL-1ra) [45]. While there is little available literature on the use of Orthokine/Regenokine and nothing to suggest it is disease modifying, Baltzer and colleagues demonstrated that Orthokine/Regenokine rendered superior improvement in patient-reported outcomes (VAS, SF-8, and all WOMAC subscales) when compared to HA and saline in a randomized, controlled trial of 376 patients with knee osteoarthritis [46].

Platelet-rich plasma (PRP) is biologic therapeutic modality derived from centrifugation of autologous blood to attain a supraphysiologic concentration of platelet and plasma proteins that accelerate the repair process. Numerous growth factors in PRP stimulate cartilage matrix synthesis and counteract the effects of catabolic cytokines like IL-1 and TNF-α. A recent double-blind, randomized controlled trial demonstrated no difference between PRP and HA in WOMAC pain score; however, the authors did demonstrate a trend toward lower concentrations of IL-1 and TNF-α at 12 weeks following injection in the PRP group [47]. A recent systematic review of 29 studies evaluating results of PRP in the setting of osteoarthritis reported that 9 of 11 studies comparing PRP with HA revealed superior outcomes with PRP [48].

Bone marrow aspirate concentrate (BMAC) has been used as both a cell source for matrix plus MSC products and for symptomatic management of osteoarthritis. As discussed previously, BMAC contains adult bone marrow-derived MSCs (bmMSCs), platelets, cytokines, and growth factors—all of which harbor unique anti-inflammatory and immuno-modulatory effects. Chahla and colleagues recently performed a systematic review of the use of BMAC for both repair of focal chondral defects and treatment of osteoarthritis [49]. Three studies demonstrated that BMAC is effective in treating osteoarthritis. The available literature demonstrated that BMAC rendered significant improvements in patient symptoms with more pronounced improvement in patients with

Kellgren and Lawrence grade II/III compared to grade IV disease; however, there is no available evidence to suggest that BMAC alters the natural history of osteoarthritis.

Lipogems (Lipogems International SpA, Milan, Italy) is a single-use system, available since 2013, designed for aspiration, processing, and transfer of adipose tissue for the harvest of adipose-derived MSCs (adMSCs). Evidence regarding Lipogems for the treatment of osteoarthritis is currently limited to case reports; however, significant improvements in pain, functional scores, and cartilage thickness have been reported in patients with osteoarthritis treated with Lipogems [50, 51]. Of note, in vitro comparison of chondrogenic potential of adMSCs and bmMSCs has demonstrated greater efficiency and quality of chondrogenesis with bmMSCs [52, 53].

Bone morphogenetic protein 7 (BMP7), marketed as osteogenic protein 1 (OP-1, Olympus Biotech, West Lebanon, NH), was the first isolated growth factor trialed for the treatment of osteoarthritis. OP-1 was shown to have reparative effects on cartilage including stimulating synthesis of proteoglycan, collagen, and HA and preventing catabolism by IL-1. While the phase I safety trial of OP1 demonstrated safety and subtle benefits relative to placebo [54], further trials were discontinued, and Olympus Biotech halted its effort to commercialize OP-1 in 2014.

Sprifermin (recombinant human fibroblast growth factor 18; rhFGF-18) binds to and activates fibroblast growth factor receptor 3 (FGFR-3) in cartilage to promote chondrogenesis and cartilage matrix production in vivo. Preclinical studies have demonstrated that sprifermin induces chondrocyte proliferation which results in increased extracellular matrix production [55]. However, a recent randomized, double-blind, placebo-controlled trial comparing sprifermin and placebo demonstrated no difference in cartilage thickness and inferior improvement in WOMAC pain scores in the sprifermin group compared to the control group [56]. A phase II multicenter, placebo-controlled clinical trial evaluating sprifermin in the setting of osteoarthritis is ongoing (NCT01919164).

Conclusion

A broad variety of new cartilage repair products have emerged over the last 20 years, designed to improve upon limitations of existing techniques. Most products combine a cell source with a matrix and/or growth factors to optimize the healing environment. Techniques that have generated excitement include augmented microfracture, matrix-assisted ACI, matrix plus stem cell productions, minced cartilage productions, off-the-shelf osteochondral implants, and injectable agents. While these products have demonstrated promising clinical and histologic results, many remain unavailable in the United States due to FDA restrictions. Additionally, while many of these techniques have compared favorably to conventional microfracture, there is very little literature comparing them to more sophisticated techniques (ACI or osteochondral grafting). Further results from ongoing clinical trials will be essential in changing the landscape of FDA-approved techniques and establishing the place for each of these techniques within the cartilage restoration algorithm.

References

1. Devitt BM, Bell SW, Webster KE, Feller JA. Surgical treatments of cartilage defects of the knee: systematic review of randomised controlled trials. Knee. 2017;24:508–17.
2. Cole BJ, Kercher JS, Strauss EJ, Barker JU. Augmentation strategies following the microfracture technique for repair of focal chondral defects. Cartilage. 2010;1:145–52.
3. Benthien JP, Behrens P. Autologous Matrix-Induced Chondrogenesis (AMIC). Cartilage. 2010;1:65–8.
4. Piontek T, Ciemniewska-Gorzela K, Szulc A. All-arthroscopic AMIC procedure for repair of cartilage defects of the knee. Knee Surg. 2012;20:922–5.
5. Schiavone Panni A, Del Regno C, Mazzitelli G. Good clinical results with autologous matrix-induced chondrogenesis (Amic) technique in large knee chondral defects. Knee Surg. 2017;26:1130–6.

6. Shive MS, Stanish WD, McCormack R, Forriol F, Mohtadi N, Pelet S, Desnoyers J, Méthot S, Vehik K, Restrepo A. BST-CarGel® treatment maintains cartilage repair superiority over microfracture at 5 years in a multicenter randomized controlled trial. Cartilage. 2015;6:62–72.

7. Trattnig S, Ohel K, Mlynarik V, Juras V, Zbyn S. Morphological and compositional monitoring of a new cell-free cartilage repair hydrogel technology–GelrinC by MR using semi-quantitative MOCART scoring and quantitative T2 index and new zonal T2 index calculation. Osteoarthr Cartil. 2015;23:2224–32.

8. Fortier LA, Chapman HS, Pownder SL, Roller BL, Cross JA, Cook JL, Cole BJ. BioCartilage improves cartilage repair compared with microfracture alone in an equine model of full-thickness cartilage loss. Am J Sports Med. 2016;44:2366–74.

9. Siclari A, Mascaro G, Gentili C, Kaps C, Cancedda R, Boux E. Cartilage repair in the knee with subchondral drilling augmented with a platelet-rich plasma-immersed polymer-based implant. Knee Surg Sports Traumatol Arthrosc. 2013;22: 1225–34.

10. Bryan W. Approval letter for biologics lincense application for autologous cultured chondrocytes on porcine collagen membrane. U.S. Food & Drug Administration. December 13, 2016.

11. Brix MO, Stelzeneder D, Chiari C, Koller U, Nehrer S, Dorotka R, Windhager R, Domayer SE. Treatment of full-thickness chondral defects with hyalograft C in the knee: long-term results. Am J Sports Med. 2014;42:1426–32.

12. Wylie JD, Hartley MK, Kapron AL, Aoki SK, Maak TG. What is the effect of matrices on cartilage repair? A systematic review. Clin Orthop Relat Res. 2015;473:1673–82.

13. Schneider U, Rackwitz L, Andereya S, Siebenlist S, Fensky F, Reichert J, Löer I, Barthel T, Rudert M, Nöth U. A prospective multicenter study on the outcome of type I collagen hydrogel–based autologous chondrocyte implantation (CaReS) for the repair of articular cartilage defects in the knee. Am J Sports Med. 2011;39:2558–65.

14. Zak L, Albrecht C, Wondrasch B, Widhalm H, Vekszler G, Trattnig S, Marlovits S, Aldrian S. Results 2 years after matrix-associated autologous chondrocyte transplantation using the Novocart 3D scaffold. Am J Sports Med. 2014;42:1618–27.

15. Kusanagi A, Mascarenhas AC, Blahut EB, Johnson JM, Murata T, Mizuno S. Hydrostatic pressure with low oxygen stimulates extracellular matrix accumulation by human articular chon-

drocytes in a 3-D collagen sponge. 51st Annual Meeting of the Orthopedic Research Society, Washington, DC, 384; 2005.

16. Kusanagi A, Mascarenhas AC, Blahut EB, Johnson JM. Hydrostatic pressure with low oxygen stimulates extracellular matrix accumulation by human articular chondrocytes in a 3-D collagen gel/sponge. Transactions of the 51st Annual Orthopaedic Research Society. 2005. p. 20–3

17. Crawford DC, DeBerardino TM, Williams RJ III. NeoCart, an autologous cartilage tissue implant, compared with microfracture for treatment of distal femoral cartilage lesions. J Bone Joint Surg Am. 2012;94:979–89.

18. Yayon A, Neria E, Blumenstein S, Stern B, Barkai H, Zak R, et al. BIOCART™II a novel implant for 3D reconstruction of articular cartilage. J Bone Joint Surg Br Vol. 2006;88-B(SUPP II):344.

19. Domayer SE, Welsch GH, Nehrer S, Chiari C, Dorotka R, Szomolanyi P, Mamisch TC, Yayon A, Trattnig S. T2 mapping and dGEMRIC after autologous chondrocyte implantation with a fibrin-based scaffold in the knee: preliminary results. Eur J Radiol. 2010;73:636–42.

20. Sampson S, Bemden AB-V, Aufiero D. Autologous bone marrow concentrate: review and application of a novel intra-articular orthobiologic for cartilage disease. Phys Sportsmed. 2013;41:7–18.

21. Bain BJ. The bone marrow aspirate of healthy subjects. Br J Haematol. 1996;94:206–9.

22. Cassano JM, Kennedy JG, Ross KA, Fraser EJ. Bone marrow concentrate and platelet-rich plasma differ in cell distribution and interleukin 1 receptor antagonist protein concentration. Knee Surg. 2016;26:333–42.

23. Kim M, Kim J, Lim J, Kim Y, Han K. Use of an automated hematology analyzer and flow cytometry to assess bone marrow cellularity and differential cell count. Ann Clin Lab Sci. 2004;34:307–13.

24. Yamamura R, Yamane T, Hino M, Ohta K, Shibata H, Tsuda I, Tatsumi N. Possible automatic cell classification of bone marrow aspirate using the CELL-DYN 4000 automatic blood cell analyzer. J Clin Lab Anal. 2002;16:86–90.

25. Gobbi A, Whyte GP. One-stage cartilage repair using a hyaluronic acid–based scaffold with activated bone marrow–derived mesenchymal stem cells compared with microfracture. Am J Sports Med. 2016;44:2846–54.

26. Gobbi A, Scotti C, Karnatzikos G, Mudhigere A, Castro M, Peretti GM. One-step surgery with multipotent stem cells and Hyaluronan-based scaffold for the treatment of full-thickness chondral defects of the knee in patients older than 45 years. Knee Surg Sports Traumatol Arthrosc. 2017;25:2494–501.

27. Calabrese G et al. Combination of collagen-based scaffold and bioactive factors induces adipose-derived mesenchymal stem cells chondrogenic differentiation in vitro. Front Physiol. 2017. https://doi.org/10.3389/fphys.2017.00050.

28. Park YB, Ha CW, Lee CH, Yoon YC, Park YG. Cartilage regeneration in osteoarthritic patients by a composite of allogeneic umbilical cord blood-derived mesenchymal stem cells and hyaluronate hydrogel: results from a clinical trial for safety and proof-of-concept with 7 years of extended follow-up. Stem Cells Transl Med. 2017;6:613–21.

29. Yanke AB, Tilton AK, Wetters NG, Merkow DB, Cole BJ. DeNovo NT particulated juvenile cartilage implant. Sports Med Arthrosc Rev. 2015;23:125–9.

30. Cole BJ, Farr J, Winalski CS, Hosea T, Richmond J, Mandelbaum B, De Deyne PG. Outcomes after a single-stage procedure for cell-based cartilage repair: a prospective clinical safety trial with 2-year follow-up. Am J Sports Med. 2011;39:1170–9.

31. Cole BJ, Farr J, Winalski CS, Hosea T, Richmond J, Mandelbaum B, De Deyne PG. Outcomes after a single-stage procedure for cell-based cartilage repair. Am J Sports Med. 2011;39: 1170–9.

32. Riboh JC, Cole BJ, Farr J. Particulated articular cartilage for symptomatic chondral defects of the knee. Curr Rev Musculoskelet Med. 2015;8:429–35.

33. Farr J, Yao JQ. Chondral defect repair with particulated juvenile cartilage allograft. Cartilage. 2011;2:346–53.

34. Farr J, Tabet SK, Margerrison E, Cole BJ. Clinical, radiographic, and histological outcomes after cartilage repair with particulated juvenile articular cartilage: a 2-year prospective study. Am J Sports Med. 2014;42:1417–25.

35. Buckwalter JA, Bowman GN. Clinical outcomes of patellar chondral lesions treated with juvenile particulated cartilage allografts. Iowa Orthop J. 2014;34:44–9.

36. Wu L, Leijten JCH, Georgi N, Post JN, van Blitterswijk CA, Karperien M. Trophic effects of mesenchymal stem cells increase chondrocyte proliferation and matrix formation. Tissue Eng Part A. 2011;17:1425–36.

37. Gracitelli GC, Meric G, Pulido PA, Gortz S, De Young AJ, Bugbee WD. Fresh osteochondral allograft transplantation for isolated patellar cartilage injury. Am J Sports Med. 2015;43:879–84.
38. Levy YD, Gortz S, Pulido PA, McCauley JC, Bugbee WD. Do fresh osteochondral allografts successfully treat femoral condyle lesions? Clin Orthop Relat Res. 2013;471:231–7.
39. Farr J, Gracitelli G, Gomoll AH. Decellularized osteochondral allograft for the treatment of cartilage lesions in the knee. Orthop J Sports Med. 2015;3(7).
40. Geraghty S, Kuang J-Q, Yoo D, LeRoux-Williams M, Vangsness CT, Danilkovitch A. A novel, cryopreserved, viable osteochondral allograft designed to augment marrow stimulation for articular cartilage repair. J Orthop Surg Res. 2015;10:66.
41. Kon E, Mutini A, Arcangeli E, Delcogliano M, Filardo G, Nicoli Aldini N, Pressato D, Quarto R, Zaffagnini S, Marcacci M. Novel nanostructured scaffold for osteochondral regeneration: pilot study in horses. J Tissue Eng Regen Med. 2010;4:300–8.
42. Berruto M, Ferrua P, Uboldi F, Pasqualotto S, Ferrara F, Carimati G, Usellini E, Delcogliano M. Can a biomimetic osteochondral scaffold be a reliable alternative to prosthetic surgery in treating late-stage SPONK? Knee. 2016;23:936–41.
43. Kon E, Robinson D, Verdonk P, Drobnic M, et al. A novel aragonite-based scaffold for osteochondral regeneration: early experience on human implants and technical developments. Injury. 2016;47:S27–32.
44. Kon E, Filardo G, Shani J, Altschuler N, Levy A, Zaslav K, Eisman JE, Robinson D. Osteochondral regeneration with a novel aragonite-hyaluronate biphasic scaffold: up to 12-month follow-up study in a goat model. J Orthop Surg Res. 2015;10:81.
45. Fortier LA, Chapman HS, Pownder SL, Roller BL, Cross JA, Cook JL, Cole BJ. BioCartilage improves cartilage repair compared with microfracture alone in an equine model of full-thickness cartilage loss. Curr Rev Musculoskelet Med. 2015;44:2366–74.
46. Baltzer AW, Moser C, Jansen SA, Krauspe R. Autologous conditioned serum (Orthokine) is an effective treatment for knee osteoarthritis. Osteoarthr Cartil. 2009;17:152–60.
47. Cole BJ, Karas V, Hussey K, Pilz K, Fortier LA. Hyaluronic acid versus platelet-rich plasma. Am J Sports Med. 2017;45:339–46.
48. Laver L, Marom N, Dnyanesh L, Mei-Dan O, Espregueira-Mendes JO, Gobbi A. PRP for degenerative cartilage disease. Cartilage. 2016;8:194760351667070.

49. Chahla J, Dean CS, Moatshe G, Pascual-Garrido C, Serra Cruz R, LaPrade RF. Concentrated bone marrow aspirate for the treatment of chondral injuries and osteoarthritis of the knee. Orthop J Sports Med. 2016;4:232596711562548.
50. Striano RD, Battista V, Bilboo N. Non-responding knee pain with osteoarthritis, meniscus and ligament tears treated with ultrasound guided autologous, micro-fragmented and minimally manipulated adipose tissue. Open J Regen Med. 2017;6:17.
51. Franceschini M, Castellaneta C, Mineo G. Injection of autologous micro-fragmented adipose tissue for the treatment of post traumatic degenerative lesion of knee cartilage: a case report. CellR4. 2016;4:e1765.
52. Reich CM, Raabe O, Wenisch S, Bridger PS. Isolation, culture and chondrogenic differentiation of canine adipose tissue-and bone marrow-derived mesenchymal stem cells–a comparative study. Vet Res Commun. 2012;36:139–48.
53. Jakobsen RB, Shahdadfar A, Reinholt FP, Brinchmann JE. Chondrogenesis in a hyaluronic acid scaffold: comparison between chondrocytes and MSC from bone marrow and adipose tissue. Knee Surg Sports Traumatol Arthrosc. 2010;18:1407–16.
54. Hunter DJ, Pike MC, Jonas BL, Kissin E, Krop J, McAlindon T. Phase 1 safety and tolerability study of BMP-7 in symptomatic knee osteoarthritis. BMC Musculoskelet Disord. 2010;11:232.
55. Ellsworth JL, Berry J, Bukowski T, et al. Fibroblast growth factor-18 is a trophic factor for mature chondrocytes and their progenitors. Osteoarthr Cartil. 2002;10:308–20.
56. Lohmander LS, Hellot S, Dreher D, Krantz EFW, Kruger DS, Guermazi A, Eckstein F. Intraarticular sprifermin (recombinant human fibroblast growth factor 18) in knee osteoarthritis: a randomized, double-blind, placebo-controlled trial. Arthritis Rheum. 2014;66:1820–31.

Correction to: Joint Preservation of the Knee

Adam B. Yanke and Brian J. Cole

Correction to: A. B. Yanke, B. J. Cole (eds.),
Joint Preservation of the Knee,
https://doi.org/10.1007/978-3-030-01491-9

Dr. Trevor R. Gulbrandsen's affiliation in the book has been updated and a typo in the city has been corrected from Lowa to Iowa.

The correct version of affiliation is below:

Department of Orthopaedic Surgery, University of Iowa Hospitals and Clinics, Iowa City, IA, USA.

The updated online versions of these chapters can be found at
https://doi.org/10.1007/978-3-030-01491-9_10
https://doi.org/10.1007/978-3-030-01491-9_14

© Springer Nature Switzerland AG 2019   C1
A. B. Yanke, B. J. Cole (eds.), *Joint Preservation of the Knee*,
https://doi.org/10.1007/978-3-030-01491-9_19

Index

© Springer Nature Switzerland AG 2019
A. B. Yanke, B. J. Cole (eds.), *Joint Preservation of the Knee*,
https://doi.org/10.1007/978-3-030-01491-9